Unapologetic Eating

Make Peace with Food and Transform Your Life

ALISSA RUMSEY, MS, RD

VICTORY BELT PUBLISHING INC.

LAS VEGAS

First published in 2021 by Victory Belt Publishing Inc.

ISBN-13: 978-1-628604-25-2

The information included in this book is for educational purposes only. It is not intended or implied to be a substitute for professional medical advice. The reader should always consult their healthcare provider to determine the appropriateness of the information for their own situation or if their have any questions regarding a medical condition or treatment plan. Reading the information in this book does not constitute a physician-patient relationship. The statements in this book have not been evaluated by the Food and Drug Administration. The products or supplements in this book are not intended to diagnose, treat, cure, or prevent any disease. The authors and publisher expressly disclaim responsibility for any adverse effects that may result from the use or application of the information contained in this book.

Author photos by Karen Obrist Photography

Cover design by Kat Lannom

Cover photography by Kat Lannom and Justin-Aaron Velasco

Interior design by Justin-Aaron Velasco

Printed in the USA
VS 0221

For all the people who have ever thought
that they were "not enough":

You are enough,
just as you are.

Contents

Introduction

A couple of years ago, I posted a series of photos on social media of me eating a sandwich. Not just any sandwich, mind you; it was a big ol' Pub Sub from Publix, the well-known southern U.S. grocery store chain. (If you are ever near a Publix, you MUST get yourself a Pub Sub. Trust me.) In the images, I'm blissfully ignorant of the fact that my partner is taking photographs. I am mid-bite, eyes closed, hunched over in my bikini, with my forehead scrunched up and my mouth open wide. Just unabashedly enjoying the *heck* out of that massive sandwich, crumbs on my face and all. When I posted the photos on my Instagram feed later that day, I wrote a quick, off-the-cuff caption asking my followers, "Why don't we see more images of women actually eating food? Not looking perfect, not talking about how 'good' or 'bad' they are being, not commenting on or criticizing their bodies, but just eating and enjoying food?"

I never expected the reaction that the series of images—and those questions—would have. Almost immediately, comments began flooding in from people telling me how validating and liberating it was to see another woman eating—and enjoying—food without offering any explanation or apologizing for what she was eating. Many people commented on how "brave" I was for posting that photo and said they could "never in a million years" post an imperfect photo of themselves that showed their rolls, their cellulite, or food on their faces. Although I hadn't thought twice about posting the photos, there was a time not that long ago when I would have been mortified to do so. Publicly post a picture of myself with no makeup, hair haphazardly thrown into a messy ponytail, visible wrinkles and stomach rolls, AND food on my face?! I never thought that I would eventually get to the point where what I looked like wasn't a factor for me when sharing a public social media post.

But why was this photo so revolutionary? Why, when you search the Internet for the phrase "women eating food," do you get served dozens of stock images of thin, young, white women posing with a salad? Why, when you do the same search but replace *women* with *men*, do you see a whole bunch of images of men eating (actually *eating*) burgers, fries, and pizza? What does it say about our society that the media we consume—whether television, movies, advertisements, or social media feeds—is almost invariably filled with thin, young, white, conventionally attractive women who never seem to be eating anything? (Or, if they are eating, it's either a) something considered "healthy" or b) something considered "unhealthy" followed by the woman apologizing or explaining, "Oh, I don't usually eat like this.") Why were the photos of me with my Pub Sub applauded, whereas similar images of Brianna Campos, a licensed professional counselor from New Jersey who is fat,* eating and enjoying food, led to her receiving dozens of body-shaming, food-shaming, weight-shaming hate messages? "I got messages saying, 'No wonder you're fat,' 'Keep eating, piggy,' and telling me they hoped no young girls followed me because I am a bad influence—just for eating!" Brianna told me.[1]

Up until this point, I had never really questioned the photos I saw daily in the media (which also speaks to my privilege as a thin, young, white woman because I was mainly seeing images of people who looked just like me), but the implicit messages that these images send to women and girls were now staring me in the face: If you're going to take a photo of yourself with food, you must look pretty doing it, and you must be thin, or else you open yourself up to commentary on how "unhealthy" (or worse) you must be. Oh, and you can't actually be *eating* the food in the photos; you must only pose with it. These societal standards were what all the women who thought I was "brave" were reacting to; they couldn't imagine sharing a photo like this of themselves for fear of being judged, teased, shamed, or bullied. It's no wonder so many women can't eat and enjoy food without feeling guilty or needing to justify themselves and apologize.

I didn't know it at the time, but posting those images marked the start of both a personal and professional transformation for me. I began to sit with, digest, and reflect upon all of the questions that I posed earlier. At the time, I had been a dietitian for almost ten years; I had embarked on this career

---

Fat is not inherently a bad word. I encourage you to read the description of the word *fat* in the "Defining Terminology" section later in this introduction.

path a decade earlier during my own disordered eating and struggles with body image. After spending most of my twenties improving my body image and my relationship to food and exercise, I had "accidentally" discovered intuitive eating a few years before my Instagram post with the Pub Sub. (I say "accidentally" because I thought I was taking a course on mindful eating, which, as you'll learn in this book, is *not* the same as intuitive eating.) That six-week course opened my eyes to a different way of approaching food, nutrition, health, and bodies. By the time I posted the images of me eating the sandwich, I had shifted my professional practice from focusing on weight loss to helping people take the emphasis *off* of weight to heal their relationship to food and their bodies.

Yet the reactions that people had to my post—and the digging that I started to do once I realized that a photo of a woman eating "real" food without explanation or apology was a big deal—caused me to begin questioning *everything*. I realized that the food and body image hang-ups that so many people face are actually symptoms of a much larger cultural problem. As I began thinking about the clients I had worked with over the years, I noticed patterns. Not only did many women feel like they needed to apologize, explain, or justify why they were eating certain foods, but this need to apologize or ask permission extended into many different aspects of their lives. I saw this pattern in my own life as well: I had spent my entire life following the "shoulds" that I had learned from society about what a woman should be and do, how she should act, and what she should look like—and apologizing when I felt like I wasn't living up to those societal expectations. From apologizing for my appearance ("I'm sorry I look awful; I didn't have time to do my makeup this morning" or "Ugh, ignore my outfit; I had planned to change"), my food choices ("I would get a salad, but I skipped breakfast, so I'm going to let myself get a burger instead" or "Oh, I know I'm being so bad, but I'm going to order dessert"), to work or personal life situations where I had clearly done nothing wrong ("Sorry I didn't respond to your text message right away" or "I'm sorry, can I add something here?"). I did it all of the time.

Food as an Entry Point to Exploration and Transformation

As I learned more about the roots of our culture's obsession with dieting and thin bodies—which I'll describe in Chapter 1—this pattern I saw in my clients (and myself) of food and body image struggles as a side effect of deeper societal issues made so much more sense. The impossible set of standards that women† are supposed to conform to have nothing to do with food, or weight, or body size. As I'll explain in this book, your struggles with food and your body have nothing to do with *you* and everything to do with the *society* that you have been raised in and now have to exist in. (This isn't to say that men aren't ever made to feel like they need to achieve certain body ideals; however, my goal in writing this book was to focus on those people who have been harmed the most by societal standards, which is primarily women.)

When I began working with clients years ago, I thought I was going to be focusing on people's relationship to food. But I quickly learned that food behaviors were the symptom—not the problem—and the relationship that really needed mending was the one people had with themselves. What presented as a problem with food or a problem with body image was more deeply rooted. The problems had nothing to do with them and everything to do with society. As my clients questioned their beliefs about food, dieting, and weight, they started to question all sorts of other thoughts, feelings, and beliefs. In the process of relearning to trust their bodies around food, I watched them start to trust themselves in many other areas of their lives.

It was then that I realized how food can be a powerful entry point into exploring more about ourselves, our beliefs, our values, and what we truly want out of life. As my friend Hana Jung, who I'll talk about later in the book, has said to me, "We are all going up the same mountain, just on different paths." This book is a compilation of the work that my clients and I have done over the years and our journey of unpacking and questioning everything we've been taught so that we can discover who we really are inside. I will break down the path that the clients I've worked with have traveled as they let go of dieting, made peace with food, and found their way back

---

†When I use the word *women* throughout the book, I'm speaking about all people who have been socialized as girls and women, including cisgender women, transgender women, feminized bodies, and gender nonconforming bodies.

to their bodies, their intuition, and themselves. And I'll show you how you can embark, or move further along, on your own path toward self discovery and transformation. This book is about food and eating, yes, but really it is a book about unlearning, questioning everything, relearning, and—ultimately—transforming your life.

Every single thing you think you "know"—about food, appearance, body size, and more—was something you were taught at some point. This book will help you begin the process of *unlearning.* You will uncover the historical and personal origins of your beliefs, thoughts, feelings, and behaviors related to food, weight, health, appearance, and other social and cultural norms. Your relationship to food is the starting point, but the real work becomes figuring out how the world has adversely affected your life and your perception of yourself. You will strip away all of the things that have been imposed upon you by society so you can find *yourself* again. Throughout this book, I'll also share how you can relearn to heal and change your perception to build back trust with your body and step into your full, authentic power.

From Unapologetic Eating to Unapologetic Living

When I began writing this book, I had no idea what title I was going to give it. But the more I wrote, the more I realized the underlying theme that was emerging. When it comes to food, body size, setting boundaries, work decisions, or life choices, I want you to be able to do what you want *without* asking permission or needing to justify, explain, or apologize. *Unapologetic eating* means eating what you want, when you want, and how you want without feeling guilty or ashamed. It is that photo of me with the sandwich: not perfect, a little messy, food on your face, clearly enjoying yourself, and fully inhabiting your body. It is the audible *mmmm* you let out when you eat something *really* good. It is being in the moment with what you are eating, and what you are doing, without feeling self-conscious or worrying about what others may be thinking. Unapologetic eating is about getting back to your roots and to who you were before society told you who you should be.

In this book, I'll walk you through the process going from trying to "fix"[‡] or change yourself to *unapologetic eating* and finally to *unapologetic living.*

I've broken down this process in four segments: fixing, allowing, feeling, and growing. In Part 1, "Fixing," you'll learn about the history of diet culture and our culture's beauty ideals. I'll also explain the real reasons why dieting and weight-control measures never seem to work and share more about why health and weight are not as inextricably linked as we've been led to believe. In this section, you'll spend some time digging deeper into your history with food and your body, including reflecting on where your food and body beliefs came from and how they have affected your life.

Part 2, "Allowing," is where you can begin to take steps to move away from dieting, sit with the thoughts and feelings that this brings up, and start to rediscover (and trust) your inner wisdom. I'll walk you through the first of two essential skills necessary for the process of unlearning: mindfulness. I recommend taking time and practicing—not just reading—the different mindfulness exercises because you will continue to return to these skills throughout the rest of the book. In this part, you will also learn more about the intuitive eating framework and several foundation elements that need to be in place as you start practicing connecting to your body and eating unapologetically.

From there, you will move on to Part 3, "Feeling." When you stop trying to "fix" yourself and begin to allow your body to just "be," many thoughts and feelings can bubble up to the surface (often ones that you may have spent years—or decades—trying to suppress). In this part, I will guide you through the process of sitting with the feelings and discomfort that can arise in this journey. You'll come up with a self-care plan and learn how to use a second essential skill in this process: self-compassion. I will also share how you can practice respecting your body by listening to it, being kind to it, and expressing appreciation for it. In addition, you will begin working through the body image healing process.

The last section is Part 4, "Growing." In the process of unlearning, you get to explore, learn, and define new truths for yourself. In the final chapters of the book, you will have the chance to do some deep self-exploration and self-discovery, learn how to become more connected to your body, and find ways to embrace your power more fully. You'll also learn how you can challenge all of the things you think you are "supposed to" do, be, act, or look like and figure out what it is that *you* really want instead.

‡I put the word *fix* in quotation marks throughout the book because, as you'll learn, you are not broken, and the problem is not with you.

I hope that you do more than just read this book and really put what you're learning into practice. To help you do that, I've included a variety of breakout boxes with reflection questions, prompts, and other helpful exercises. I encourage you to take some time with these reflections and have a journal or something else on hand to write down your thoughts, feelings, and memories; doing so will help you get the most benefit possible out of this book. Try to complete the reflection questions in writing and practice the techniques that I reference in the chapters. I wrote this book to be both educational *and* practical so that you understand the concepts intellectually but also integrate them into your day-to-day life.

Sitting with Discomfort

Many of the things that you read in this book may make you uncomfortable, unsettled, defensive, or even outright angry. Over the years, I have learned that discomfort and defensiveness serve to alert me that there is something deeper to unpack and explore. The moments in which I've felt the most uncomfortable or defensive are the times in which I have grown and evolved the most. I hope that you can notice any discomfort that arises throughout this book and use that as an invitation to sit back and be open to what comes up for you. As Sassy Latte (@sassy_latte), a political creative whose work constantly challenges me to think critically, says, "Finding out that you were wrong, mistaken, or ignorant aren't attacks on your character. These discoveries are chances to course correct values, beliefs, and behaviors."[2] Unlearning and confronting your biases comes with discomfort, but it is within this process that you can grow, evolve, and rediscover who *you* really are.

In this book, I talk about the various systems of oppression that exist in our society. When groups of people are oppressed—for example, fat people and Black[Ω] communities—people who are not in those groups hold privilege that does not force them to experience oppression based on the size of their body or their skin tone. The word *privilege* can make some people bristle, so I want to explain that I'm talking about privileges at the *societal* level rather than on a *personal* level. The privileges that you may hold have nothing to

---

[Ω] I capitalize the B in Black to recognize the ethnic identity of Black folks in the United States. Read more in the "Defining Terminology" section

do with how *you* feel about yourself but about how *society* treats you. That means, for example, that a person can have thin privilege and still struggle with their body image. Just because a person has size privilege or white privilege doesn't mean they haven't suffered; it means that they haven't suffered *because of* the size of their body or the color of their skin. As I'll discuss later in the book, oppression is used as a tool (both overtly and covertly) by the people and/or groups in power to marginalize people across various intersections of identities, including gender, sexual orientation, religion, ability, immigration status, and much, much more.

Try to be gentle with yourself and show yourself compassion as you read, learn, explore, and practice the concepts from this book. This process of moving from dieting to unapologetic eating and unapologetic living is a continuous, ever-evolving journey. Allow yourself permission to not know everything, to be uncomfortable, to get it wrong, to make mistakes, to not be "perfect." By doing so, you'll then have more space to learn and grow. You may find it helpful to read this book in starts and stops to give yourself time to digest, think, reflect, and practice the tools and concepts you are learning. The intention for this journey is not "read, learn, and then do it perfectly." In fact, it's pretty much the opposite. Perfectionism, as I'll share more about, doesn't allow you any space to learn and grow, so I want you to commit to showing up, trying new things, experimenting, and making mistakes because that's the process in which learning and growth occur.

In the spirit of constant learning and growth, I want to acknowledge something: This book is not perfect. When I read the published version months from now, I know that I will notice all sorts of things that I would have done differently had I known what I have learned by that point. But that's the thing: It could never be perfect, and perfection should never be our goal (which I have continued to remind myself as I've been writing this book). I—just like everyone else—am constantly unlearning and relearning, continuing to make mistakes, and (with the help of the phenomenal equity consultants McKensie Mack and Lindley Ashline) naming and uncovering my implicit biases. The goal is not perfection; the goal is to show up, put yourself out there, and then, when you get it wrong and are corrected, learn better and do better the next time. It's a constant evolution of unlearning and relearning, unlearning and relearning—and being open and committing to doing so. I'm committing to this right alongside you.

One final (but very important) note: Although I have struggled with my relationship to food and my body, I hold a lot of privilege that has made this journey much easier for me than for others. As a white, thin, heterosexual, cisgender, able-bodied, middle-class woman who grew up in a small, primarily white town in Connecticut, my lived experiences are but a small and limited view of the overall human experience (as shown in the very different reactions to thin and fat body sizes showing up online that I shared earlier). Disordered eating, disconnected eating, eating disorders, and body image struggles show up differently in people of different identities and lived experiences. Throughout the book, I've done my best to identify my privilege and tell stories using a variety of clients whose identities are different than mine in the hope that you will be able to see yourself and relate to them. You're also going to see me quoting and citing Black and Brown women of color, fat women, and genderqueer people because they have been at the forefront of the body liberation movement for decades, and it's with them that so much wisdom lies. They paved the way for us to learn how to let go of dieting and embrace our bodies as a form of courageous resistance, self-love, and collective care, and I thank them for their labor.

No matter who you are or what identities you hold, I wrote this book intending to encourage more people to think outside of the arbitrary boxes that society has put us in. To make peace with food, feel at home in your body, understand your inherent worth, and move closer to unapologetically eating *and* living. Because true freedom and liberation come from rejecting all the instances of "I should" and "I'm supposed to" to find—and trust—who you really are deep inside.

Defining Terminology

Before you go any further, I want to pause to define some terminology that I use throughout this book because some words and concepts may be new to you. Where I use those terms, I have attempted to include them alongside examples, descriptions, and stories, but I have also defined them here. I encourage you to read through these definitions and come back to them as needed while you are reading the book.

- **anti-Blackness:** According to Charlene A. Carruthers, anti-Blackness is "a system of beliefs and practices that destroy, erode, and dictate the humanity of Black people."[3] It is a form of racism that specially targets Black people.

- **BIPOC (Black, Indigenous, People of Color):** A more inclusive and specific term than "people of color," the addition of Black and Indigenous helps to "account for the erasure of Black people with darker skin and Native American people," according to Cynthia Frisby, a professor at the Missouri School of Journalism at the University of Missouri.[4] Throughout the book I use the term "BIPOC people," even though the word "people" is already in the acronym, to make it clear that I am talking about groups of people.

- **Black:** I capitalize the B in Black to recognize the ethnic identity of Black folks in the United States. As Alexandria Neason of the Columbia Journalism Review writes, "I view the term Black as both a recognition of an ethnic identity in the States that doesn't rely on hyphenated Americanness (and is more accurate than African American, which suggests recent ties to the continent) and is also transnational and inclusive of our Caribbean [and] Central/South American siblings."[5] The Associated Press style guidelines were updated in June 2020 to include capitalizing the word Black when used to describe a person's or people's race or ethnicity; the w in white is not capitalized, in part because white people are not discriminated against because of their skin color and to avoid legitimizing white supremacist beliefs.

- **capitalism:** An economic system in which private individuals and corporations control the production of and access to goods and services. The profits that come from the production of the goods and services are also controlled by private companies, instead of by the people who provide labor to the companies. A focus is typically placed on economic growth, profits, private property, and limited government intervention over social issues like access to safe housing, income equality, healthcare, and education.

- **cisgender:** When a person's gender identity (that is, how someone experiences their own gender—i.e., as male, female, both, in between, or neither) matches their sex that was assigned to them at birth.

- **Eurocentric (or Eurocentrism):** Centered around or specifically highlighting European culture and Western civilization. Often this means favoring Western civilizations over non-Western ones.

- **fat:** A word used to describe a person's body size. Despite the negative connotations that society has assigned to it, *fat* is not inherently a "bad" word. Many people within the fat acceptance and body positivity communities use the word *fat* as a neutral adjective to describe their body size (similar to descriptors like short or tall). As Stephanie Yeboah writes in her book *Fattily Ever After,* "We deserve to re-claim the very word used to harass and hurt us."[7] Due to the negative associations that society has linked to the word *fat* and the baggage that may come with it, not everyone may feel ready to use it to describe themselves. We never want to assume how someone identifies or put a label on them. That said, I have chosen to use the word *fat* throughout the book as a neutral descriptor of body size in solidarity with the fat acceptance movement, in an effort to destigmatize the word, and because size oppression is a real thing, and we need to be able to describe the groups of people who experience size oppression if we hope to eliminate it.

  There is no fixed or consistent meaning to what constitutes a "fat person," and it can represent a wide range of body sizes. Some people consider "fat" to apply to any person with a body mass index (BMI) above "normal" (i.e., people with "overweight" or "obese" BMIs). Others consider "fat" to apply at the point where body size begins to significantly limit access to seating, public infrastructure like plane seats and turnstiles, and high-quality healthcare. Still others consider "fat" to be when a person wears plus-sized clothing, which can vary among clothing retailers, but in the United States is considered a size 14 to 28 (above a size 28 is usually referred to as "extended plus size").

- **fatphobia (also includes anti-fat beliefs):** The fear of and/or hatred of fat bodies. Can include a fear of becoming fat or fear of being fat.

- **healthism:** When health and disease are positioned as an individual person's problem and as something they must be obligated to "fix." With healthism, "health" becomes solely about one's personal practices without acknowledgment of the very real systemic and structural barriers that can impede health and well-being. Healthism's version of health does not incorporate any of the myriad social factors that, as you'll soon learn, have a much larger impact on the health of both the individual and the population as a whole. Healthism also assumes that all people want to or should pursue health; it makes health an obligation rather than a personal decision.

- **healthy/healthier:** Throughout the book, I often put these words in quotation marks to signify how the words are complicated, subjective, and often problematic. Our culture has assigned moral implications to these words. In our society, *healthy* tends to be thought of as *good*, whereas *unhealthy* tends to equal *bad*. (For this reason, I put *unhealthy* in quotation marks throughout the book, too.) Throughout the book, I talk more about how these connotations can have a harmful impact on our relationship to food.

- **homophobia:** Fear of, hatred of, and/or discrimination against people who are lesbian, gay, or bisexual. There are also people who use the term *queerphobia,* which can mean the fear of, hatred of, and/or discrimination against anyone who doesn't identify as heterosexual or cisgender and includes homophobia, biphobia (fear of, hatred of, and/or discrimination against people who are bisexual), transphobia (fear of, hatred of, and/or discrimination against people who are transgender), and more.

- **inclusive/inclusivity:** Being inclusive means honoring people's lived experiences and realities, even if they (or especially if they) differ from your experience or your reality.

- **intersectionality:** A term coined by Kimberle Crenshaw to describe the ways in which people with varying identities encounter the world.[8] Everybody holds various identities that intersect with one another, including their race, class, gender, physical ability, sexuality, age, nationality, religion, body size, socioeconomic status, and more. Intersectionality explains how the combination of several different identities will affect a person more than if they were living with just one at a time.

- **marginalized people:** Those people or groups of people who are relegated to the outskirts of society by systems of power and the people who hold power in a society. Marginalization involves confining a group of people to a less-important, less-powerful position in society. I also use the term "marginalized body" or "marginalized bodies"; by doing so I am not objectifying the person, but speaking to the ways in which systemic injustice specifically attacks (and marginalizes) certain bodies.

- **obesity and overweight:** While these words are commonly used to describe larger bodies, they have been developed and co-opted by the medical community to medicalize and pathologize a person's body (which means "to represent something as a disease" or treat someone as if they are "abnormal"). These words themselves are fatphobic and stigmatizing. *Overweight* is a word that assumes that there is a "correct" weight that a body should be and that if you are "over" that weight, then you are abnormal or different. The word *overweight* is rooted in the BMI charts, a problematic and flawed measure that assumes health is based on size (which, as I explain in the book, is not the case). Meanwhile the word *obese* comes from the Latin word *obesus*, meaning "having eaten until fat." The term assigns illness based on size, not on any other parameter, and places blame on the individual, which is not only incorrect but is stigmatizing. For this reason, naming people as "overweight" or "obese" isn't just talking about their body mass; it is by definition designating them as "atypical" or "unnatural," which further marginalizes a person to the outskirts of society. This is why I do not use those terms to describe people and why, when I do reference them, I put them in quotation marks to signify that I don't recognize them as official terms or agree with what they usually signify.

- **oppression:** When individuals or groups of people are subject to social, economic, and political burdens and perpetual disenfranchisement because they belong to a certain social group (because of their gender, race, sexual orientation, socioeconomic class, and more). In the textbook *Introduction to Community Psychology*, the authors state, "Typically, a government or political organization that is in power places these restrictions formally or covertly on groups so that the distribution of resources is unfairly allocated—and this means power stays in the hands of those who already have it... We can conclude that oppression is the social act of placing severe restrictions on an individual, group, or institution."[9] Oppression is a tool that is used to marginalize people across various intersections of identity.

- **patriarchy:** Refers to a social system where men hold most of the power, authority, and control in society.
- **privilege:** Refers to the social, economic, and political advantages or rights that the dominant group of people hold based upon their gender, race, sexual orientation, social class, etc.
- **racism:** The prejudice against, and the oppression and/or marginalization of, BIPOC people based upon the socially constructed racial hierarchy that privileges white people. Systemic racism includes the social systems, structures, and institutions in power that cause disparities in access to resources and opportunities for BIPOC people.
- **relationship to food**: How you regard food and behave toward it. A positive or "healthy" relationship to food can mean regarding all foods as neutral, allowing yourself to eat the foods you enjoy (and then move on), and trusting your body to tell you what and how much it needs. Many people have a damaged or disordered relationship to food, which may include behaviors like dieting, restricting, and bingeing; preoccupation with food; rigid behaviors or rituals around food; oppressive feelings of guilt and shame associated with eating; and/or feeling out of control around food. When we can shift how we regard and behave toward food, we can improve our relationship to food and find freedom and liberation.
- **sizeism:** The prejudice and discrimination against, and the oppression and/or marginalization of, people based on their body size. Most often is directed toward people who are fat. Closely linked to weight stigma.
- **thin:** There is no fixed or consistent meaning as to what constitutes "thin"; however, it is often used to describe anyone who fits into "straight-sized" clothing which is a U.S. size 12 and smaller (that is how I use it in this book as well). Although you may not feel thin (which speaks more to our screwed up society standards than your body), if you can buy clothing directly off the rack from any store, you are straight-sized and therefore benefit from certain social privileges. Although body image issues impact people of all sizes, thin/straight-sized folks are not the targets of structural or institutional sizeism (i.e., you're not assumed to be "unhealthy" just because of your size, you

can go to the doctor without having weight loss recommended as a fix for everything, and your health insurance rates aren't higher because of your body size).

- **transgender (also abbreviated as trans)**: A term that describes people whose gender identity and/or gender expression is different than the sex they were assigned at birth. Gender identity is a spectrum with many identities between the cisgender and transgender identities.

- **weight-centric or weight-normative**: An approach to health and well-being that views body weight as a determinant of health and emphasizes weight management (i.e., weight loss and the maintenance of a "normal" body mass index) when promoting health and well-being. In a weight-centric approach, a person who goes to the doctor for any type of medical issue is usually evaluated first based on their weight, regardless of whether their weight is relevant to what they are presenting with. A weight-centric or weight-normative approach assumes that weight and disease are related in a linear fashion and places an emphasis on "personal responsibility" for diet-, exercise-, and other health-related choices and outcomes (i.e., healthism). In this approach, a "normal" body mass index is conflated with health, whereas an "overweight" or "obese" body mass index is conflated with disease.

- **weight-inclusive**: An approach to health and well-being that does not focus on weight or weight reduction as a prerequisite for or measure of health and instead views health and well-being as multifaceted. Specific weights and body mass indexes are not idealized or pathologized. A weight-inclusive approach acknowledges that weight is not a behavior, but rather an outcome over which a person has very little control. This approach seeks to provide nonstigmatizing care and holds that everybody is capable of pursuing health and well-being independent of weight. The focus is taken off of weight and put upon modifiable lifestyle behaviors and the social determinants of health, including improving access to healthcare and reducing weight stigma.

- **weight stigma**: The negative attitudes and beliefs about fat folks and the assumptions made based upon their body size. It is a form of discrimination and oppression toward fat people in which they face daily barriers in society that thin people do not. This may include fewer job opportunities, lower pay, less respect, fewer clothing options, and more. Closely linked to fatphobia. Also known as sizeism.

PART 1

Fixing

CHAPTER 1

It's Not About the Food

What would our lives—and our world—look like if everyone could feel worthy in their bodies? If we could live our lives outside of the constraints of who we are told we *should* be or what we are *perceived* to be, and just be who we are? If, instead of having others trying to control our bodies, and us, we could be able to be guided by our internal wisdom? What if we could eat, and live, on our terms, without apologizing or offering explanation?

Every day I hear from women who tell me that they can't stop thinking about food or worrying about their bodies. They spend so much time thinking about what they're eating, what they're going to eat, and how much of it they're going to have. Every day is judged as "good" or "bad" based on what they ate (or didn't eat) and often by the number they see on the scale. As one client said to me, "My first thought when I wake up in the morning and my last thought before I go to bed is 'What did I eat?! Ugh, I'm so bad.'"

These women appear to have everything "together" in every other aspect of their lives. But under the surface, there is a recurring theme: Thoughts of food and what their bodies look like take up *so much* of their brain space that there's little room for anything else. Yet when we take a step back, food is just the tip of the iceberg. What presents as a problem related to food is, in reality, much deeper and more complex. Our screwed up, oppressive relationship to food is a symptom of the problem, not the cause. Body image struggles are not a personal flaw; they're a symptom of a bigger, more complex system that has been in place for centuries.

Western culture is hostile to women's bodies (the same can be said for many cultures around the world). From a very young age, we are taught—either directly or indirectly—that the value we have in the world is closely linked to our appearance and to other people's evaluation of our appearance. We are taught to diet and shrink ourselves to assimilate and be accepted. So many of us do. We spend a huge portion of our time, money, and energy attempting to "fix" ourselves to fit into the status quo. And no wonder: We live in a culture that venerates thinness. Our society places a premium on bodies that are thin, young, white, heterosexual, cisgender (meaning one's gender identity matches their sex assigned at birth), able-bodied, and conventionally attractive. To be anything else is to risk very real threats to your physical, psychological, and emotional health (though not necessarily for the reasons you may think).

We've been taught that women are supposed to look, act, and live a certain way. This indoctrination keeps us caged. Dieting and being made to feel shame about our bodies hold us back from fully living our lives because they keep us stifled, distracted, and dissatisfied, not to mention hungry. Dieting dampens our personalities, our relationships, our creativity, our joy, and our life experiences. It costs us time with friends and family, blunts connection to ourselves and to others, and affects our ability to work, lead, and parent.

This loss begins early. According to data from the National Institute on Media and Family, girls begin giving up activities because they don't like how they look as early as age ten.[1] More than 50 percent of thirteen-year-old American girls are unhappy with their bodies; that number grows to 80 percent by age seventeen and remains that high throughout adulthood.[2] So if you thought you were alone with your food and body image struggles, you most certainly are not.

Think of all the missed opportunities that come from waiting until you get to your "goal" weight or waiting until you feel happy about your body before you're willing to do certain things. I've seen women put off traveling, dating, switching careers, applying for promotions, and having children—all because they felt like they needed to lose weight first. It's really hard to be your full, authentic, empowered, unapologetic self when you are trying to live up to the ideals that society puts on women. As I will explain, society's unrealistic expectations are by design.

The good news is you can take an alternative path that doesn't involve dieting, self-loathing, or self-control. When you stop pursuing weight loss and cease numbing yourself with dieting, you can begin to transform your life. As you stop trying to control your body and give up attempting to fit yourself into the box (and body) that our dominant white, Eurocentric society deems "acceptable," you can turn inward toward the wisdom deep inside of you. You can begin to celebrate who you are instead of apologizing for what you are not. As you learn to trust your body with food, this trust transfers to other areas of your life. And thus begins the process of unlocking your true self and the ability to live your most authentic, meaningful, liberated life. But first, let's explore how the heck we got to this place.

Dieting as a Controlling Force

A cultural focus on body size and appearance (and therefore dieting) teaches us to deny what we truly want in favor of something that someone else says we should have or should be. We are taught to ignore our body's signals, and our body's wants and needs, in pursuit of a rigid, narrow definition of beauty and health. Dieting is controlling and oppressive by nature and also by design.

Western culture equates thinness to health, happiness, attractiveness, and worthiness, a system of beliefs that is often referred to as *diet culture*. In our society, to be thin is to be morally superior, whereas to be fat is to be unhealthy, lazy, and a failure. We are taught from a very young age that body size and the foods that someone chooses to eat reflect their worth as a person. Eating "bad" or "unhealthy" foods makes you a bad person, whereas eating "good" foods and trying to diet down to a smaller size is seen as virtuous. In this way, our culture promotes dieting and weight loss as a way to achieve a higher status in society. People are told that they have to eat a certain way and be a certain size to be "healthy." Therefore, certain foods and certain body types are inherently elevated while others are vilified. These cultural beliefs about body size and morality, worthiness, and even health didn't come out of nowhere. They were specifically created to establish social hierarchies.

The Colonialist Roots of Diet Culture

Diet culture, and the belief system that equates *thin* to *good* and *fat* to *bad*, may seem like a new phenomenon, but it has existed for centuries. For much of history, humans' main concern was getting enough food. For centuries, fat, round bodies were deemed beautiful, healthy, and desirable (though you can find examples of fatphobia—a fear of fatness—as far back as Ancient Greece and Rome).[3] The more modern origins of the diet culture we know today are rooted in colonialism, racism, classism, and sexism. That might sound far-fetched, but stick with me—I promise you it's not.

Our culture was built upon the control of Black, Indigenous, and People of Color (BIPOC) communities, which allowed white people to rise to the top and hold the power. To establish social hierarchies where white people (especially white men) could remain at the top, white Europeans and Americans linked being Black and/or being fat to negative traits like greediness and laziness. As Sabrina Strings, author of *Fearing the Black Body*, explains, "Two critical historical developments contributed to a fetish for svelteness and a phobia about fatness: the rise of the transatlantic slave trade and the spread of Protestantism. Racial scientific rhetoric about slavery linked fatness to 'greedy' Africans and religious discourse suggested that overeating was ungodly...In the United States, fatness became stigmatized as both black and sinful. Slenderness served as a marker of moral, racial and national superiority."[4] White men effectively created a societal "other"—marginalizing Black people and, in their efforts to do so, relegating fatness as something to fear and avoid. This fatphobia, rather than any concern of health or well-being, is what began our culture's fixation on weight. As I'll talk more about in Chapter 3, the link between health and weight was established as a result of fatphobia—not the other way around.

In the United States, food and body size have always been closely tied to morality. This association is due in large part to religious rhetoric that held pleasure as sinful and believed that denying the body's appetites was a way for a person to get closer to God. From that concept came the idea that "overeating" or eating "bad" foods signified a "bad" or "immoral" person. This idea that anything "impure" must be avoided explains almost all popular diets. It also explains the common stereotypes that exist about fat people: that they are lazy, uneducated, and lack willpower. These negative terms—linked directly to body size—denote immorality.

The Sexist Roots of Diet Culture

In addition to colonialism and racism, diet culture also has its roots in sexism and the desire for female obedience. We live in a patriarchal society, a social system in which men hold the majority of the power and have historically dominated leadership roles at every level of society. So, who benefits from women being preoccupied by dieting and conforming to body ideals? Men (white men in particular).

When we examine history, especially in the nineteenth and twentieth centuries, each time women gained more power and advancement, society responded with the creation of more and more beauty and body ideals. As Naomi Wolf describes in her book *The Beauty Myth*, "A cultural fixation on female thinness is not an obsession about female beauty but an obsession about female obedience...Dieting is the most potent political sedative in women's history; a quietly mad population is a tractable one."[5] Obsessing over weight, size, and appearance is not only harmful physically and mentally (as you'll see in Chapter 2), but it holds women back in society. Once again, society's emphasis on thinness is not about women's health or well-being but about their submission.

Creating a culture that elevates thinness and demonizes fat bodies serves as an oppressive force to keep women and BIPOC people down and white men and their institutions in power. (Note: This isn't to say that men are not affected by diet culture but, by and large, people who have been socialized as women, including cisgender women, transgender women, and people in feminized and/or gender nonconforming bodies, have historically been the prime targets.) Those in power have, over time, conditioned society as a whole to believe that certain groups can't be trusted. Our culture teaches us that our bodies aren't to be trusted, which we then internalize as the message that we can't trust ourselves.

When we don't trust ourselves, we are more apt to look to others to measure how we are "doing." When it comes to food and body size, this lack of trust often shows up in the form of frequent weighing (to make sure we are staying "on track") or counting calories (to make sure we are staying "in control"). But this also shows up in many other facets of our lives. Whenever we look for external approval rather than relying on internal body signals and self-trust, others can then define us. When you don't trust yourself, it becomes easy to be influenced by societal expectations versus pursuing what you really want. In this way, diet culture—and therefore dieting—serves as a way to control people. When you are concerned with fulfilling a societal "ideal" of thinness, you are distracted from fully living your life and are not able to step into your full power. Dieting distracts people from doing other, more important, things, which is exactly what those in power want.

To be clear, I do not say this to shame anyone who attempts to conform to these societal body ideals. Very real oppression exists for people who hold marginalized identities, and it's understandable that someone would want to protect themselves from this injustice. The blame does not rest on the individual but on the societal systems and structures put in place to make things convenient for men while subjugating women, fat people, BIPOC people, and queer people. We've all been existing in these systems since day one, so it makes sense that we would participate in working to achieve these ideals. But these are the same systems that disconnect us from our bodies and ourselves and teach us to deny what our bodies want and need in favor of what society deems "acceptable." To move forward, we must become critical consumers and objectively assess all of the systems in which we take part.

Reflection Questions

What has dieting or your pursuit of weight loss gotten in the way of?

What is it costing you not to improve your relationship to food and your body?

What would you do if you weren't spending as much time thinking about food or your body?

The History of Beauty Ideals

Thinness is just one social beauty standard that we have been indoctrinated to believe we must adhere to. In addition to body size, there are dozens of other beauty ideals in our culture—most often directed at women. These standards of beauty are anything but accidental. The beauty ideal is the socially constructed idea that a woman's appearance, "prettiness," and desirability are her most important traits. Society rewards those who work to achieve, maintain, and adhere to the "ideal," a practice that takes a good deal of time, money, and energy. Convincing women that they must pursue certain beauty ideals also serves as a distraction. When women are busy trying to achieve these "ideals," they are less likely to have time to pursue liberation, equality, and power.

What was thought of as "beautiful" used to vary considerably between cultures, but as Western beauty (and body) ideals overtake more of the world, we are unfortunately seeing more cultures conform to these ideals. History shows us that beauty ideals (including body size) are in constant flux. In Western society, women's "ideal" body has shifted every decade or so throughout the twentieth century. Again, this is by design.

Before the twentieth century, the "ideal" woman's body in white American culture was typically voluptuous, with full breasts, hips, and a soft belly. In the early 1900s, women wore corsets to emphasize their waist and curves. During the tail end of the first wave of popular U.S. feminism in the 1920s, which was primarily centered upon white women, a skinny, curveless body shape came into fashion as women took to binding their chests and wearing straight, flapper-style dresses to de-emphasize their curves. In the 1940s and '50s, a fuller body type returned, as the "glamorous

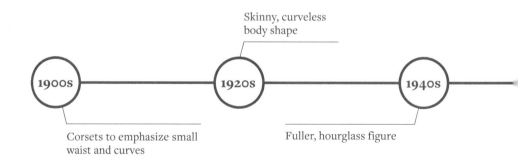

housewife" with an hourglass figure became popular. The second wave of feminism in the 1960s and '70s brought back the thin, androgynous body as a beauty ideal. In the 1980s, we saw the rise of "fit" and "toned" bodies, à la Jane Fonda and Jazzercise. The ideal was still slim but now strong as well. The 1990s saw a reemergence of the "waif" look, with an uptick in white models who were thin, pale, and young-looking. Big breasts also began to be fashionable, and plastic surgery for breast augmentation became popular.

The beauty ideal today is similar to the 1990s, but it's become even *more* unattainable, and in some cases literally impossible, given the prolific use of minimally invasive surgery, Photoshop, and filters. The "ideal" woman's body in the U.S. as of 2020 is thin, with a small waist, muscle definition, and a thigh gap but also with big breasts and a large round butt.

Because most women don't naturally fit that description, products like shapewear—those tight undergarments that make a body look smooth under clothing—were created to make a woman look "better" by getting closer to the standard of beauty. The explicit purpose is to "smooth" the body and therefore make it look more "acceptable" by society's standards. Although it's understandable if you think you look "better" in shapewear, often when you feel as though you "have" to look a certain way, it's due to conditioning from being *taught* that this way looks better. That's not to say that you're wrong for wearing it or that you have to give it up. There are folks who understand the history of shapewear and still wear it because they like it and enjoy how it looks. But, as I'll discuss more shortly, thinking critically about what prompts us to use shapewear (and to try to meet other beauty ideals) then makes us more aware of our motives for using it and, in the end, everyone is able to make the choice that feels best for them.

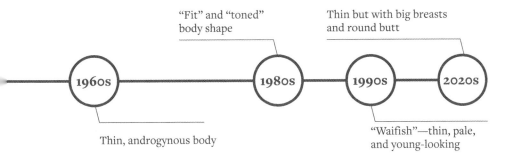

Chapter 1: It's Not About the Food

Eurocentrism and Whiteness

Something important to note about all of the beauty standards that I just described is that they are overwhelmingly Eurocentric. The default concept of "beautiful" aligns to the white person's features. So while beauty ideals are harmful to all women, women of color carry a much larger burden. Achieving greater proximity to whiteness means becoming more valuable to society and can function to improve one's social status. Society is full of subtle and not-so-subtle messages telling women of color that the more white they look, the better. As activist Sonya Renee Taylor writes in her book *The Body Is Not an Apology,* "In Western societies hair is often tied to notions of femininity, beauty, and gender...Hair should have a certain texture, should be a certain color. For Americans, the rules for hair (like most of our body rules) come with a default aesthetic: long, straight, fine...and, if possible, blonde...Short, dark, kinky hair...would never be the default and by extension never be normal. In our society, normal is the pathway to worthy and beautiful."[6] Just as we see with body and weight ideals, beauty ideals were shaped against a racist (classist, sexist, ableist) backdrop.

Ageism

Several years ago, when I first started noticing deepening wrinkles on my forehead and around my eyes, I panicked. I bought all sorts of antiaging creams and researched the cost of Botox. As soon as I noticed gray hairs, I immediately started plucking them. I was terrified of getting older and was ashamed and embarrassed of my aging face and body for giving me away. And it's no wonder. In our culture, youth is prized, and this value is reflected in the standard beauty ideals. Also, women are taught that our most highly valued social asset is our looks, so it's not surprising that so many of us are afraid to age.

The message of youth being better is conveyed in ways both subtle and not so subtle. Women who age "well" or "gracefully" (i.e., who still look young) are celebrated. In an era where injectables like Botox and fillers are marketed to younger and younger women and retouching a photo is as simple as downloading an app, the smooth, ageless face is ubiquitous. This is reflected in the media, where we rarely see women over the age of 35. (The same can't be said for older men, who show up in the media at least ten times more frequently than older women.) When a woman inevitably does age, her visibility and value plummets. No wonder women are terrified of any sign of aging and try to do whatever they can to "fix" it.

Our fear of aging—and our worship of youth—is handed down to us via capitalism and the patriarchy. A capitalistic society needs labor and productivity to increase profits. Young people have more ability to be productive and more labor-generating years in them, so they are valued more than older adults. Also, with age comes power. As Kelly Diels, an educator, writer, and coach, shared with me, "Wrinkles and gray hair are a function of age, and with age comes wisdom. That's why women aren't allowed to show age—because it telegraphs internal power."[7] Power, in our male-dominated culture, isn't meant to be wielded by women. Whenever a woman has something that conveys power, including signs of aging, society often tells her she should be ashamed of it and try to cover it or keep it hidden. In the end, "men don't age better than women, they're just allowed to age."[8]

Are They Really "Flaws"?

Similar to my experience with my first wrinkles and gray hairs, when I began to notice cellulite on my legs I immediately tried to find a "fix." I thought cellulite made me look unattractive, and I spent years (and lots of money) on creams and lotions to try to make it go away. Never for a minute did I stop and think about *why* I believed that cellulite, wrinkles, and gray hair were not attractive. If I had, I would have realized that I had learned these beliefs rather than being born with them.

Many of the things that we consider "flaws" today were not actually seen as such until society—and then advertisers—made them out to be. As Jes Baker says in her book, *Things No One Will Tell Fat Girls*, "You hate your body because Don Draper told you to."[9] Although it's not quite as simple as that, private corporations do set out to make us feel insecure so that beauty product manufacturers can sell us a "cure" (and make money). Let's look deeper at a few of these so called "flaws."

Body Hair

Although it is now a societal norm for women to shave their armpits (or else risk being labeled "gross"), women never thought to do so until the early 1900s when sleeveless dresses became en vogue, and a company that sold men's hair removal products decided to target women. They launched a multiyear ad campaign geared toward selling hair-removal cream to women by convincing them that smooth underarms were the latest must-have beauty trend. In the advertisements, underarm hair was called "embarrassing," "unsightly," and "unclean." Meanwhile, the ads suggested that women with hairless underarms were "refined," "dainty," and "perfectly groomed."

This hairless ideal soon extended to women's legs as well. Up until the 1930s, most women didn't shave their legs because they typically wore pantyhose. But during World War I, when silk and nylon manufacturing was forced to slow down, more and more women began to remove their leg hair. Advertisers jumped on board, positioning smooth, hairless legs as the epitome of womanhood. Fast-forward eighty years and most women today consider hair removal a necessary evil. Almost all the women I know wouldn't dream of putting on shorts or a skirt without first shaving their legs; the same goes for a bathing suit and their bikini lines or a tank top with their underarms. It's a beauty ideal so ingrained in our society that it's hard to imagine a time when it wasn't the case.

Cellulite

Biologically, cellulite occurs naturally for 80 to 90 percent of women. That's right: Basically, *all of us* have it, no matter our body size. The dimples and bumps are a result of natural subcutaneous fat poking through connective tissue (men's cellular structure is slightly different, which is why it's not as prevalent on their skin). Cellulite doesn't discriminate between body sizes or types—women big and small get cellulite—and it's not harmful to your health. Nowadays, it's thought of as an unsightly skin condition to be fixed, but before the 1960s and '70s, it was just considered normal skin. Then in the late 1960s, the term *cellulite* was first referenced in *Vogue* magazine, introducing its readers to the word and creating yet another beauty standard to try to achieve. Once cellulite was seen as a "problem" to be fixed, skin care companies began creating cellulite-elimination products to profit off another beauty ideal.

Gray Hair

In Western cultures, gray hair signifies a loss of youth. And with beauty ideals being firmly planted in "youthfulness," anything that signifies old age becomes taboo—at least for women. As with most beauty ideals, a double standard exists for men and women. Men who let their hair gray are called "silver foxes," and their hair color is referred to as "salt and pepper." Women, on the other hand, get the message from a young age that we'd better cover up the gray. It's almost impossible to find a woman with naturally gray hair in the media; women must "age gracefully" by disguising their graying hairs, whereas a man with graying hair is called "distinguished." However, until the 1940s and '50s, most women didn't dye their grays (though not because it wasn't a beauty ideal but because it was considered something that only "loose" women did, and at that point, there was no way for a woman to change her hair color without going to a salon). That was until Clairol, a hair-coloring company, revamped the image of hair coloring to appeal to women's anxieties over aging. They ran advertisements telling women that their gray hair caused them to be old and "not fun," that it confined them to wearing clothing in "subdued colors," and that they could only have friends from the "older set." And a new hair-related beauty ideal was born.

Shiny White Teeth

I was watching an old episode of *Grey's Anatomy* recently (yes, I am still a devoted fan) and was struck by how not white, and not perfect, the actors' teeth were. This show was filmed less than twenty years ago, yet the difference was startling to me. Watch any television show or movie that was filmed before the early 2000s, and you'll see the same thing: everyone's teeth are a natural bone-white color and vary in size. In the mid-1990s, in-office teeth-whitening products first came to dentists' offices—closely followed by over-the-counter do-it-yourself products—and shiny, bright white teeth were advertised as the new beauty must-have. If you look at social media, magazines, or TV today, you'll find that all teeth are blindingly white, perfectly straight, and the same size. This "Hollywood smile" is now considered the norm in our youth- and status-obsessed society, even though white, straight, symmetrical teeth are not natural and only attainable at a cost.

Wrinkles

I've had many similar ah-ha moments watching the faces of people in television shows and movies from ten or twenty years ago. Take Carrie Bradshaw in *Sex and the City*. In the iconic opening scene, Sarah Jessica Parker, the actress who plays Carrie, is thirty-two years old and has fine lines around her eyes and on the bridge of her nose (not to mention her forehead—it actually moves!). The scene was filmed in 1998, before Botox and cosmetic fillers became ubiquitous and fine lines on the face were considered normal. The FDA officially approved Botox Cosmetic for use on facial lines in 2002, giving the green light to Allergan, the maker of Botox, to begin a multi-million-dollar marketing campaign for the facial injectable. The company capitalized on the cultural pressure for women's bodies and faces to remain looking young and put out ad campaigns targeting middle-aged women.

Today almost 60 percent of Botox users are between the ages of forty-five and fifty-four. But the age of "selfie" culture, the proliferation of Photoshop and retouching, and the 24/7 stream of smooth jawlines, chiseled cheekbones, and wrinkle-free faces has spurred a younger demographic of women to use injectables. According to the American Society of Plastic Surgeons, from 2010 to 2018, Botox procedures increased 28 percent among people between the ages of *twenty and twenty-nine*.[10] Botox is now being marketed toward younger women as a *preventative* measure—something they should use before fine lines or wrinkles even start to show. The thirty- to thirty-eight-year-old demographic now makes up almost 20 percent of all Botox injectable treatments annually. Unsurprisingly, women make up 94 percent of all Botox treatments (and 92 percent of cosmetic procedures overall).[11] The fact that young, wrinkle-free women are spending time and money getting Botox to freeze their faces preventatively says a lot about the demands that Western culture places on us to stay young.

Questioning and Experimenting with Beauty Ideals

It's not a bad thing to take part in any of these beauty ideals. They aren't inherently evil or wrong, and you may really enjoy partaking in certain beauty rituals. Not to mention that privilege, power, respect, and even higher salaries can come from conforming to these standards. That's right: Studies have found that women who wear more makeup and are "well-groomed" make significantly more money than women who wear less makeup.[12] (Meanwhile, grooming doesn't come into play for men's salaries—surprise, surprise.) This is a problem because although some women enjoy beauty rituals, others do not. When opting out of adhering to societal beauty and body norms affects your paycheck, it stops being about choice and starts being about the control and oppression of women, fat folks, and BIPOC people.

At the same time, there is power in knowledge and in questioning: Are you taking part in certain beauty rituals because you want to or because you feel you have to? When you understand the roots of beauty ideals, you can begin to decenter appearance as the most important aspect of a woman's—and your—character. All women—and all humans—are worthy and valuable, no matter what they look like. When you can internalize this belief, then you don't *need* makeup or hair color to feel beautiful or visible or worthy. You don't *need* to cover up your skin. You don't *need* to avoid wrinkles. Instead, you get to *choose* which beauty products or ideals you want to partake in and which ones you don't. That's what freedom and liberation is: having a choice about what you want to do or not do; what you want to look like or not look like. For some, this could mean wearing makeup, using Botox, shaving their legs, or whitening their teeth. For others, freedom may mean opting out of these ideals. In the end it comes down to having the choice to do what makes you feel good.

Now, that doesn't change the fact that we are all a product of our upbringing and culture, and we don't make any decisions inside a vacuum. As long as women are held to unattainable beauty standards, and as long as it affects our earning potential, the urge and even the need to partake in beauty rituals will continue to persist. But when you are conscious of where these oppressive beauty ideals came from (i.e., they were created by white men and/or companies who profit from the ideals), why they continue to evolve and change (i.e., to continue to keep women and BIPOC people down and/or make money), and know that you have options outside of what society considers "normal," then you can make the decision that feels best for you.

Beauty rituals like makeup and hair grooming can be an empowering form of self-expression and identification. At the same time, if you're looking to move away from using certain beauty ideals on autopilot, it can be freeing and liberating to experiment with rejecting certain social beauty norms. I, for one, found this to be the case when I began trying to go makeup-free a few years ago. (Important disclaimer: I hold a lot of privileges that made this experiment easier for me than it may be for other people. Despite my ever-multiplying face wrinkles, I am young, thin, white, and, even on my makeup-free days, I naturally fit into many conventional beauty ideals. So an experiment like this is going to be easier for me than it will for a person who is not thin, white, or young. But the end result— that is, how you feel—can be similar.) Although I have never been a huge makeup person, I, like many women, rarely used to leave the house with a naked face. Makeup made me feel prettier and more accepted. If I did go out of the house without makeup, I never felt as attractive or as confident. As I began learning about the origins of beauty ideals, I realized that I wanted to be able to feel comfortable and confident with or without makeup. At first, it was really hard. Going out to a restaurant in New York City on a Friday night without makeup felt like walking naked on a fashion runway. So I started slowly—first by leaving off foundation and then, gradually, cutting back on my eye makeup.

It took almost a full year, but I eventually got to a point where I felt 100 percent myself, comfortable and confident, makeup or not. I am now able to go out in public without hiding or camouflaging or covering any part of myself up, which—aside from taking way less time to get ready—feels really freaking liberating. Could I have gotten to the same place while still wearing makeup? Probably. But for me, going barefaced allowed me to get there much faster. It pushed me to work through the discomfort of feeling different, of not feeling like I looked "perfect." And it showed me that I can allow myself to be seen and be loved and be open as just me. Because my choosing to go barefaced was about way more than the makeup. Experimenting with this beauty ideal helped me to know what my full, true self is under the makeup. And I can let that shine through with or without any on—whichever I choose.

In the end, you get to choose what beauty ideals you partake in, whether that's wearing high heels and fashionable clothes, using hair dye, getting a blowout, shaving your legs, and even having plastic surgery. I get it—legs look fabulous in high heels, and a little mascara can work wonders. Plastic surgery can be life-changing for many people, including trans folks, people with disabilities, and people who want to use surgery to make changes to their bodies. But we need to question why the vast majority of women feel obligated to spend their time and money on all of these external trappings, whereas very few men do. We also should wonder why the beauty and dieting industries target women far more than they do men. So I challenge you to dig deep and start to question the "why" behind your choices. Then maybe, if you feel comfortable, you can begin to play with letting some of those beauty ideals go—even if it's for just a little while. As one of my clients said, "I know now that I can wear whatever I want, not use makeup (or use it if I want), and be confident in who I am without letting other people's opinions sway me. It feels so empowering."

Explore Your Beauty Rituals ───────────

Make a list of the different beauty rituals you participate in and reflect upon why you do these things. Which of them do you do for yourself? Are there any that you do for others? Perhaps there is some overlap? Which of these do you enjoy? Are there any that you do because you feel like you have to?

Dieting as a Way to Belong

As our culture's body and beauty ideas were created, conforming to them was not only a way to achieve status or worth but a way to belong. The need to belong has a strong evolutionary benefit.[13] Way back when, belonging to a group was essential for human survival. Humans hunted together, cooked together, and protected the others in their group. When enemies would attack, or when it was difficult to find food or shelter, people who were part of a group were more likely to survive. If you didn't belong to a group, your chances of survival were low. In modern times, this is not necessarily the case, but humans still have a strong desire to belong to a social group and be accepted by others.

In present-day society, there is a strong negative bias against fat bodies (which I'll discuss in more detail in Chapter 3). As I mentioned earlier, body size is intertwined with morality, and we're programmed to believe that thin bodies are inherently "good," whereas fat bodies are "bad." People in fat bodies are marginalized and "othered," which means they're relegated to the outskirts of society. As human beings with a strong need to belong, we are taught that we can avoid this marginalization if we make our bodies smaller—or at least *try* to make our bodies smaller. So belonging, for many people, requires dieting and food restriction. Dieting can also be a way that BIPOC people assimilate into Western society. To protect themselves against oppression, they may seek weight loss or pursue other white beauty ideals.

Much of the time, people are accepted by Western society only when they are thin, or when they are in the pursuit of thinness. As Noreen,* a former client of mine shared, "By dieting and making an effort to lose weight, I was attempting to show people that I deserve to be seen as valuable and to be treated well. When I was actively trying to no longer be fat, I fit into the box that society liked: I was being a 'good' fat person, and I was congratulated for doing the 'right' thing. Now that I have given up dieting and have chosen to embrace my body, rather than attempt to shrink it, people don't know what to do with me. I can no longer pretend that I'm trying to fit in, within a society where striving for the thin ideal is so ingrained."

Bonding Over Diet-Talk

What is seen at a larger societal level is also experienced within smaller social groups. These days, *not* dieting can feel like not belonging. In many families, workplaces, and social settings, it is considered normal to talk about what diet someone is on. Almost every single person that I work with tells me that they are the only person in their social group who is trying *not* to diet. This lack of community and outside pressure from friends and family makes taking an alternative path that much more difficult.

When I first began dieting in high school, I immediately got attention for eating "healthy" foods. Eating foods that were deemed "healthy" and "good" made me feel better than people who didn't seem to pay attention to what they ate; I felt morally superior. I loved the opportunity to talk about my diet and what I was (or was not) eating. As more and more of my peers got caught up in dieting, it became a form of bonding to talk about our diets and our weight loss and our bodies.

---

* All current and former client names and identifying details have been changed to protect their privacy.

Fast-forward twenty years to a recent dinner out in New York City. I was dining with several smart, successful, interesting women, but the conversation was dominated by what they were eating. One of them had eliminated gluten and dairy; another one was midway through her third time with Whole30; yet another was raving about her experience with the keto diet. Years ago, I too would have joined in with the diet talk, happy to talk about what I was or wasn't eating. Instead, I sat there, frustrated that such successful women were wasting their time dieting, but also feeling somewhat left out that I couldn't (or wouldn't) contribute to the conversation. Even me, a firm anti-diet dietitian, still could feel a sense of not-belonging when the conversation turned to dieting.

Body Bashing

Body bashing is another phenomenon that frequently occurs when groups of women get together. Women often bond over their body shame, sharing the parts of themselves that they dislike, with each person chiming in with her own tales of body-hate. A scene from an episode of *Sex and the City*, a television show centered around four thin, white, wealthy, conventionally attractive women, illustrates this:

> Charlotte: "I hate my thighs."
> Miranda: "Well, I'll take your thighs and raise you a chin."
> Carrie: "I'll take your chin and raise you a [points at nose]."
> *They look expectantly at the fourth woman, Samantha, who refuses to participate.*
> "What?" Samantha says, "I happen to love the way I look."[14]

Another phrase that commonly arises in social circles (not to mention in every single form of media) is, "I feel so fat." This type of statement is invariably followed by someone else—a friend, a family member, a partner—reassuring them, "Oh no, you're not fat—you're beautiful." These types of comments have become so normalized, and even expected, that we don't even notice them for how damaging and fatphobic they are because those "reassurances" are saying that if someone is fat, they aren't beautiful. Body bashing only serves to reinforce the beliefs that thin is better than fat and that the most valuable aspect of a woman is her appearance.

Dieting as a Coping Mechanism

When Susann, now thirty-nine, was growing up, her home life was chaotic and unreliable. She never knew what kind of mood her parents were going to be in, and she never knew when the adults in her life were going to be there for her. "As a kid, I had so many big feelings, but there was no support and no one modeling how to cope with emotions," she shared with me. "So I started to eat in order to not feel those very big feelings." At eight years old, Susann began to use food to numb and cope with the emotions she was having because she was never taught any other way. "Having 'big feelings' was not okay in my family," she said. "The message that I received was that intense feelings were for 'crazy people,'* and I wanted to be better than that, so I kept my feelings inside and stayed 'in control.'"

At the same time, Susann was getting messages from her family members, as well as from the media and through friends, that being a "big girl" was not good and not desirable. "Since I didn't know how to cope with my feelings outside of eating, I went straight to intense food restricting and exercising, starting when I was ten years old," Susann explained. "Looking at the numbers on food labels and on the scale gave me a sense of control and pride. I ended up losing weight and got a ton of praise and attention for it. I felt like by controlling my body, I could control how other people viewed me."

When things feel out of control in life, many people turn to dieting. Trying to control something, like the food they eat or their body size, can provide a false sense of security. This sense of control can, in the moment, make someone feel more stable and safe. Neuroscience explains this phenomenon. Our brains are wired to keep us safe. Each time you go through some type of "threat," your brain is wired to remember that threat and—the next time it arises—old thought patterns and behaviors emerge as coping mechanisms. This means that, in response to stress or chaos, negative body thoughts can arise, and the urge to perform dieting behaviors, whether through food restriction or exercising, increases. Therefore, dieting can be a

---

* The word *crazy* is an ableist term. When we call someone crazy, we are basically saying that that person's lived experience doesn't make sense or isn't valid. The word *crazy* has been used as a tool of oppression to make marginalized folks question their reality so that they think they are the problem or that something is inherently bad about them. Read more at https://www.npr.org/2019/07/08/739643765/why-people-are-arguing-to-stop-using-the-words-crazy-and-insane.

way to feel safe and in control while it distracts from the other, more over-whelming emotions that may feel hard to deal with.

Another client of mine, Nina, experienced this firsthand. "When I look back, my periods of dieting almost always coincided with me feeling out of control in another part of my life. I first started dieting around the time that my parents announced they were getting a divorce; another phase of diet-ing coincided with my husband losing his job. Whenever life feels chaotic, I notice more of an urge to restrict my food or to try a new diet. Instead of dealing with the issue, I cope by turning to dieting and exercise."

Dieting is the ultimate coping mechanism because it keeps us distracted from difficult feelings and helps us feel like we have control even when we really don't. But dieting is a counterproductive coping mechanism because, eventually, it doesn't work. (I'll share the reasons why in Chapter 2.) The next distraction tactic we tend to jump to is judging ourselves as having "failed." Then back to the diet, to try to get "control" again, and round and round it goes.

Although controlling what you eat may feel good in the short term, it doesn't help to address the actual problem, *and* it causes more issues in the long run. The reality is that you don't actually have control over much of what happens in life. That means trying to control things will keep you in a loop of continuing to feel unsafe and anxious. In Chapter 10, I'll share more on ways you can safely give up the need to control, but for now, remember that having an urge to diet probably means something bigger is going on.

While dieting itself is often used as an oppressive force, it can also be a way that folks in marginalized bodies cope with the oppression they ex-perience daily. As Carolina Guízar, a Mexican-American dietitian based in New York City, explains, "Diet culture can be a positive distraction from the oppression that people of color and people in larger bodies face on a daily basis. Dieting can be a way of coping with the pain of constantly being 'othered' and judged by the color of their skin or the size of their body, while also helping one assimilate into a culture that prizes smaller, white bodies and specific foods."[15] When it comes to people in larger bodies, dieting may be a way in which they gain access to healthcare or physical infrastructure (like chairs or airplane seats) that is denied to them because of their size. For example, many surgeons require people to be below a certain weight before they'll perform lifesaving surgeries. In many ways, for folks in larger bodies, dieting can be a way (if only in the short term) of coping and assimilating into a culture that is so centered upon, and built for, smaller bodies.

Our culture feeds us messages that certain bodies are "not enough," and that there is something wrong with us if we don't fit the ideal. The diet and beauty industries capitalize on this, marketing to people who believe they need to lose weight to become a "better" version of themselves. Most people have not processed all of the ways in which they've been told that their body is "wrong." So, very often, dieting is a way to cope with these messages rather than face deep wounds.

Body and Beauty Ideals Steal Our Time, Money, and Energy

Society encourages people to change *themselves* to better fit into the (white and male-dominated) world. Conforming to body and beauty ideals is time-consuming and expensive (not to mention futile). The more time we spend trying to "fix" ourselves, the less time we have for other things. Years ago, a group of friends and I were discussing our getting-ready rituals before a night out. For most of us, it went something like this: wash and blow dry hair, shave legs and underarms, make sure to get a bikini wax *just in case,* apply makeup, and decide on the "right" outfit (which often entailed at least a few phone calls or texts to get a friend's opinion). One of our guy friends sat there listening with his jaw open—he could not believe the amount of time we spent getting ready. When we asked him what he did before a night out, he said, "Well, I take a shower and put on a clean shirt." That was it. Meanwhile, we women were spending several hours prepping—just for one night out. And we weren't even considering the time, money, and energy we had spent on dieting, diet plans, "healthy" food, or gym memberships.

When you extrapolate this one scenario to a lifetime of trying to comply with society's body and beauty standards, just think of all the time, energy, and money that is spent. As society's marginalized groups continue to push back against the thin ideal and other white, Eurocentric beauty standards, the definition of "beautiful" and "desirable" continues to change and evolve. In doing so, it keeps us continually striving for an arbitrary "ideal" and costing us much of our time, money, and energy.

Once again, this is not to shame anyone who attempts to conform to these body or beauty ideals. For many marginalized folks, working to achieve these ideals may be a way of protecting themselves against the oppression that they face. But the more you can work to not let how your body looks or what size it is hold you back from living out your values and being fully yourself, the more you can be free. And the more of us who are free, the more social and political impact we can have both individually and collectively. Because no one is free from oppression until all bodies are liberated.

Body Autonomy and the Power of Choice

There is power in knowledge and in understanding how our society's different beauty and body standards came to be. Although the knowledge doesn't negate the oppression that anyone in a marginalized body faces, it shifts the blame to the true culprit. You are not to blame for "failing" to lose weight or maintain a certain size body. The blame sits squarely on the shoulders of the system that was set up to overpower you.

All behaviors are adaptive and begin for a reason. At some point in your life, dieting was probably something that served you. Perhaps it made you feel safe, accepted, or in control. And you may still find that, to this day, dieting is something that keeps you feeling safe. I can't and won't ever tell someone what to do with their body. However, I *can* encourage you to unpack and dismantle the beliefs about food and body size that society has programmed into you. You may begin to recognize how suffocating it has been to prioritize the look and size of your body above all else. Then you can reject the messages, beliefs, and behaviors that keep you in that cage. When you step out of that cage, you can begin the process of coming home to yourself and redefining what self-acceptance means to you. This is when magic happens.

If there is still part of you that is unsure about all of this, that is okay. My goal is to support you, if and when you decide that you're ready, to explore a life without dieting or attempting to shrink your body. If you've gotten this far, my guess is that there is at least part of you ready to walk down this new path. So let's begin the unpacking, unlearning, and redefining.

CHAPTER 2

Your Brain on Diets

Each year, more than 50 percent of American adults try to lose weight. The diet industry in the United States makes more than $70 billion per year. (Yes, that is *billion*.) Yet research shows that 90 to 97 percent of people who lose weight through dieting will regain it within two to five years.[1] How is this possible? Turns out it has nothing to do with people "failing" the diets, and everything to do with diets failing the people.

Before I dive into this more, I want to pause to define *diets* and *dieting*. *Merriam-Webster Dictionary* defines the word *diet* as follows:

1. food and drink regularly provided or consumed
2. habitual nourishment
3. the kind and amount of food prescribed for a person or animal for a special reason
4. a regimen of eating and drinking sparingly so as to reduce one's weight

Merriam-Webster also defines the word *diet* when it is used as a verb:

1. to cause to take food
2. to cause to eat and drink sparingly or according to prescribed rules[2]

The word *diet* was historically used to refer to what a person usually eats; it was a neutral descriptor. Since the diet industry has co-opted the word, it is most often used to describe the *absence* of eating something. We now most often see the word used when it's linked to weight loss or certain food rules.

I'm going to talk a lot about diets and dieting in this book, so let's make sure we're on the same page as to what I am referencing when I use these terms. Most people understand the words *diet* or *dieting* to mean diet programs such as the Atkins Diet, the South Beach Diet, Jenny Craig, the keto (or ketogenic) diet, and the Paleo diet. Although I definitely consider those diets, my definition of a *diet* or *dieting* is much broader. When I use those terms, I'm referring instead to any way of eating that is dictated by external forces rather than internal ones. A diet is when someone or something outside of yourself determines *what* you eat, *when* you eat, or *how* you eat. It is any activity, system, company, person, or program that promotes its way of eating (and/or exercising) as one that helps you lose weight. By this definition, the word *diet* expands to include activities like counting calories, macros, or points and measuring or weighing food; terms like *portion control, clean eating, watching what you eat;* labels for foods such as "good" or "bad"; and cheat meals or cheat days. The word *diet* also includes programs or ways of eating that identify themselves as (or are identified by others as) "wellness" related, including WW (formerly Weight Watchers) intermittent fasting, and Whole30, as well as apps like Noom or MyFitnessPal. These diets may be marketed as a way to manipulate your body size or appearance, or they may not—or at least not overtly.

This is where it gets tricky because many of these diets and their promoters claim that they are *not* diets. In fact, many people I work with tell me that they've never "really" dieted. Then, when I ask them about their food history, they tell me about cutting out all sorts of foods and food groups, trying to "watch" what they eat by not having too much sugar or carbohydrate, or doing Whole30 every January. These behaviors *are* dieting. No matter whether you call it wellness, a lifestyle change, or something else, if it involves external control and the hope or promise of weight loss, then it is a diet. Now a part of you may be thinking, "Well, I'm really doing this for health reasons." That is all well and good, but if you still harbor the hope—either conscious or subconscious—of losing weight or gaining "control" of your eating or your body, then you're still dieting.

Diet Culture Is Everywhere

As I explained in the previous chapter, everyone in the United States (and many other countries) is indoctrinated into a culture of dieting and weight "control" from a very early age. Diet culture is pervasive in almost every aspect of our society. We are exposed to it throughout our medical system, education system, public health entities, and all forms of media, including news programming, advertising, television, and films. It's so insidious that it can often be difficult to identify. We are so used to its existence that we don't even question it. Yet when you start paying attention, you'll notice how pervasive diet culture is. Here are some examples of diet culture:

- Commenting on a meal, "Oh, I could never eat that; if I did, I'd be huge!"
- Describing a weekend of eating as being "off the wagon."
- Planning to "start over on Monday."
- Using terms like *bad, naughty, guilty pleasure,* or *indulgence* to describe food.
- Looking in the mirror and saying, "I feel so fat."
- Hearing someone else describe themselves as fat and responding with, "You're not fat; you're beautiful!" (The subtext: Fat is bad, and fat is not beautiful.)
- A grocery store clerk complimenting a shopper for being "so good" for having so many "healthy" foods in their grocery cart.
- Going to see a doctor for an earache and being told you need to lose weight.
- Exercising to "work off" a meal or compensate for your eating.
- Mentioning the "obesity epidemic" (without the quotation marks).
- Portraying fat people on TV or in movies as the "bad guy" or the lazy, stupid, and/or funny sidekick.

On the surface, many of these examples may not seem all that bad, but, as you'll see shortly, this ever-present diet culture has a huge effect on our bodies, our minds, and our lives. Not to mention that it objectifies and elevates thin, white bodies while oppressing and marginalizing fat, BIPOC bodies. This diet culture—and the resulting diet industry—was birthed by a patriarchal, Eurocentric culture that rose to power through exploiting, oppressing, and controlling other people's bodies. In other words, diet culture, and the dieting industry, is inherently sexist, racist, and ableist—even if people don't realize it.

In the United States, the diet industry takes advantage of the insecurities and lack of self-trust instilled in us by diet culture. It then makes more than $70 billion per year capitalizing off of our shame.[3] Each year, as many as 50 percent of Americans aged twenty and older try to lose weight. Diet culture affects all people, but women are more likely than men to report trying to lose weight: 56 percent said they'd tried to lose weight compared to 42 percent of men.[4] A 2008 survey of more than 4,000 American women aged twenty-five to forty-five found that 67 percent of women were trying to lose weight.[5] Dieting has become so common and normalized that we even see high rates of it in children and adolescents. A survey of high school students in 2017 found that 60 percent of females and 34 percent of males were attempting to lose weight, while 46 percent of nine- to eleven-year-olds are "sometimes" or "very often" on diets.[6] These numbers were even higher in college-aged women: 91 percent of women surveyed on a college campus had tried to control their weight by dieting.[7]

The dieting industry continues to grow year over year, making billions of dollars by convincing us that our bodies need to be changed and that we can't trust ourselves to determine how to eat. It preys on people's insecurities, which have developed as a result of growing up in a diet culture, and compels millions of people every year to spend massive amounts of time, money, and energy trying to lose weight. The diet industry makes its money by persuading you that the next time you try will be different. That if you just buy its product or service, you will finally lose weight, get "healthy," and get "in shape." As people catch on to the diet industry's BS, diet culture changes its form to keep us ensnared.

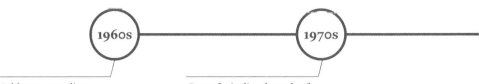

Cabbage soup diet;
launch of Overeaters
Anonymous; first
iteration of Weight
Watchers

Grapefruit diet; launch of
Slimfast; low-fat diet in
the Dietary Goals for the
U.S.

Diet Trends in the Twentieth Century

Over the years, the diet trend has shifted. The 1960s gave us the cabbage soup diet, the launch of Overeaters Anonymous, and the first iteration of Weight Watchers. In the 1970s, we got the grapefruit diet and the launch of Slimfast, as well as the first endorsement by the federal government of a low-fat diet in the Dietary Guidelines for the United States. In the 1980s, Jenny Craig opened its first weight-loss clinic, and Oprah Winfrey popularized the liquid diet when she went on national TV to announce her dramatic weight loss. The low-fat craze took off even more in the 1990s, and fat became the most demonized component of our meals. The pendulum swung in the opposite direction a decade later, as Dr. Robert Atkins released the third version of his high-fat, low-carb *Atkins Diet* book, followed closely by low-carbohydrate diets like The South Beach Diet and The Zone Diet. The early-2000s saw low-carb foods overtake the fat-free and low-fat products on shelves, in diet books, and in media around the world. Carbohydrates became the new diet devil, whereas fat made a comeback. In the last decade, the Atkins Diet and the South Beach Diet have fallen out of favor to be replaced by other (very similar) low-carb diets like the ketogenic and Paleo diets. Now people are all about fattier foods such as avocados, whole eggs, and nuts as they shun bread, pasta, and fruit. Diets continue to shape-shift with one goal: continue to hook people onto dieting and make money (to the tune of $70+ billion per year).

In recent years, the diet industry, sensing consumers' changing attitudes about dieting, has begun to pivot away from selling restrictive, weight-loss-focused diets. As more and more people start to view "traditional" diets

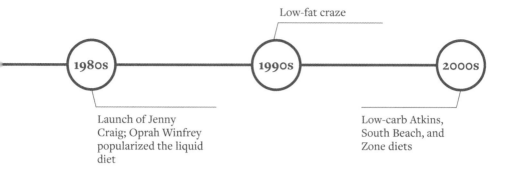

as old-school, and millennials see most fad diets as something of their parents' era, the diet industry has had to change gears to stay relevant. So the industry has reinvented itself as the champion for wellness and health—a "lifestyle change" instead of a weight-loss diet. For example, in 2019, Weight Watchers rebranded as WW to take the word *weight* out of its name. The company declared that its focus was no longer weight loss but overall health and wellness. The rebranding even included a new tagline: "Wellness that works." Yet the same systems still remained in place: counting points, weekly weigh-ins, and setting "goal weights." The program isn't really about wellness, and it *is* still about weight loss; the company's business model hasn't changed. So why the name change? Simple: Company leadership was trying to reach more people and increase profits.

The Wellness Diet

Christy Harrison, MPH, RD, author of the book *Anti-Diet* and host of the podcast *Food Psych,* calls the shift from weight-focused diet programs to wellness-centric ones *The Wellness Diet.* Under the umbrella of The Wellness Diet, you can find things like "clean" eating, detoxes, cleanses, gluten-free, dairy-free, and other elimination diets. As Harrison explains, "*The Wellness Diet* is my term for the sneaky, modern guise of diet culture that's supposedly about 'wellness' but is actually about performing a rarefied, perfectionistic, discriminatory idea of what health is supposed to look like."[8] The diet industry is taking the same system of body oppression and renaming it under the pretense of "health and wellness." Health and wellness then become just another way to oppress and control groups of people, especially women, BIPOC people, and fat people.

On the surface, these wellness diets may not explicitly say that they promote weight loss, but it is still the underlying theme. Look no further than the popular elimination diet plan, the Whole30. This thirty-day program claims to help you transform your "health, habits and emotional relationship with food" and discover "food freedom."[9] Scroll a bit further down the page, though, and the website touts the benefit of "losing weight healthfully and sustainably"—proof that this program is still about weight loss, just under the guise of wellness. The Whole30 organization tries to argue that it's not a diet, yet if you go back to my original definition earlier in this chapter, this is exactly what it is. There are extensive "rules" that you must follow, including the removal of several primary food groups and a whole list of ingredients that are "not allowed." It advocates for not weighing yourself during the thirty days, yet allows "photos and/or measurements on Days 0 and 31." Now, perhaps weight loss is not everyone's primary reason for trying the Whole30 plan, but if you were to look underneath this guise of "wellness" and "finding what foods work for you," you still get the implied message: *and you'll lose weight.*

Almost everyone I've worked with over the past decade has done Whole30 at least once, if not multiple times, and every single person has told me a version of the same story. As one of my clients shared with me, "I loved the structure and the rules of the Whole30; they made me feel safe and less anxious. I always feel great when I start it, then I eat one 'off-plan' food, and I spiral out of control. It is so restrictive that at the end, I always end up out of control, eating everything in sight. Then I end up with worse food habits than when I started." This experience is not exclusive to Whole30. There is an entire market of new diet plans, companies, and apps created with the promise of the ability to "stop dieting" and "still get results." Even if weight isn't mentioned upfront, the subtext is still that this will be the plan that helps you lose weight "for good." But this isn't even close to the truth.

Dieting Doesn't Work

With revenue of $70 billion per year, you'd assume that the dieting industry offers effective products. Yet, as I shared earlier, at least 90 to 97 percent of people who lose weight through dieting will regain it within two to five years, which means that most of the time, diets *do not* result in long-term weight loss.[10] Despite all the ads that say otherwise, it is very rare for people to lose weight and keep it off "for good." Not only that but one- to two-thirds of people who diet regain *more* weight than they originally lost, ending up at a higher weight than where they started. A review of more than thirty long-term studies showed that going on a diet actually *causes* weight gain. The more diets someone has tried, the more they weigh.[11] So, not only does dieting not work for long-term weight loss, but it is also associated with increased risk of binge-eating, eating disorders, and long-term weight gain.[12] Weight loss programs have more than a 90 percent failure rate, yet we continue to blame ourselves and our willpower rather than placing the blame where it really belongs: on the product (aka the diet) that doesn't do what it's advertised to do.

In reality, less than 5 percent of people who attempt to lose weight will keep it off in the long run; even then, the average amount of weight loss maintained is only about 2.4 pounds.[13] Those who do maintain their weight loss are usually engaged in very disordered food and exercise behaviors—ones that, if they were in a thin body, would be considered an eating disorder.[14] Yet in people at higher weights, these behaviors are considered to be "healthy" and are encouraged. Diet culture strikes again.

Diets Make People Unhealthier

Not only do diets fail at making us thinner, but they also make us unhealthier. Dieting and intentional weight-loss efforts lead to food and body preoccupation, overeating and bingeing, lower self-esteem, weight cycling, and disordered eating behaviors and eating disorders.[15] The 2008 survey I mentioned earlier found that 65 percent of women aged twenty-five to forty-five had some form of disordered eating, and another 10 percent met the criteria for eating disorders.[16] That means that three out of four women eat abnormally or think about or behave abnormally around food, including skipping meals, restricting major food groups, binge-eating, and restrained or controlled eating. Feelings of guilt and stress over food are also common. Dieting is the most common type of disordered eating. And consider this: A child is 242 times more likely to have an eating disorder than they are to have type 2 diabetes.[17] If you took a sample of 100,000 children, only 12 would have type 2 diabetes, whereas 2,900 would meet the criteria for an eating disorder. Yet the vast majority of our public health education is spent warning parents about "childhood obesity," which has led to a generation of dieters and is a sign that dieting is not really about health.

Although not all dieters progress to eating disorders, the majority of people diagnosed with an eating disorder have a history of dieting. The best-known environmental contributor to the development of eating dis-orders is our society's idealization of thinness and the stigmatization of, and discrimination against, fat bodies.[18] The prevailing belief is that eat-ing disorders primarily affect young, thin, affluent, white women, but this generalization couldn't be further from the truth. Eating disorders affect people of all sizes, races, and gender identities. Transgender people are much more likely to experience symptoms of disordered eating and eating disorders compared with those who are cisgender.[19] A 2018 survey found that the prevalence of eating disorders in transgender youth is as high as 71 percent.[20] When it comes to race, there is a huge disparity in how women are diagnosed and treated. One study had clinicians read a description of disordered eating patterns, with race as the only variable factor.[21] While 44 percent of clinicians identified the white women's behavior as prob-lematic, only 17 percent identified the same behaviors as problematic in the Black women. These disparities affect people of color and indigenous folks as well. In 2016, Gloria Lucas founded Nalgona Positivity Pride, a Xicana-Indigenous body positive and eating disorder awareness organiza-tion, in response to the lack of resources that exist for low-income people of color and indigenous-descent people. "Eating disorders have been seen as mainly impacting white, privileged women and therefore awareness and treatment have been centered on this demographic," she said in an inter-view with the National Eating Disorders Association. "The violent estab-lishment of this country created multi-generation legacies of disparities, economic inequality, and historical trauma all which impact health, repre-sentation, and resources."[22]

The eating disorders of people at higher weights often go undiagnosed as well, and this group is less likely to receive treatment for their eating disorders. Eating disorder treatment centers are notorious for having a fatphobia and weight stigma problem. I've heard so many stories from fat folks who were in treatment for eating disorders, yet were fat-shamed, limited to a certain number of calories, and prohibited from eating between meals. As Deb Burgard, PhD, a psychologist who specializes in eating disorders, says, "We prescribe for fat people what we diagnose as disordered in thin people."[23] Almost every one of my clients has been shamed for their weight or praised for losing weight. And all of their disordered eating behaviors started when they went on a diet or tried to "eat healthier."

Weight cycling, or repeated cycles of intentional weight loss followed by unintentional weight gain (also known as yo-yo dieting), is also very common among dieters. This was the case for Alex who, at thirty-six years old, had been dieting since she was ten years old. She lost large amounts of weight a few times on different diets: once in high school, again in her mid-twenties, and then once more in her early thirties. However, the weight always came back, and each time she regained more weight than she had lost. "I would go on a diet and lose the weight, but then the second I got praise from people I would just start eating again," she told me. The majority of my clients share similar stories of repeated attempts to lose weight, only to regain it. I've had multiple clients report gaining and losing hundreds of pounds over their decades of dieting. This pattern of repeatedly losing and regaining weight has a negative effect on a person's health. It increases the risk of heart disease, high blood pressure, diabetes, chronic inflammation, certain forms of cancer, and even death.[24] Weight cycling is an *independent risk factor* for poor health outcomes, which means that losing and regaining weight is worse for a person's health than staying at a higher weight. Not to mention that weight cycling may explain some, if not all, of the increased disease risk and poor health outcomes we see in people who have a higher BMI.[25]

It's important to note that I am *not* saying weight gain itself is bad, nor is the inability to lose weight a problem. Despite what our society has programmed us to believe, fat bodies are not bad. Plus, as I'll discuss in Chapter 3, weight and health are not as inextricably linked as diet culture has led us to believe. Weight is not a good indicator for health (let alone human worth or value), and being at a higher weight has not been shown to directly cause health problems. Most of the differences we see in health outcomes between thin people and fat people probably have to do with weight stigma, rather than weight itself. I'll get into this more soon; for now, I just want to be clear: *There is nothing wrong with being fat.*

Dissecting the Problem

Make a list of every single thing that you have tried to do to "fix" your body. This could include diets, exercise plans, medications, supplements, food delivery services, spa treatments, etc. Then evaluate these strategies:

- How far did each of these strategies take you toward "fixing" your food and body image issues?
- What happened after you stopped using these strategies?
- What did using these strategies cost you when it comes to your time, money, energy, brain space, emotional or physical state, etc.?

Why Diets "Fail"

The dictionary defines *willpower* as "the ability to control one's own actions, emotions or urges." It shares how one can use willpower in a sentence: "The dessert buffet tested my willpower."[26] What a perfect example of diet culture, right within the dictionary. Diet culture likes to make you think that it is your lack of willpower that causes you not to be able to eat "correctly" or lose weight. It places the blame on the individual, saying that if only you had the self-control to eat "right," then you'd be able to keep the weight off. That idea couldn't be further from the truth, yet the dieting industry wants people to believe this because it keeps them going back to dieting, which means more money in companies' pockets. Think about it: If dieting *really* worked, then the entire dieting industry would tank overnight. My anti-diet colleagues and I often say that our goal is to get to a place where we're out our jobs because it would mean that our society's sexist, racist body ideals would be dismantled, and people would be able to be accepting of their bodies no matter what their size.

The reality is that the vast majority of people are unable to lose weight not because they lack willpower but because the human body is wired for survival. Our bodies are much smarter than we give them credit for. We have a complex biological system that works to ensure we get enough food to stay alive. When you restrict or limit certain types of food or cut back on the amount of food you eat, your body gets the message that you are starving, so it switches into survival mode. It doesn't matter if you are surrounded by enough food to feed you for weeks. Your body is still biologically wired as it was centuries ago when food was truly scarce, and the ability to store extra calories as fat and burn fewer calories at rest was a genetic survival mechanism. Now, any threat of restriction or food scarcity (like a new diet or setting food rules) feels to your body like starvation is coming. And when your body senses starvation, it does everything it can to try to keep you alive and to keep you within your set point weight range.[27]

Set Point Theory

Set point theory describes the idea that an individual body is genetically programmed to stay within a certain weight range. As a person loses or gains weight, their body compensates to get back into that set point range. It's estimated that the average person's set point range can vary by 10 to 20 pounds, though it's often a much bigger range if you're constantly dieting.[28] Your set point weight range is not set (no pun intended) in stone. It can change over time due to things like genetics, weight-loss attempts, hormonal shifts, and aging. That's because, despite what diet culture says, you aren't meant to stay the same weight for your entire life.

Everyone's set point is different. For many people, their set point weight falls on the higher end of the spectrum, into the "overweight" or "obese" BMI categories.[29] This is completely normal. We are not all meant to have the same size body, just as we are all not meant to have the same height, foot size, or hair color. Body size diversity is inherent within a population and is something that we can—and should—respect rather than trying to change.

At this point, many people ask, "Well, how can I figure out my set point weight?" or "How long will it take for my weight to stabilize in my set point range?" If I were to put my nutrition therapist hat on, I'd be curious to understand *why* you want to know what your set point is. This is a great place to dig deeper to uncover your beliefs about body size (which you'll do in Chapter 5). The thing is, whenever you try to control your weight—even to "get to" your set point—you're still doing a form of dieting. There is no objective way to determine what your set point weight is (and anyone who says there is is telling you some total BS). Trying to "figure it out" or worrying whether you are above or below it only keeps you stuck in the dieting cycle and disconnected from your body.

That disconnect is one of the reasons why I find set point *not* to be a helpful concept to most people. It continues to put the focus on weight. I introduced set point theory here because it helps explain why trying to "control" weight doesn't work. My hope is that you won't get caught up in whether you're at your set point. Instead, just know that when you eat based on internal cues and stop trying to interfere by dieting, your body will *eventually* settle within your set point weight *range*. Emphasis on *range* because, even when you're not dieting, your weight will naturally fluctuate and change over time. Also, I put emphasis on *eventually* because when you stop dieting, it's common to initially gain some weight as you go through a period of food habituation, which I talk about more soon.

Without any external interference, our bodies respect our set point weight range (even if society and the culture at large do not). In their book *Body Respect*, Lindo Bacon and Lucy Aphramor offer a helpful analogy around set point. "Your set point is controlled similar to a thermostat. Imagine you set your home thermostat to 65 degrees. Every thermostat is programmed to maintain a certain acceptable range. Let's suppose your range is 4 degrees. This means your temperature control system won't get too aggressive as long as the house stays between 63 and 67 degrees. However, if the temperature drops below 63 degrees, the heat turns on...Likewise, if it gets hotter than 67 degrees, the air conditioning comes on."[30]

Similar to a thermostat, your body pulls out all the stops to try to keep your weight within its genetically programmed set point range. Whenever you drop lower than your set point, your body feels threatened, so it does everything it can to help you regain weight. It does this in a variety of ways, including the following:

- Decreasing your metabolic rate (aka the number of calories your body needs each day to stay alive)
- Decreasing thyroid activity (which is involved in regulating metabolism)
- Decreasing levels of your fullness hormones
- Increasing levels of your hunger hormones
- Increasing your cravings for calorie-dense foods[31]

This system only works the way it is supposed to if you let it. If you keep messing with the thermostat by dieting or manipulating food and exercise to "control" your weight, it breaks down. Your body fights even harder to regain control of your weight-regulation mechanism. This is why two-thirds of people not only regain the initial weight they lost but also put on some "extra" pounds post-diet. The body increases weight a bit higher than it was before to protect against subsequent attempts of thermostat fiddling (that is, future diets). With every attempt to diet, the rate of weight loss slows down, which is the reason you might find that the weight comes off easily during your first diet, but subsequent attempts don't have the same results. Over time, chronic dieting can increase your set point weight range, and these biological responses kick in even if you are at a higher weight than "usual."

The Deprivation-Binge Pendulum

Your body responds in much the same way whenever it feels like starvation is on the horizon, even if your weight hasn't changed. To your body, dieting feels like starvation. Your body doesn't want you to starve, or die, so it responds by increasing your appetite, lowering your fullness signals, and increasing your cravings, especially for energy-dense foods like those high in sugar and fat. This happens even if you are not actively dieting. I often see people who say they've given up dieting but are still thinking like dieters—still conscious of everything they eat, still judging their food choices, still feeling bad when they feel they've eaten the "wrong" thing or "too much," still trying to control themselves around food even if they're not technically following a specific diet. Although you may not be depriving yourself through traditional diets, the threat of future deprivation is implied when you aren't letting yourself have certain foods, aren't keeping all kinds of

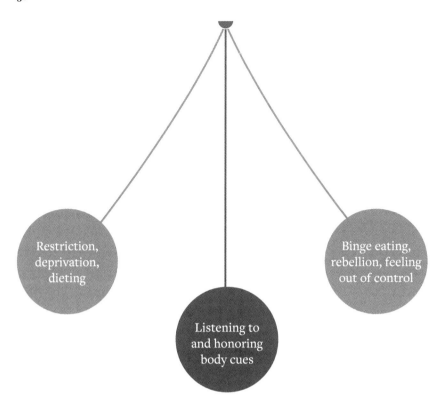

foods around, or feel guilty or ashamed about what you're eating. You send your body the conscious or subconscious message, "Tomorrow, I'll try not to do this again," which your body hears as, "Better get food in now." This type of sneaky diet mentality will cause the same outcome as traditional dieting: a bigger appetite and more food cravings.

Biologically, this makes sense: If you really were in a famine, energy-dense foods and an increased appetite would be a great way to save your life. But what ends up happening is you enter into the deprivation-binge pendulum.

On one side of the pendulum is deprivation. When you begin to restrict your food intake, whether it's through cutting out certain foods, counting calories, "flexible dieting," or any other type of external control, your body senses deprivation. To your body, even the most nonrestrictive diet can feel like starvation. You end up swinging all the way to the left side of the pendulum. And maybe you can stay there for a little while, but eventually, your body's starvation mechanism (increased hunger and cravings) kicks in, and you end up swinging all the way to the right: to the binge side.

Those of you who've been in this pendulum know what it feels like to swing from restriction and its intense hunger and cravings to a sense of being out of control around food, which usually leads to overeating and bingeing. Often what happens at this point is that people feel guilty and out of control and think they need to diet again to get "back on the wagon," which sends them all the way back to the left side of the pendulum: to deprivation.

The swinging motion of a pendulum is controlled by gravity. In our bodies, this deprivation-binge pendulum is controlled by genetics and biology. Pull the pendulum to one side; what does it do when you release it? Swings wildly over to the other side, then back and forth, back and forth. It's impossible to stop that pendulum by exerting control over your eating behaviors. It will just keep on swinging.

Here's what can happen: You decide to cut back on sugar and plan to "allow" yourself to have sweets only on occasion. You get rid of all the sugar in your house and stock up on all sorts of "healthy" food and dessert alternatives. For a few weeks, everything goes great, and you're able to stick to these rules. Then, you start to notice more cravings for ice cream, cookies, and candy. You try to eat a "healthier" version, but the craving doesn't go away. Finally, you break down and buy a pint of ice cream and eat it all in one sitting. Afterward, you feel guilty, ashamed, and down on yourself and vow that you'll never eat any sugar again.

The Dieting Cycle

Another helpful concept in explaining why diets don't work is the dieting cycle.

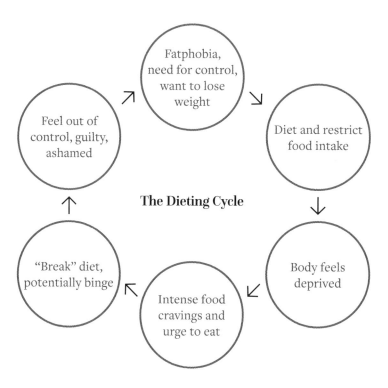

When you restrict certain foods or food groups, you may be able to avoid eating those foods for several days or even several weeks, but eventually, your body feels deprived. This deprivation feels to your body like starvation, so you end up getting cravings, "breaking" the diet, and, often, overeating and bingeing. This can cause you to feel out of control, ashamed, and guilty, and so, to regain control, you start dieting and restricting again. Which eventually leads to deprivation, breaking the diet, bingeing, followed again by guilt. And the cycle continues.

Now let me be clear: This isn't your fault—it is the fault of the diet, the restriction, and the deprivation. Your biological system makes it nearly impossible to eat less than you need, willpower or not. The only way to get out of the dieting cycle is to let go of restriction and stop trying to control your eating. When you do this, your body can move out of its feast or famine mode, and the pendulum will come to a gentle swing close to the middle of the arc. I'll talk more about how you can go about this in Part 2.

The Science of Habituation

Another phenomenon at play is *habituation,* which means that the more you are exposed to something—whether that be a food, a noise, or a certain smell—the less you notice or respond to it. After living in New York City for more than twelve years, I've become habituated to the near-constant noise. The car horns, the ambulance sirens, the garbage trucks at all hours of the night—at this point, it's mostly background noise. Yet whenever a friend from out of town comes to visit, they always comment on how *loud* it is. It is always funny to me because I hardly hear it anymore; I have almost no response to it. However, my out-of-town friends who live in quiet suburbs are not used to these sounds, so their heart rate jumps whenever a siren goes off, and they barely sleep, kept awake by the sounds of the city.

Habituation also happens with food. If you restrict certain foods or try to keep them out of your house, it makes these foods more exciting and desirable. You tell yourself you can't have them, and then your brain fixates on them. It makes sense that, when you finally get access to those foods, you find it hard to control yourself or stop eating. Your body has no idea when you'll allow yourself to eat that food again, so it keeps driving you to eat more and more.

On the other hand, when you allow yourself to eat all sorts of foods and keep these foods around you, they become less exciting, and the desire to eat them diminishes.[32] One of my clients went through this with macaroni and cheese, a meal she had loved but kept mostly off limits because she could never stop eating it and always ate to the point of being uncomfortably full. During our work together, she decided to permit herself to eat it whenever she wanted so she could work on habituating to it. At first, she ended up having it three or four nights a week and often ate until she felt uncomfortably full, but she continued to keep it in the house and allow herself to have it. One day, after several weeks, she checked in with her body to see what she wanted to eat and realized, "Wow, mac and cheese doesn't sound good right now!" She had habituated to it. She still allowed it to be an option for meals, but she found that, after the first few weeks of eating a lot of it, she rarely wanted it. When she did choose to eat it, she was usually able to stop at the point of comfortable fullness, without exerting any control. To this day, several years later, she continues to keep mac and cheese stocked in her pantry to make sure it is always allowed and available.

I know you're probably thinking something to the effect of, "But if I allow myself to eat *<insert commonly demonized "junk" foods>* whenever I want, I'd just eat it all the time." Look, I know this *feels* like the truth, and likely it would be if you still have a dieting mindset. But if you start to shift your mindset from the binary of dieting, restriction, and scarcity to the spectrum of abundance and allowance, then food habituation can happen, and the deprivation-binge pendulum can stop. Now this process, which I'll discuss more in Chapter 9, is not easy, but it is possible. Food habituation has been studied with all types of food, including those that most people consider "binge" foods, such as pizza, potato chips, and chocolate. When a certain food becomes familiar and is not kept off-limits, and you know you can eat it whenever you want, it becomes less compelling. You get used to knowing it will be there today, tomorrow, and the next day, and you actually end up eating it less often. It also gives you the space to eat and enjoy the food without scarcity thoughts like, "I better enjoy this now; starting tomorrow, it's back to eating clean." Remember, thoughts like that end up triggering the diet-binge pendulum.

Interestingly enough, we see very similar eating behaviors between dieters and people who suffer from food insecurity, those who don't have consistent access to affordable, nutritious food. Several studies have shown that people with food insecurity have an increased likelihood of eating disorders and binge-eating behaviors.[33] This is another example of our bodies trying to protect us from famine, whether it's due to a diet or socioeconomic issues and lack of access to food. It also goes to show that the myth of eating disorders only affecting wealthy women is false.

What About Food Addiction?

If I had a nickel for every time I've heard someone say they're addicted to food (sugar in particular), I'd be rich. People regularly toss around statements like, "Once I start eating ice cream, I can't stop," or, "If I even open a bag of cookies, I'm a goner." Maybe you have even uttered something similar yourself.

The idea of food addiction has been around for a while. (In 1960, Overeaters Anonymous started with the premise of helping people who suffered from addictive behavior with food.[34] Spoiler: OA is a diet.) There is even a food addiction screening scale, which was created by adapting drug and alcohol addiction screening tools. There is a lot that is wrong with this, not the least of which is the fact that we can abstain from drugs and alcohol and still survive just fine, but there is no possible way that we can live without food.[35]

Nowadays, ever since carbs, sugar, and processed foods have become demonized, it's common to hear people complain about their "sugar addiction." And yes, technically we can live without some types of sugar (though really, who would want to?), so many people who try to cut out sugar also try to restrict carbs, something that our bodies do need.

When people describe feeling "addicted" to food, what they are usually describing is a mix of intense cravings, a feeling of being out of control around food, and frequent overeating or bingeing on certain highly palatable foods. The experience of being out of control around food is a very real one, and the language of addiction ("this is a biological drive that I can't control") fits with this feeling. But that does not mean that food, or sugar, addiction is real, even if it *feels* real. There has been no evidence that food has a pharmacological effect on the brain the way drugs do. In fact, there is little to no evidence to support sugar (or food) addiction in human or animal studies.

What the studies have shown is that addiction-like behaviors occurred only when people had their sugar intake restricted or limited. As the authors of the review state, "These behaviours likely arise from intermittent access to sweet tasting or highly palatable foods, not the neurochemical effects of sugar."[36] This is the pendulum swing again: When you cut out sugar, you end up wanting it more; and when you finally eat it, you feel out of control and end up bingeing. There is no proof that food itself is addictive; and when you look at the food addiction screening tool questions, it's quite possible that what they are actually screening for is disordered eating behavior.

Animal studies corroborate these findings. Rats that only have intermittent access to highly palatable foods end up developing compulsive eating behaviors. But the rats that have continued access to the same foods don't show any addictive-like behaviors.[37] So it's the uncertainty of when you'll be able to get the food (or sugar) again that makes these compulsive eating behaviors occur, not a true physical addiction.[38]

Then there is the "but sugar lights up the same brain pathways as drugs" argument. Well, yes, sugar does light up those same pathways and increases the release of dopamine, which makes us feel good. But do you want to know what else lights up those same pathways? Music. Smiling faces. Winning a prize. Finding something funny. Being in love. All of these pleasant and enjoyable events activate the same pathways, but this doesn't mean we are addicted to them.

Not only is there limited research on food and sugar addiction but the research that does exist doesn't account for restricted eating patterns (like diets and dieting behaviors). And given what we see from the research—that intermittent access to food causes more addictive-like behaviors—we can safely assume if you have dieted, you're going to feel that compulsive eating tendency. This doesn't mean that you are addicted to food or that you need to abstain from highly palatable foods, like those high in fat or sugar. It means that you need to stop dieting.

CHAPTER 3

The Truth About Health, Nutrition, and Weight

When I was in school to become a dietitian, everything I was taught linked weight to health. Someone has diabetes? Help them lower their blood sugar by losing weight. Heart disease? Prescribe a cardiac diet and weight-loss counseling. At the time, I truly believed I was helping people. If only I could educate people about nutrition and calories, then they would lose weight and—because of this—be healthier. I mean, calories in/ calories out, right? As it turns out, no. How wrong I (and our weight-centric education system) was.

Current health guidelines and public health policies in the United States, and many other countries around the world, evaluate health through a *weight-centric* or *weight-normative* lens. A weight-normative approach views body weight as a determinant of health and emphasizes weight management (i.e., weight loss and the maintenance of a "normal" body mass index or BMI) when promoting health and well-being. When a person goes to the doctor for any type of medical issue, they are usually evaluated first based on their weight, regardless of whether their weight is relevant to what they are presenting with. For example, a client of mine once went to see her doctor for a persistent earache, only to be told that she needed to lose weight and should go on a diet. This is a prime example of weight stigma, which I'll share more about shortly.

Despite mainstream medical advice, weight and health are *not* as inextricably linked as diet culture has led us to believe. It is impossible to tell anything about someone's health based on their body size. Neither body weight nor BMI are good indicators of health and, despite what you've probably heard, being at a higher weight has not been shown to *cause* disease.[1] Although certain diseases may be *associated* with higher weights, it is important to distinguish between *correlation* and *causation,* as I will explain later in this chapter.

I've talked about the concept of a *diet culture,* or a society in which thinness is prized and equated to health, happiness, and worthiness. Nowadays, it's easy to assume that the link between health and weight has always existed. But interestingly (and infuriatingly) enough, the roots of diet culture predate any scientific "evidence" connecting weight and health. In fact, until the early 1900s, weight loss was not part of most physician or public health recommendations. When the medical community started to advise weight loss, it wasn't because there was any scientific evidence linking weight to health but because our culture had already created a desire for thinness and a bias against fatness. Fatphobia, the dislike of and fear of fatness and fat people, came way before any public health messages about weight or body size. In this way, fatphobia has never been about health at all; instead, it's a means to justify race, class, and gender prejudice.

The Impact of Weight Stigma

Brianna Campos, a licensed professional counselor from New Jersey, had been working out at her gym for years when a man approached her and shook her hand. He said to her, "I just want to let you know that it gets easier. You're doing a great job." In reflecting on this interaction, Brianna said to me, "Would he have done the same thing if I was in a thin body?" Because of Brianna's body size, the man assumed that Brianna was not fit and new to exercise. "Despite the fact that I have been exercising for years, and that I know all the muscle groups and what machines and weights to use, he assumed that I had just started working out," she recalled.

Unfortunately, Brianna is not alone. Fat people face these types of comments (often referred to as *microaggressions*) daily. Comments like these are a form of weight stigma—also referred to as weight bias—which is a form of discrimination or stereotyping based upon someone's weight.[2] It encompasses the negative attitudes and beliefs about fat folks, and the *assumptions* made based upon their body size. For example, a common stereotype in our society is that fat people are lazy, sloppy, uneducated, and/or unattractive— all of which show weight bias and fatphobia. Weight stigma is in the workplace, schools and universities, and healthcare facilities; it's perpetrated by members of the community, friends, and family in all sorts of public and private places.

Here are some examples of weight stigma:

- People who have an "obese" BMI make less money than thin people and are less likely to get promoted.[3]
- The average American woman is a size 14—and 67 percent of American women wear a size 14 or larger—but most retail clothing stores don't carry anything larger than a size 12.
- Fat jokes are considered socially acceptable.
- People in larger bodies pay more for many goods and services, like airline tickets, insurance, and clothing.
- Kids are routinely shamed and bullied by other children as well as by teachers and family members because of their body size.
- People assume that someone who is "obese" doesn't eat healthy or exercise.
- It's considered a "kindness" to compliment someone on their weight loss and tell them how great they look "now."

The media perpetuates weight stigma and fatphobia to the point that it's been so normalized that most people don't even recognize it as a problem. Take weight-related compliments. On the surface, they may not seem like an issue—you're just letting someone know that they look good, right? Although this may be your intention, complimenting someone on their weight loss and telling them how great they look is in effect saying that they didn't look good *before* and that, if they gain weight (as we've already established that most people will), they won't look great again. Weight-related compliments also reinforce the thin body ideal and the myth that being smaller is better. A comment like, "You look so great; did you lose weight?" implies that the person only looks good if they look thin. Plus, you never know what is really going on with someone. A client of mine received frequent compliments on her weight loss during a period when she was struggling with a severe eating disorder. "People telling me I looked so good was reinforcing my disordered eating behaviors," she says now. A simple way that we can all stop perpetuating weight stigma is to not comment on anyone's body, especially without their consent.

Weight Bias and Healthcare

Weight bias has been documented in a variety of healthcare providers, including doctors, nurses, psychologists, and dietitians. In some studies, healthcare providers reported that they viewed "obese" patients as non-compliant, lazy, undisciplined, dishonest, and unintelligent. This weight bias leads to worse care for fat people, does little to promote health, and is linked to *worse* health outcomes.[4] For patients with higher BMIs, doctors spend less time with the person, have less patience with them, take them less seriously, provide less health education, and are less likely to perform certain interventions and screenings, including pelvic exams, mammograms, and cancer screens (compared with patients with "normal" BMIs).[5] Weight stigma also puts the focus on the individual's responsibility for health, which prevents us from looking at the social determinants of health (which, as I talk about shortly, impact health outcomes more than behaviors).

For example, a thirty-two-year-old client of mine went to see her physician for an annual physical. Everything looked great: Her blood sugar was normal, her cholesterol had gone down since the previous year, and her blood pressure was in a normal range. Her doctor then told her, "You should consider weight-loss surgery, even though you're otherwise healthy." A perfectly healthy thirty-two-year-old with a BMI that just crossed into the "obese" category, being recommend weight-loss surgery? This is weight stigma (and fatphobia).

The Health Effects of Weight Stigma

It's no surprise to learn that people with higher BMIs put off going to the doctor because, when they do go, they experience weight stigma and often receive substandard medical care.[6] Brianna Campos recalls doctors lecturing her on the dangers of being "overweight" without even asking about her health habits. Over time, this shaming caused her to avoid going to the doctor. "Even when medically necessary, I would avoid going," she says. "And I still get anxiety before going to a new doctor." Clearly, avoiding the doctor can have significant health consequences for people of any weight. The fact that weight stigma causes fat folks to put off visiting the doctor means that, by the time they do visit the doctor, their illness or disease may have progressed. For this reason, and others that I'll get to shortly, weight stigma may explain some, if not all, of the health differences we see in people with higher body weights.

Experiencing weight stigma raises people's risk of chronic diseases and death, no matter how much they weigh.[7] Weight stigma has a range of negative physical and mental health consequences, including an increase in stress, blood pressure, chronic inflammation, diabetes, cardiovascular disease, anxiety, depression, low self-esteem, and disordered eating behaviors, including binge-eating.[8] One study found that people who experienced weight stigma had a 60 percent increased risk of dying, regardless of their BMI.[9] Experiencing weight stigma causes chronic stress, which has a huge impact on our bodies and our health.[10] When you consider all the daily weight discrimination someone in a larger body faces (e.g., comments from family members or strangers, hearing fat jokes, anxiety about finding clothes that fit or having a chair they can comfortably sit into, and so on), the amount of stress they may experience every day is way more than someone in a smaller body. And we know that stress is an independent risk factor for a whole host of diseases, including heart disease, diabetes, high blood pressure, anxiety, and depression. Combine this with the fact that people with higher BMIs are more likely to avoid going to the doctor and it's no wonder that people who experience weight stigma have worse health outcomes.

Here's another thing that is important to remember as we look at weight science research: In the late nineteenth and early twentieth centuries, when doctors and scientists started to study nutrition and health, fatphobia and weight stigma influenced what they researched, how they designed the studies, and how they interpreted the results. We still see this same trend today. The vast majority of studies focused on weight and "obesity" do not control for weight stigma or the biases of the researchers themselves. Yet we know that weight stigma is an independent risk factor for health outcomes, disease risk, and risk of death—no matter what someone's weight is.

It's not just external weight stigma that is involved here. Living in a weight-centric society, many fat people have *internalized* weight stigma, meaning they have bias and stigma toward themselves. Internalized weight stigma has negative effects on your mental and physical health. In fact, one study found that "identifying oneself as overweight, irrespective of actual body mass, predicts impaired physical and psychological health outcomes long-term."[11] This means that when someone thinks of themselves as "overweight" or "obese," they are likely to have poor health outcomes down the road—*no matter what their weight or BMI actually is.*

But Isn't It Important to Know Your Weight or BMI?

One concern people often voice to me is that if they are too "easy" on themselves and accept their body size, then they won't be motivated to change their health behaviors. In reality, the opposite is true: When weight-related feedback is given, people are *less* likely to make long-term health behavior changes.[12] Telling people that they are "overweight" or "obese" and that they need to lose weight for health is *not* a good motivator. So, all those BMI screenings in schools, at doctors' offices, or in community settings not only don't help get people to change their behaviors, but they can actually cause health behaviors to worsen.

Words like *overweight* and *obese* are a type of weight stigma, as is the term *weight management*. The underlying message is that something is wrong with your body. When people experience weight stigma, studies have found that behaviors related to food and exercise get worse. One study showed that 79 percent of women who experienced weight stigma ended up coping by eating more food *and* by refusing to change their diet.[13] Also, women in the "overweight" or "obese" BMI categories who have internalized weight stigma report more frequent binge-eating compared with women with the same BMI who have not internalized stigma.[14] The same outcomes are seen when we look at physical activity: Adults who experience weight stigma are more likely to avoid exercise.

As I've outlined here, the long-term consequences of weight stigma, including chronic stress and worsening behaviors related to food and exercise, mean that weight stigma is an independent risk factor for both disease and mortality (or death), no matter what someone's weight is. Most of the differences we see in health outcomes between people in smaller bodies and larger bodies likely have to do with weight stigma, rather than weight itself.

A Note About the Terms *Obese* and *Overweight*

You'll notice that throughout this book I put the words *obese* and *overweight* in quotes. Although these words are commonly used to describe larger bodies, they are words that have been developed and co-opted by the medical community to medicalize and pathologize a person's body (which means "to represent something as a disease" or treat someone as if they are abnormal). These words themselves are fatphobic and stigmatizing.

Overweight is a word that assumes that there is a "correct" weight that a body should be and that if you are "over" that weight, then you are abnormal or different. The word *overweight* is rooted in the BMI charts, a problematic and flawed measure that assumes health is based on size (which, as I'll explain shortly, is not the case).

The word *obese* comes from the Latin word *obesus*, meaning "having eaten until fat." The term assigns illness based on size, not on any other parameter, and places blame on the individual, which is not only incorrect but is stigmatizing and can cause stress, anxiety, and shame. As I've just discussed, people who are stigmatized based on their size can have profoundly negative mental and physical health effects.

Calling people "overweight" or "obese" isn't just naming their body mass; it's designating them as atypical or unnatural, which further marginalizes a person to the outskirts of society. This is why I do not use those terms to describe people and why, when I do reference them, I put them in quotes to signify that I don't recognize them as official terms or agree with what they usually signify.

The History of the BMI

To discuss the Body Mass Index, or BMI, we have to begin in Belgium during the year 1832. That was the year that Adolphe Quetelet, a Belgian astronomer, mathematician, statistician, and sociologist, developed something called the Quetelet Index (QI), which was the ratio of a person's weight in kilograms to their height in square meters.[15] He developed the QI to categorize a population of human beings and to define the characteristics of a "normal man." Quetelet had no interest in measuring health or "obesity"; he was a *statistician* looking at population models rather than a medical practitioner studying individual human health conditions. Not to mention that he developed the QI equation based on data from a white, European population, which means that it doesn't take into account body sizes and diversity in other populations. Nevertheless, the QI eventually became what we know today as the BMI.

Fast-forward to the early 1900s in the United States, where diet culture (rooted in racism, classism, and female obedience) had a firm foothold, and people were starting to ask doctors to help them lose weight. Up until this point, weight loss was not part of most medical or public health

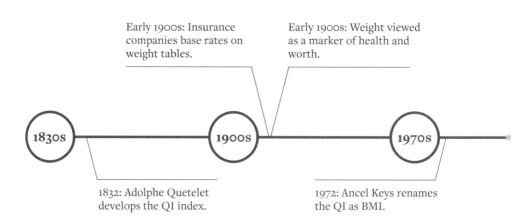

Early 1900s: Insurance companies base rates on weight tables.

Early 1900s: Weight viewed as a marker of health and worth.

1830s   1900s   1970s

1832: Adolphe Quetelet develops the QI index.

1972: Ancel Keys renames the QI as BMI.

recommendations. As diet culture swept through the medical community, doctors started keeping scales in their offices and regularly weighing people.

Simultaneously, U.S. life insurance companies started using weight and height metrics to determine their rates.[16] They noticed that their data (again, based exclusively upon a population of white, wealthy men) showed a higher rate of death for "overweight" people. Although later studies of larger, more diverse samples of the population showed the opposite—that the "overweight" people actually had a *lower* risk of death—insurance companies took their early data and, to save money, promoted weight as a determinant of early death. Soon, doctors (and the federal government) started using data from life insurance companies to evaluate people's "health," and more and more doctors began promoting weight loss for health.[17]

At this point, BMI was still not intended to be used to evaluate a person's health. However, in 1972 researcher Ancel Keys, who disagreed with the insurance weight tables and sought to find a different way to evaluate body mass, proposed that the Quetelet Index now be called the Body Mass Index (BMI) and that it be used to study and link health, disease, and "obesity."[18] This brings us to the measurement that is still widely known and used today.

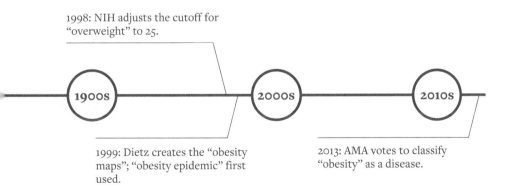

1998: NIH adjusts the cutoff for "overweight" to 25.

1900S   2000S   2010S

1999: Dietz creates the "obesity maps"; "obesity epidemic" first used.

2013: AMA votes to classify "obesity" as a disease.

Why the BMI Is BS

The BMI calculation uses a person's height and weight to categorize them as *underweight, normal weight, overweight, obese,* or *morbidly obese.* This measurement has become the de facto way that government agencies, medical professionals, drug manufacturers, and health researchers classify people's weight to evaluate, and even diagnose, health. Yet the BMI has been widely recognized as a problematic measurement for several reasons:

- It's based on height and weight data primarily from white, middle- to upper-class Europeans, which means it's not a representative sample of the general population and does not account for differences in "average" body sizes in other ethnic groups.[19]

- It does not take into consideration differences in age, sex, bone structure, body fat versus muscle, fat distribution, or how muscle mass changes with age. For example, people who have a high percentage of muscle mass end up being classified as "overweight" or "obese," even if they have low amounts of body fat.

- The differences between BMI classifications—i.e., between "normal" weight and "overweight" or "obese"—are largely arbitrary.[20] They are not based upon any scientific data but defined instead by a handful of people with ideas of what a "normal" weight should be.

- In 1998, the National Institutes of Health, in a controversial move, adjusted the cut off for "overweight" down to 25.[21] So 37 million Americans went to bed having a "normal" BMI and woke up the next day considered to be "overweight." (Read more about this in the next section.)

- BMI isn't a good indicator of health status. A 2016 study of more than 40,000 people found that 47 percent of people classified as "overweight" and 29 percent classified as "obese" were metabolically healthy (meaning that their blood pressure, cholesterol, triglycerides, glucose, and C-reactive protein [a measure of inflammation] were all normal). Plus, 30 percent of people who were in the "normal" weight BMI category were found to be metabolically *unhealthy.*[22]

Let's dig deeper into a few of these points.

BMI Categories Are Largely Arbitrary

In 1998, the National Institutes of Health (NIH) decided to lower the "overweight" BMI category threshold to 25 for all genders. Previously, it had been 28 for men and 27 for women.[23] The committee based this decision on a World Health Organization (WHO) report from 1996, which was written by the International Obesity Task Force (IOTF), which recommended the BMI category of "overweight" be lowered. The primary funders of the IOTF report? Hoffmann-La Roche and Abbott Laboratories, two pharmaceutical companies that make weight-loss drugs. Not to mention that various weight-loss drug companies were paying many of the researchers and scientists who were on the WHO and NIH committees. These companies had an active interest in having more Americans classified as "overweight" so that they would have a much larger market for their weight-loss drugs.

The "Obesity" Paradox

More evidence to support that BMI is BS: The BMI category with the highest risk of death is actually people who are classified as *underweight.* In fact, if you're "underweight," you are twice as likely to die than someone in the "normal" weight category. Not only that, but the BMI category with the lowest risk of death is people who have a BMI of 25 to 29.9 and are classified as "overweight." Known as the *obesity paradox,* people who are "overweight" live the longest out of any group, including people who are "normal" weight. Meanwhile, people who have a BMI between 30 and 34.9 (in the "obese" range) have the same risk of death as a person with a "normal" BMI.[24] (Side note: It's considered a "paradox" only because researchers, with their weight bias, expected the opposite to be true.) The following illustration shows least risk of death to greatest risk of death based on BMI.

Obesity Paradox

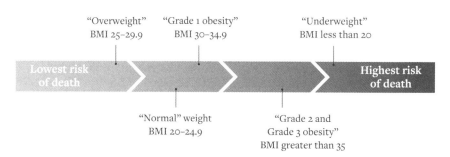

If people who are "underweight" have the highest risk of mortality, why is it that people rarely accuse models or other thin people of "promoting death"? Yet fat people are constantly trolled for this exact thing and are forced to "prove" their healthfulness. Oh right: fatphobia (aka, not health).

In addition to conferring a lower risk of death, a higher BMI also appears to be beneficial in many instances. For example, in people with type 2 diabetes, high blood pressure, cardiovascular disease, and chronic kidney disease, those who have a BMI in the "obese" range live longer than thinner people with the same conditions. A high BMI also seems to have some protective effect as we age, with research finding that in people older than age 55, those with a BMI in the "overweight" and "obese" categories had decreased risk of death compared to people with "normal" and "underweight" BMIs.[25]

The BMI Misclassifies Large Swaths of the Population

Some doctors find BMI useful as a screening tool to indicate when to check people for things like high cholesterol or elevated blood pressure. Although this may be helpful in certain cases, the BMI is not a perfect measure given that 30 percent of people with a "normal" BMI have health conditions like diabetes or high cholesterol.[26] Also, having a higher BMI doesn't automatically mean a person is in poor health (like my client who was perfectly healthy but was told to get weight-loss surgery based only on her BMI). Although a higher BMI may be *associated* with health risks in certain people, it does not mean that a high BMI itself is a health state. A great example of this can be found in professional athletes: Due in large part to their high muscle mass, many pro football players have BMIs of 30 or greater, putting them in the "obese" category, even if they are healthy. This mismatch isn't just in athletes: Research has found that almost 50 percent of people who are in the "overweight" BMI category and 30 percent of people with an "obese" BMI are actually healthy, showing no signs of disease.[27]

The BMI was never meant to be used as a proxy for health, yet it is now used as exactly that when people visit their doctor's office, when scientists conduct research studies, and when the government makes policies at the population level.

The Makings of the "Obesity Epidemic"

Not a day goes by without a media outlet reporting on the growing toll of the "obesity epidemic" in America, defined by—you guessed it—the BMI. But this is misleading for several reasons (not to mention, it's harmful). Although Americans' weights had been increasing for decades (interestingly enough, this increase occurred simultaneously with the rise of dieting, which, as you learned in Chapter 2, increases weight gain), "obesity" wasn't widely reported by the media, or even thought of as a disease, until 1999. That was the year that William Dietz, the director of the Division of Nutrition, Physical Activity, and Obesity of the Centers for Disease Control (CDC), created the series of infamous "Obesity Maps." Although the CDC had data on changing American weight patterns for some time, it wasn't until Dietz repackaged the numbers into color-coded maps that people took note.

You've probably seen these maps. I learned about them in college and even used them in presentations early in my career. They are a series of maps of the United States showing the prevalence of "obesity"—the number of people with a BMI greater than 29.9, from 1990 through today. The maps start with most states colored blue, signifying rates of "obesity" as less than 15 percent. Over time, the states' colors shift from light blue to dark blue to yellow to red, signifying increasing rates of "obesity" from less than 15 percent to more than 30 percent of a state population. The maps are striking when you watch them advance over time, and with their creation, Dietz effectively was able to convince people that there was an "obesity epidemic" spreading across the country.

Although the maps may seem impressive, they're misleading. The maps use state borders as the boundaries for the shifting colors, which overstates the extent of "obesity" because the size of a state doesn't have any relation to the size of its population. For example, Alabama and New York are almost the same size geographically, yet Alabama has a population of only 4.9 million compared to New York's 19.4 million. When you look at the states in which the rates of "obesity" first increase—like Mississippi, Alabama, Louisiana, and West Virginia—it shows us that BMI increased more in places that had a higher percentage of poor people and minorities. Although the maps made it seem as though "obesity" was spreading like a disease, it was more indicative of places that had larger rural and lower-income populations.[28]

Around the same time, a study that named the economic effect of "obesity" to be upward of $100 billion per year was published.[29] This figure was extremely misleading. Authors of the study calculated all of the healthcare expenses that occurred in people with a BMI in the "overweight" or "obese" range and named this number as the total "cost of obesity." They did not take into account what factors may have caused any of the health issues, such as genetics, socioeconomic factors, stigma, or diet or exercise behaviors. They assumed that if you got breast cancer, gallbladder disease, or had a heart problem, it was a result of your weight. Needless to say, as we'll explore more shortly, weight has not been shown to *cause* any of these diseases.

At this point, many scientists, researchers, and physicians used the "obesity epidemic" rhetoric to push forward their agenda of classifying "obesity" as a disease. Why would they want to do this? As J. Eric Oliver outlines in his book *Fat Politics,* the people who were trying to convince the public that the "obesity epidemic" was a thing to be fearful of had financial incentives to do so. The pharmaceutical companies who made weight-loss drugs, as well as various weight-loss and diet companies, paid many of the health researchers and government committee members who were making these public health decisions. As Oliver writes, "What I thought was an epidemic began to look a lot more like a politically orchestrated campaign to capitalize on America's growing weight."[30]

If "obesity" were classified as a disease, these organizations would benefit financially by having their drugs or weight-loss procedures subject to insurance reimbursement and because more of the American public would be convinced that they needed the companies' drugs or programs to "cure" their "obesity" to be healthy. Organizations with a financial incentive in the "obesity epidemic" soon got their wish. In 2013, the American Medical Association (AMA) voted to classify "obesity" as a disease, going *against* the recommendation of their own committee that had studied the subject.[31] The committee recommended that "obesity" *not* be classified as a disease, mainly because it is difficult to define, and the measure used to categorize "obesity" (the BMI) is flawed. Yet the AMA went ahead and did so anyway, paving the way for drug companies and surgeons to benefit financially. Although Americans' weights were increasing, no actual science existed to show that the rise in BMI was causing people harm. Yet this "causation" was, and still is, consistently stated as fact.

Weight Science: Correlation Versus Causation

Despite what healthcare professionals, government agencies, and popular media may say, there is no research to prove that higher amounts of weight or body fat *cause* diseases like heart disease, cancer, diabetes, or stroke. Although some of these health conditions are more common in people at higher weights, there is no evidence that the conditions are caused by "excess" weight. So although there may be a *correlation* between weight and health, this is not the same thing as *causation*.[32]

The book *Body Respect* describes correlation versus causation using cigarettes as an example.[33] Smoking cigarettes causes yellow teeth; it also causes lung cancer. Although yellow teeth are *correlated* with lung cancer, it doesn't mean they *cause* lung cancer. The same holds true for weight. Higher weights are *correlated* with certain diseases, but it doesn't mean they *cause* the disease. Blaming weight, or "obesity," for poor health is like blaming yellow teeth for lung cancer. Weight and health are associated, but weight isn't the underlying cause for poor health—a person's weight may simply be an effect of other variables that are the *actual* causes of health, such as genetics, environmental causes, weight stigma, and factors like what we eat and our physical activity level. Yet in our weight-centric society, "weight loss" is often prescribed as a way to achieve health.

This recommendation is made despite extensive research that shows that in terms of modifiable health risks, a person's behaviors—not weight— impact health most. When a person eats more nutritious foods and starts moving more, disease markers like blood sugar, heart rate, and blood pressure decrease. This decrease happens even when a person doesn't lose any weight.[34] For example, a study about high blood pressure and physical activity found that blood pressure and resting heart rate decreased *regardless* of whether the person lost weight.[35] One group of people in the study lost weight, whereas another group did not, but both groups saw a similar improvement in their blood pressures—meaning that the improvement came from the behavior change (in this case, exercise) rather than the weight. This shows us that health can be improved regardless of whether someone loses any weight.

Viewed another way, we also don't have any evidence that weight loss *alone* improves a person's health or lowers their risk of disease. If that were the case, we'd all be prescribed liposuction to suck the fat from our bodies. But, as one study showed, liposuction alone does not lower any markers of disease, including blood glucose and inflammatory markers.[36] Or if you look at research in people with type 2 diabetes, one review found that after an initial drop in blood glucose and insulin levels, six to eighteen months later those markers had increased to where they started, *even when people maintained their weight loss*, which again means that behaviors (along with several socioeconomic factors, as we'll talk about shortly) most impact our health.[37]

Note that nearly all the studies that link "obesity" with diseases are epidemiological studies, not experimental trials, which means researchers are surveying the population and relying on self-reported data (including self-reported weights) to draw conclusions based on BMI and health. Many of these do not account for or control for other factors that may be contributing to diseases, such as access to medical care, genetics, socioeconomic status, weight cycling, and weight stigma. Yet all of these criteria do play a role in the development of diseases, independent of what someone weighs. Even if these surveys show higher rates of disease at higher weights, many other factors could be contributing to the increase in disease.

If Not Weight, Then What?

In her book *Gentle Nutrition*, Rachael Hartley includes a chapter on redefining health. In it she writes, "When most people say they are 'getting healthy,' they don't mean seeing a therapist, meditating, getting enough sleep, or spending more time with family, driving the speed limit, getting vaccinated, practicing safe sex, purchasing better health insurance, getting a job that pays more money, or moving to an area with less pollution. For most people, 'get healthy' is code for losing weight. It means exercising more, eating less, and eating 'healthier,' according to whatever diet is currently in vogue."[38]

As I've mentioned, weight is not a good indication of health status and, when people focus on weight, it ends up causing weight stigma, which leads to more health problems. If the goal is to improve health, focusing on weight clearly backfires. As my client Sarah described it to me, "If I try to eat better or exercise more and then the scale doesn't change, it makes me feel completely defeated, and all my hard work feels useless, so I give up." I hear this all the time—people start to make positive behavior changes, like eating more fruits and vegetables or being more physically active, and when they don't see the scale budge, they immediately feel like what they're doing isn't working, so they stop.

Sarah also found that stepping on the scale and weighing herself would be the thing that determined whether she'd feel good about herself or bad about herself that day, *regardless of her behaviors* with food. I can relate. For almost ten years, I got on the scale several times a week. If the number was something I (arbitrarily) considered "good," then I'd breathe a sigh of relief. If it was a "bad" number, my mood would immediately change, and I'd feel guilty and ashamed, like I had "messed up." Weighing oneself can also fuel disordered eating behaviors, as my client Monica found. "If I got on the scale and the number wasn't what I wanted to see, I would immediately start restricting my food intake for the next few days," she said.

Focusing on weight detracts from the real source of health problems and can promote unhealthy behaviors related to food and exercise. So, if we don't focus on weight, how do we go about measuring and promoting health? Simple: The focus should be placed on the modifiable health behaviors that affect our risk of disease (along with supporting policies that improve people's access to resources, safe housing, good healthcare, and more). Weight is not a behavior and, as I discussed in Chapter 2, it's not something that we as individuals can have much impact on, especially in the long term. What we *can* change are our health behaviors, which include eating habits, physical activity, smoking, alcohol use, sleep patterns, and stress management. These behaviors are not only things we can modify but also what more accurately predict our chance of developing a certain disease.

When it comes to measuring physical health, instead of tracking weight loss and BMI, which don't address the real source of health problems, we can look at health markers such as cholesterol level, blood pressure, blood glucose, or insulin level to predict physical health more accurately. It's also important to emphasize, as I'll explain shortly, that health is about much more than just physical health and lab values.

Health at Every Size®

One approach that can be useful to take the focus off of weight is the Health at Every Size® framework (HAES®). The HAES approach is a registered trademark of the Association for Size Diversity and Health, a nonprofit that began in 2003 to promote size acceptance and end weight discrimination and stigma. But the tenets of the HAES framework had been around for decades in the work of fat activists and the fat liberation movement than began in 1960. (You will learn more about that subject in Chapter 13.)

The HAES framework rejects the use of weight or BMI as a proxy for health and instead works to support people of all sizes in finding compassionate ways to take care of themselves, no matter what their size. The focus is on health and well-being, rather than weight, and promotes positive physical and mental health behaviors through five principles:

- Weight inclusivity
- Health enhancement
- Respectful care
- Eating for well-being
- Life-enhancing movement[39]

HAES accepts and respects the inherent diversity in body sizes, supports health policies that provide better access to care, works to end weight stigma, promotes flexible eating based upon internal signals, and encourages people to partake in whatever forms of movement feel enjoyable to them. HAES has been extensively researched, and the approach has been associated with a multitude of health benefits, including improved cholesterol levels, lower blood pressure, no weight cycling, better body image, and increased physical activity (all independent of weight changes).

HAES can be a useful tool when opting out of viewing health through a weight-centric lens. For many people, especially those in very fat bodies, it has been a life-saving way to center their health needs and advocate for themselves. However, recent critiques of the approach have noted that the framework may not be helpful for everyone. It tends to center white people and, especially in the last several years, be promoted by thin practitioners (despite being founded by marginalized fat folks). Others note that HAES relies on Western science, which does not typically consider the social factors involved in health. (I'll speak more about this shortly.) Although there is certainly room for HAES to evolve, many professionals and activists apply an intersectional lens and center the liberation of *all* bodies—regardless of race, gender, ability, or sexuality—as part of their HAES practices.

Health Is More Than Just Physical

In talking about health, it's important to note that physical health is just one component of overall health and well-being. Mental and emotional health are both components of how healthy we feel, but they are often overlooked. Indeed, dieting and weight-centric approaches to health often have negative side effects on a person's mental health, including increased anxiety and depression and decreased self-esteem and self-confidence.

Aside from the markers that the medical community typically looks at for physical health (like lab work and blood pressure), you can often get a better understanding of "how you're doing" based upon how you feel physically, mentally, and emotionally. For example, some ways that my clients and I measure their health progress include

- Being more attuned to their body's hunger and fullness cues
- Not stressing about food as much and constantly thinking about what to eat (or not eat)
- Having more energy
- Improved sleep quality and quantity
- Finding more ways to cope with stress and other emotions

- Less frequent bingeing behaviors
- Experiencing a decrease in food cravings
- Having more trust in your body and less second-guessing food choices
- Improving flexibility, strength, and/or endurance

As I discuss more in Parts 2 and 3, you can do plenty of things to take care of your body (no matter what its size) and promote physical and mental health. But although these modifiable health behaviors are a better focus than weight, there are many factors related to our health that are out of our control.

The Social Determinants of Health

As someone with three degrees in nutrition, exercise science, and health, I got into this line of work with the belief (due to my schooling and thanks to diet culture) that what largely determines a person's health is what they eat and how much they exercise. Oh, how wrong I was!

Health is influenced by many factors, most commonly grouped into five broad categories: genetics, behaviors (also consider lifestyle factors), environmental influences, medical care, and social factors. Genetics and lifestyle behaviors contribute to only a fraction of the health differences among groups of people. According to the CDC (and others), a person's individual behaviors and modifiable risk factors such as diet, exercise, smoking, and alcohol consumption account for around 36 percent of the difference in health outcomes observed among groups of people.[40] Diet and exercise probably make up less than 15 percent within the lifestyle behaviors group. So, yes, nutrition and activity level can have an effect on health, but the contribution is much less than we'd like to believe, and those criteria are certainly not the main contributors to a person's health (physical or mental).

The WHO defines the social determinants of health as "the conditions under which people are born, grow, live, work and age."[41] The organization names twelve factors that are largely unmodifiable and strongly influence a person's health outcomes. The main determinants of health (that account for 65 to 70 percent of health outcomes) are a variety of social factors, including

- The type of job a person has and the working conditions at that job
- How much education a person has
- How much money a person makes
- Access to enough food (i.e., food security)
- Access to healthcare services and the quality of that care
- Access to safe housing, clean water, reliable transportation, and public safety
- The level of discrimination a person faces (like weight stigma or racism)
- Social support and coping skills
- Language and literacy

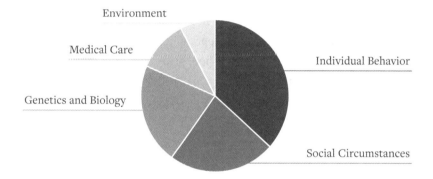

Health improves in line with a person's socioeconomic status; in other words, the more money, power, and resources a person has, the better their health. If you make enough money to support your basic needs, have access to safe housing, education, and good healthcare, and don't experience oppression or discrimination regularly, then you are much more likely to have better health outcomes than someone who faces regular discrimination, has to live paycheck to paycheck, or who doesn't have access to enough affordable, nutritious food.

Much of this disparity has to do with the body's stress response. People who are poor, live in unsafe neighborhoods, or suffer from discrimination like racism or sizeism have greater exposure to daily stressful life events. When an acute stress response is turned on briefly, it can save your life (think running from a tiger or dodging a bullet), but when that stress response becomes chronic and is activated day over day for years on end, it increases a person's risk for a whole host of diseases. Even if these people eat healthy and exercise regularly, their risk of disease and early death is much greater compared with people who are higher up in the social hierarchy. As we discussed with weight stigma, when the body experiences chronic stress, the risk of many diseases—including diabetes, high blood pressure, stroke, heart attack, and depression—can increase. For example, Black Americans have higher rates of high blood pressure that are not explained by genetics or lifestyle alone; their experiences of racism are a contributing factor. Similarly, people who experience poverty also have increased rates of high blood pressure, much of it related to the impact of stress.[42]

The social determinants of health also affect health behaviors related to food and exercise. One theory that is helpful to consider is Maslow's hierarchy of needs, a model that describes five-tiers of human needs displayed in a pyramid. (Note: Maslow's hierarchy of needs was informed by the beliefs of the Blackfoot Nation and the time he spent with them in Canada. In this way Maslow's hierarchy has been whitewashed, prioritizing the individual rather than the collective community and spirituality that the Indigenous perspective included.)[43]

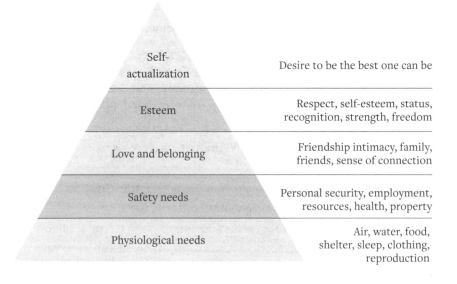

Physiological needs, which include access to enough food, water, and shelter, are the foundation of the pyramid. Next up are safety and stability needs, such as secure employment and safe housing. If these basic needs are not met, then people are more likely to have worse health outcomes. If you suffer from food insecurity and are not sure where your next meal is going to come from, how are you supposed to worry about how healthy that food is? Or if you are working several jobs to make ends meet, are you going to have time to hit the gym after work? Probably not.

When we focus only on an individual's weight or behaviors, we neglect to address the structural and systemic issues that contribute to health (and life) inequalities. Those of us who are lucky enough to be born into a family with secure housing and who live in a safe neighborhood, have enough money to afford food, and can get a good education have a huge leg up when it comes to our health outcomes.

Healthism and Morality

Along with thinness, diet culture puts health on a pedestal. In our culture, if you're not actively pursuing health (even outside the weight-centric paradigm) then something is "wrong" with you. Health and morality are closely intertwined. As my client Maya shared, "As a chubby adolescent, I was rewarded for eating 'good' foods. As I got older, I knew that a surefire way to gain praise from others was to eat as healthy as I could and constantly be partaking in dieting or weight-loss efforts."

Economist Robert Crawford explains that "healthism situates the problem of health and disease at the level of the individual."[44] In this way, "health" is about one's personal practices without acknowledgment that very real systemic and structural barriers can impede health and well-being. Healthism's version of health does not incorporate any of the myriad social factors that have a much larger impact on the health of both the individual and the collective.

Just as diet culture equates weight to health, healthism equates health to value and morality. But no one is morally obligated to pursue health. For many people, our culture's rigid, narrow, biased version of "health" is not even accessible. The definition of health as "absence of disease" becomes unattainable and ableist, in many ways preventing certain people—like those who suffer from chronic illnesses—from pursuing health. In the end, no one owes anybody else their health. Your health—and your definition of health—is something that you get to determine and (re)define for yourself. Plus, as you will see in the next chapter, a person's desire to be healthy—in addition to their desire to be thin—is not something that they are born with; instead, it's something that is imposed upon them through specific societal and cultural norms.

CHAPTER 4

Diet Culture Is Insidious

In the United States (and many other countries around the world), we are indoctrinated into diet culture from a young age. From the day you are born, you are exposed to direct and indirect messages about food, appearance, and body size. You learn associations like *thin is good* and *fat is bad*. Sometimes you get this message directly, like when a caregiver makes a comment about their weight. Other times, this message is more indirect and insidious, like when the fat character in a TV show or movie is the villain and the popular characters are thin, young, and conventionally attractive.

When we live and breathe diet culture all our lives, we inherently form biases—whether we want to or not. Recall that diet culture rose out of a patriarchal, racist society that purposefully oppressed and disempowered bodies that those in power deemed "inferior," which has influenced our society to have a preference for a certain type of person and an aversion toward "others" who don't fit that mold. These preferences are handed down through books, movies, television shows, advertisements, news media, politicians, and even healthcare providers. From day one, we are programmed to elevate certain bodies and devalue others, which is why it is almost impossible to remain neutral toward different people; stereotypes and beliefs are instilled in us from the very beginning.

Diet culture has created an arbitrary expectation of what we are supposed to look like and how we are supposed to act. Our culture has caged us. We've been conditioned and programmed to believe that to be loved, accepted, and valued in society, we must strive to be thin (and young and white and beautiful and perfect). On an individual level, this cage makes us lose sight of ourselves, to abandon our intuition, wants, and desires. We spend our lives punishing ourselves and trying to make ourselves smaller to comply with society's expectations of what an "ideal" and a "good" body is. On a collective level, diet culture functions as a way to oppress large swaths of the population. Getting out of this cage and rediscovering our true selves starts by confronting and challenging our beliefs (instead of blindly following them, as we've been taught to do). Certain things that we have taken as norms need to be turned upside down and questioned. Let's begin this process of unlearning, starting with diet culture.

Bringing Awareness to Diet Culture

Diet culture is all around you *and* internalized within you. Yet, before now, you may not have even been aware that it existed at all. It is so deeply embedded into the fabric of society that it usually just feels completely normal. Often, we don't even notice when something that we see, hear, or do is perpetuating or reinforcing diet culture. These unconscious biases are referred to as *implicit bias,* meaning you are unaware of your biases or how they may affect your understanding, actions, and decisions. You have formed these biases without even realizing it.

Diet culture is so normalized that identifying it is tough to do. The first step in moving away from diet culture is becoming aware of all the pervasive ways that it shows up around you and within you. This includes both extrinsic, or external, instances of diet culture as well as internal manifestations, often referred to as *diet mentality.*

Extrinsic Examples of Diet Culture

Several overarching themes signal diet culture:

- Conflating body size with health, well-being, and/or happiness
- Intentionally controlling eating behaviors to try to affect your body size
- Anything or anyone who tells you what to eat, when to eat, or how much to eat—i.e., any way of eating that is not based upon your internal body signals
- Whenever certain foods or ways of eating are denoted as "bad," while other foods or ways of eating are elevated and promoted as "good"
- Any message that creates or profits from your insecurities by offering you the "solution"—i.e., a product or plan
- Anything that positions a certain diet, "lifestyle change," or style of eating as the answer to your problems
- Using exercise to compensate for, "burn off," or earn food
- Any message that tells you that you are not enough and need to change your body or yourself in some way, shape, or form

Some types of diet culture are easier to recognize than others—for example, fad diet plans or programs such as Weight Watchers (now WW), the keto or Paleo diet, Jenny Craig, or the Atkins Diet, which all openly promise weight loss. These types of diets tell you what to eat, when to eat, or how to eat and often eliminate certain foods or food groups. However, you also need to be aware of other, sneakier forms of diet culture. The following forms of it are less explicit and may not immediately scream "diet culture":

- Intentionally controlling your eating to "maintain" your weight
- Letting any external factors—like your weight or your clothing size—dictate your eating decisions
- Eating plans promoted as a "lifestyle change," "balanced eating," or "everything in moderation" (yup, that's diet culture too!)
- "Clean eating," cleanses, and detoxes
- Describing certain foods as "treats" or "indulgences" (the message: this is something you shouldn't have as often)
- The idea of "cheat" meals and "cheat" days (see the preceding bullet)
- Food marketing that uses terms like "guilt-free" or "sinfully delicious" (which assign morality to food)

- Messages that conflate food choices and healthy eating to personal willpower or lack thereof
- Treatments that claim to "shrink" or "tighten" parts of your body
- Gyms or exercise plans that promise to "tone" your body
- "Fitspiration" on social media that promotes fit, toned, thin bodies

These more insidious forms of diet culture may not overtly promise weight loss. Often they market "eating healthier" under the guise of well-being, which can make them tougher to sniff out. Yet the message is still the same: Follow this plan, do these things, and you'll be "healthier" (subtext: thinner). It's still about making money by feeding into society's (and therefore our) fear of being fat and all the moral implications that our culture assigns to food choices and body sizes.

Sneaky diet culture also shows up often on social media in the form of so-called health and nutrition "experts" who espouse a certain perfectionistic idea of what health and wellness are supposed to look like. These people are most often young, thin, white, fit, and middle- to upper-class. They talk about eating the "right" foods and removing those that are not "clean." Elimination diets, fasting, detoxing, cleansing, and clean eating are common among these "wellness" influencers. They show off a supposed "ideal" for people to subscribe to. It may be delivered with "love and light" or under the guise of "self-love," but the wellness influencer (and industry) is still diet culture. These people perpetuate (and make money off of) the system that upholds impossible standards of health and beauty.

The images and messages of diet culture are also displayed via the media that we consume. The majority of images we see of women in the media are thin, young, and white—even though 67 percent of women in the United States are sized 14 and up and nonwhite women make up around 40 percent of the population. What we see—and what we don't see—makes a huge difference in how we learn what is worthy and what is not. In this way, the media—TV, movies, books, advertisements—all continue to share and perpetuate diet culture messages and beliefs.

Diet culture can (and will) show up in casual conversations as well. You might hear any or all the following in daily conversations:

- People discussing what diets they are following or what foods they are (or aren't) eating
- Fat shaming and fat jokes

- Complimenting weight loss
- Expressing fear of weight gain or of being fat
- Commenting on or judging another person's food choices
- Justifying what they are eating

As you start to notice and recognize how much diet culture is normalized and baked into our society, you'll realize how often people talk about it.

> Oh, you're ordering a salad? You're being so good and healthy!

> I wish I could eat like that, but I'd be huge if I did.

> I'm going to be bad today and get the fries.

As you become more aware of diet culture, you will probably start to notice it everywhere, and you may feel really frustrated; this feeling is common and expected. One of my clients came into a session annoyed that no matter where she went, she was faced with diet culture—in her grocery store (where only fat-free yogurt was available), during a workout class at the gym ("Let's get beach body ready!"), on a magazine rack (every cover featuring a thin, beautiful, young, white woman), in the lunchroom at work (where everyone talked about what diet they were on). It was everywhere! Feeling annoyance, frustration, and even anger is normal and completely justified. Not only is the frustration warranted, but it will help as you work to resist and reject diet culture. I'll talk more about that shortly.

Internalized Diet Culture and Diet Mentality

When you take any societal beliefs regarding food, exercise, and body size that you learn and apply these standards to yourself, you're internalizing diet culture or *diet mentality*. A person's diet mentality is honed via years of swimming in diet culture's messages and through countless attempts at different diets and eating plans. Even if you've never formally gone on a diet, you most likely have certain external eating rules or food rules that you believe you "should" follow. Plus, even if you don't think of it as dieting, anytime you let an external measurement (like weight) or someone else (like a nutritionist or someone you follow online) govern your eating decisions, you still have a diet mentality. It may be very subtle, but diet culture is still dictating what and why you eat rather than your body being your guide.

Diet mentality includes your internal thoughts and feelings, as well as your behaviors. The following are some examples:

Behaviors

- Following a specific diet plan with external rules of what, when, and how much to eat
- Avoiding foods "high" in calories, carbs, fat, or sugar
- Eliminating or restricting certain foods or entire food groups
- Measuring your food
- "Watching" your portions
- Trying not to eat "too much"
- Ignoring your body's hunger cues
- Avoiding social situations because you're afraid of being around certain types of food
- Exercising to compensate for eating or to earn your food
- Weighing yourself

Thoughts and feelings

- Labeling foods as "good" or "bad"
- Having a feeling of "messing up" and needing to start over tomorrow (or Monday)
- Thinking you "should" or "shouldn't" eat something
- Feeling guilty after eating
- Judging yourself for not having enough willpower or being out of control
- Fearing others' judgment about your food choices

Just like external diet culture, this internal diet mentality serves to disconnect you from your body's intuition. It keeps you in the cycle of seeking external validation and confirmation that you're doing things "right" rather than paying attention to internal signals and tuning into your own deep, unique wisdom.

Practice Noticing Diet Culture and Diet Mentality

For one day, pay attention to instances of both external diet culture as well as internal diet mentality. Make a list of all of the different forms that you notice throughout the day. Review your list. Are there any that surprise you? Can you think of some other forms of diet culture or diet mentality that you may have overlooked?

How Diet Culture Undermines You

Looking back at the statements and examples I just gave about diet culture and diet mentality, you may be wondering why some of these things are harmful. As a new client said to me recently, "But certain foods *are* better for us than others. I *do* eat better and feel differently when I am paying attention to what and how much I'm eating."

I understand this sentiment and why it may seem confusing that certain aspects of diet culture are harmful. Yes, certain foods *do* have more nutrients than others. And yes, eating certain things *may* make your body feel better or worse. However, although food rules and beliefs I shared may not seem harmful on the surface, they're all grounded in the belief that our food choices affect our worth and that a thin body is better than a fat body. These beliefs and rules—and the diet culture that reinforces and perpetuates them—are what keep you disconnected from your body. It's impossible to honor your body and give it what it needs—nutritionally or otherwise—when you're caught up trying to follow external rules or diet mentality.

People often say to me, "But if I'm not hard on myself, or if I don't force myself to eat a certain way, then I'll never make healthy decisions. That judgment actually *helps* me make changes." This type of thinking is very common (hint: because diet culture has programmed us to believe this!). Although it may seem as though you would never make a healthy decision if you weren't hard on yourself, in reality, the opposite occurs.

I explored this recently with my client Tabitha. She had a lot of guilt and judged herself harshly when she didn't make a "healthy" food decision. So I asked, "What ends up happening when that judgment arises?" She shared that she would feel awful about herself for a few days, then she'd gather up her "discipline" and try to be "really good" about everything. Her attempt would work for a few days, but then she'd inevitably lose control and "fall off the wagon." This cycle of "good" days followed by "bad" days would continue—there was never a middle ground. "I would tell myself, 'I'm in control, I'm in control' until eventually, I would feel out of control. Then I'd go right to the thing that I had told myself I shouldn't eat," said Tabitha. She realized that the diet mentality rules around eating were setting her up for failure.

Shame does not help us to embrace ourselves and our bodies in ways that make us feel free. Shame does not liberate us; in fact, it most often does the opposite. I'll talk about this more in Chapter 5, but for now, know that guilt, shame, or judgment may work in the short term (emphasis on the *may*), but in the long term, those things only serve to disconnect us further from our bodies. Diet culture breeds shame and guilt. Diet culture is what makes you feel like you're not thin/pretty/good enough and causes you to spend a lot of time, money, and energy chasing these made-up standards of health and beauty. Diet culture, and likewise, your internal diet mentality, perpetuates an unrealistic beauty, body, and health ideal.

Understanding the Effects of Diet Culture

By keeping us focused on an external body ideal, diet culture undermines our ability to understand, listen to, and trust our bodies. This is why diets or "lifestyle changes" feel easy at first but end up impossible to stick to. They're never sustainable, but not because you lack willpower. Instead, diets fail because diet culture disconnects you from your body, and dieting and diet mentality triggers the starvation response that I spoke about in Chapter 2. Diet culture keeps you on the restrict/binge pendulum, so you're always either on a diet and being "good" or off it and being "bad." There is rarely an in-between.

Diet culture and diet mentality also have a host of other negative side effects, including the following:

- Increased preoccupation with food and your body
- Lower self-esteem
- Higher rates of disordered eating behaviors and eating disorders
- Increased stress
- More frequent bingeing
- Increased cravings
- Decreased confidence
- Higher rates of weight cycling or yo-yo dieting (linked to increased risk of certain diseases)

Not only can diet culture harm physical and mental health but it can interfere with many other facets of life. Diet culture undermines your true self and can cause you to miss out on so many things. I can't tell you how many women I know who have avoided dating and intimacy because they were afraid of what the other person would think of their bodies. Or who canceled plans because they were on a diet or were worried about being around so much food. Or who find themselves less present around family and friends because they are worried about what others may be thinking. Diet culture steals our time, money, and energy. But you can take that all back.

Assessment: How Has Diet Culture and Diet Mentality Affected You? _____

Check all that apply:

- ☐ I don't feel my hunger cues.
- ☐ I'm not able to tell when I'm full until I'm stuffed.
- ☐ I have canceled plans or avoid certain social situations.
- ☐ My relationships have suffered.
- ☐ I've been distracted or less present with friends and family.
- ☐ I've had mood swings.
- ☐ I've experienced strong cravings.
- ☐ I worry about what other people think about me.
- ☐ I worry about how my body looks.
- ☐ I have avoided intimacy.
- ☐ I compare my body to others.
- ☐ I compare my eating to others.
- ☐ I compensate for eating with exercise or skipping meals.
- ☐ I have exercised to burn a certain number of calories.
- ☐ When I break a food rule, I end up saying "screw it" and going off the rails.
- ☐ I feel guilty when I eat certain foods.
- ☐ I spend a lot of my day thinking about food or my body.
- ☐ Breaking a food rule or stepping on the scale has caused me to feel awful about myself all day.
- ☐ I feel anxious when I'm not able to control what I eat.
- ☐ I'm not able to trust my body to tell me what I want or need.
- ☐ I have trouble listening to my intuition.
- ☐ I often second-guess my decisions.
- ☐ I've stopped myself from doing something because of my weight or how my body looks.

What else has diet culture taken from you? How else has it interfered with your life? What have you stopped doing or enjoying because of diet culture, fat-phobia, or fear of judgment?

_____

Examining Your Dieting History

In Chapter 1, I described how dieting can serve as a way of coping and as a way to belong. Think back to when you first began dieting; what was going on in your life? Linda, a forty-five-year-old mother of three, always tied her history of dieting with her engagement and wedding. "I wanted to be thin for my wedding day," she told me. Yet when we started unpacking what was going on in her life around that time, she realized there was more to the story. At twenty-two, Linda's then-boyfriend had a close friend pass away from lymphoma. One year later, when they were twenty-three, Linda's best friend died of cancer; the following year, another one of Linda's friends died suddenly. Linda had been with all three people when they passed away. "Looking back now, I can see that dieting and attempting to lose weight was a form of coping for me. In a point of life where everything seemed random and impossible to comprehend, it allowed me to feel some semblance of control over what was happening to me."

Although dieting initially served to help Linda in a moment of deep pain, over the next fifteen years, the negative side effects had become glaring. When asked what her focus on weight loss had done to her, Linda replied, "The more I dieted, the more obsessed and out of control around food I became. I never used to be like that; I never binged." Not only did dieting affect her relationship to food, but it had caused her to miss out on many aspects of life. "No matter what size my body was, I was still never happy," Linda shared. "I barely had any photos of myself with my kids, and I didn't use social media because I was too ashamed to be tagged in photos. I said no to so many social things—last summer, I refused to go swimming at my sister's house because I didn't want to be in a bathing suit."

For many people caught in the dieting cycle, their emotional state is grounded in the success or failure of their efforts to change their bodies. When Linda didn't lose weight, she'd berate herself and go down a shame spiral. She'd end up being moody, depressed, and short with her husband and kids. If she saw a number on the scale that she liked, her mood would improve, and she'd feel better about herself. But that only lasted so long. "When I was at my smallest, I constantly thought about and worried about food. I was still not happy with how I looked, even though my body now was the weight I thought I wanted."

Dieting and the pursuit of an "ideal" body take up so much time and energy. It can leave you with little energy for other pursuits, including connection to yourself and others. A focus on shrinking your body or altering your appearance to fit into the societal norms can end up causing you to hide your true self. Attempting to make your body smaller often results in making your life smaller too.

Explore Your Experience with Dieting

Think back to the first time you dieted or tried to restrict your food intake. What was going on for you then? What may have played into your decision to want to lose weight? How has dieting affected you, mentally and physically? How has dieting affected your food behaviors? What have you given up or not done because you were dieting?

Resisting Diet Culture

It can be frustrating, infuriating, and downright painful at times to be so conscious of diet culture and the many, many ways in which it is displayed in our society. Comments from friends, family members, or strangers can be annoying at best and traumatic at worst. Yet this awareness is also the first step in a journey toward something bigger. There is an alternative anti-diet or non-diet path—one that you'll be learning more about in this book—that allows you to tap into your body's deep wisdom and intuition and step fully into your power. This path that enables you to live in freedom, take up space, and be your complete, expansive self.

Think of all the time you have spent dieting, exercising, and shrinking yourself to try to fit into a mold deemed "acceptable" by society. What else could you do with that time? What would it be like to get all of that time back? Instead of asking, "What is standing in the way of me being thinner/smaller/prettier?" I propose you ask new questions:

- What are dieting, food- and exercise-obsessing, and body anxiety standing in the way of?

- Who are you, deep down, and who do you want to be?
- Do you want to have more fulfilling relationships?
- Do you want to be a more involved friend, sibling, or parent?
- Do you want to grow mentally, emotionally, or spiritually?

This topic came up within an online community that I run. "Prior to my anti-diet journey, I never considered having a true hobby," a woman posted. "I used to think, 'How does anyone have time for that?' I spent most of my free time at the gym, meal prepping, or home cooking 'healthy' meals." She went on to share that now that she had stopped dieting, she had a lot more time on her hands and was looking for suggestions on what others on this journey had done. Many women chimed in sharing similar experiences, and the hobbies and activities and relationships they wanted to spend more time on. One person posted this inspiring reflection:

I want to spend time discovering myself. I want to find out what I'm harboring that makes me short-tempered with my family sometimes. I want to read 30+ books (and to stop reading Harry Potter over and over). I want to pray more, give more compliments, and try a few new recipes each month. I want to do another philanthropy project. And YES, I want to eat both tasty and healthy food and get on my elliptical 'cause it feels good to move and play Beat Saber on the Oculus cause it's freaking fun and exciting and I'm pretty good at it. I want to do those last few things without worrying about the size of my butt.

We'll be diving into this more in Chapter 5, but for now, take a minute to reflect. Has dieting or focusing on your weight and appearance helped you live a truer, more meaningful life? Or has it led you further away from yourself?

Take a Time Inventory

Grab a pen and answer the following questions:

- How much time do you spend each day thinking about food and your body?
- How much time do you spend each day feeling guilty or second-guessing your decisions related to food and exercise?
- How much time do you spend each day planning, prepping, or preparing "healthy" foods?
- How much time do you spend each day, on average, reading or research-ing about changing your body or actively trying to change your body?

Take the daily amount of time from the four questions above and multiply it by 365. This is (approximately) how much time you spend each year focused on food and your body. How would your life be different if you felt confident and calm in your relationship to food and your body, and you weren't spending this time trying to change yourself? What would you do with all of that time instead?

Reject the Diet Mentality

To move away from dieting, you first need to be aware of all of the ways diet culture is present, both outside you and within you. Once you are aware of the behaviors, thoughts, or feelings that constitute *diet mentality*, you can begin to give them up. *Reject the diet mentality* is the first principle in the intuitive eating framework, as described by Evelyn Tribole and Elyse Resch.[1] It involves the following:

Step 1: Reflect upon and acknowledge the harm that diet culture and diet mentality have caused.

Step 2: Bring your awareness to the ways diet culture and diet mentality show up.

Step 3: Call it out for what it is—"This is diet mentality talking" or "That is diet culture."

Step 4: Begin to challenge your thoughts and beliefs and shift your behaviors.

You won't necessarily move through these four steps linearly. Step 1, in particular, is one that most people will need to return to throughout this process (and honestly, throughout their lives). Diet culture is sneaky and persistent. As you do the internal work to move away from dieting, diet culture will continue to pop up in a multitude of ways. Whether it's a well-meaning family member sending you information about a new diet, a doctor recommending that you lose weight for "your health," or an Instagram ad sneaking its way into your feed—diet culture is everywhere. All of these situations may trigger a small (or large) part of you to consider, "Well, maybe just *one more diet*...and then I'll do this intuitive eating thing." This reaction is completely normal. You will almost certainly have times of wanting to go back to dieting or trying dieting again. That impulse doesn't make you a bad person; it's the reality of living in a society that prizes young, thin, heteronormative, able-bodied people. Moving away from diet culture in a society like this is tough, which is why it's helpful to continue to return to your reflection from Step 1: What has your history with dieting shown you? How has it been damaging? How have you been held back because of dieting?

Remind yourself that the dieting industry is a $70 billion per year monolith with the sole purpose of making you feel "less than" so that you fork over your money, time, and energy to try to lose weight. The dieting industry profits from your shame and oppression. Remember, the dieting industry was not born out of a desire to make us all healthier. It began as a way to oppress Black people and to keep anyone other than white men down and "othered." Today, diet culture and the dieting industry continue to oppress fat people and harm people of all sizes, especially women and people of color, who live in a world where disordered eating behaviors are normalized.

You may also find yourself continuing to reflect and bring awareness to all the sneaky forms of diet culture as you move through this process. This is why Step 2, which I spoke about early in this chapter, is a step you continue to return to. There will always be new and varied forms of diet culture popping up, so you have to keep your radar active and alert. Over time, it will get easier and easier to identify these sneaky types of diet culture.

Call Out Diet Culture

I covered the issues in Steps 1 and 2 earlier in this chapter, so let's dive into Step 3: Call it out. Once you are aware of the various ways diet culture and diet mentality are appearing, bring it into your consciousness by actively identifying problematic thoughts as "This is diet mentality." For example, if you go to choose something for breakfast and notice that you think, "That's too many calories," or, "That's too many carbs," call that out as diet mentality. Or if you are at a restaurant and feel like you "should" eat a salad, remind yourself, "This is diet mentality." The more awareness that you raise, and the more you call diet culture or diet mentality out, the easier it becomes to start moving away from it.

Challenge Your Thoughts and Shift Your Behaviors

As you notice food rules or thoughts pop up, challenge them by doing the opposite of whatever your diet mentality is telling you. You may still have thoughts to restrict or not to eat a certain food, but can you change your behavior anyway? Behaviors are the easiest things for us to change. (I use "easiest" relatively: I know for many people, especially those with active eating disorders, it can be quite difficult to practice new behaviors.) Thoughts and feelings take longer to shift. You can start the process by actively working on challenging the thought by changing your behavior. For example:

Diet Mentality Thought $\longrightarrow$ Behavior

"I should only order a half sandwich" $\rightarrow$ Order the full-size sandwich.

"I'm hungry, but it's too soon to eat, so I'll wait" $\longrightarrow$ Eat something right now.

"I want a cookie, but it's a lot of sugar" $\longrightarrow$ Eat the cookie.

Challenge the diet mentality by taking the opposite action, then notice what happens. Get curious without judging yourself for doing something "good" or "bad" (which is also diet mentality!). How does the food taste? Is it satisfying? You are not evaluating; you're listening. The judgmental or guilty thoughts may still be there ("I can't believe you ate that; what were you thinking?!"), but over time, the more you challenge those ideas, the quieter they will get. I'll share more tools related to shifting your thoughts and feelings in later chapters. For now, practice rejecting the diet mentality by calling it out and working to challenge your behaviors related to food.

Let Go of the Tools of Dieting

Another step toward rejecting the diet mentality is to get rid of what Tribole and Resch refer to as the *dieter's tools*. Dieting involves eating based on external cues, like calorie counting or measuring portions. As you work to reconnect with your internal cues, start to let go of any of the external "tools" that you may be using, including

- Food tracking apps
- Calorie, macro, or point counting
- Avoiding, limiting, or restricting certain foods or food groups
- Low-calorie or low-carb recipe sites or cookbooks
- Following a meal plan
- Measuring or weighing your food
- Using exercise to compensate for eating or to burn a certain number of calories
- Eating less early in the day to compensate for a big evening meal
- Using cheat days or cheat meals
- Using a scale to weigh yourself

It may feel scary to give up some of these tools. If you notice any anxiety or fear arise at the thought of giving these up, dig into that some more. What does thinking about letting go of these tools bring up for you? Does it worry you? If so, what worries you specifically about giving up these dieting tools? Common responses that I hear include the fear of being out of control and not being able to stop eating. The reality is that dieting—i.e., any type of food restriction, both physical and mental—is what causes you to feel out of control around food and/or binge-eat. It's really hard to stop eating when you've been restricting food; remember—eating more is the body's normal response to feelings of "starvation." But once your body learns and trusts that you will honor the cues it's sending you and that you'll keep feeding it, the intense drive to eat will decrease. (I'll talk more about this in Chapter 7.)

What About the Scale?

I find that it can feel especially anxiety-provoking for people to think about giving up stepping on the scale. If weighing yourself is part of your weekly (or daily) routine, it can feel scary to give up. Many people use the scale as a way to reassure themselves that they are "on track," so giving it up feels like giving up control. But is the scale truly helpful? Think about it: How do you feel after weighing yourself? What happens if you see a "good" number? What about if you see a "bad" number—what happens then?

For most people, the number on the scale—despite being just a number— is anything but neutral. It's an emotional trigger that sets the tone for the day. Seeing a "good" number can make a person feel great, whereas seeing a "bad" number can trigger feelings of shame and anxiety that affect the whole day. The number that appears becomes a criterion for self-judgment. That judgment can affect everything from the way you eat to the way you dress to the way you interact with others. Often clients tell me that the number on the scale—whether it's "good" or "bad"—leads to disconnected eating like overeating and bingeing. A "good" weigh-in can be cause for celebratory eating ("I've been so good this week, I should get myself an ice cream!") whereas weight gain—or lack of weight loss—can set off a binge ("Screw it, I tried so hard this week, and didn't lose any weight, so what's the point?").

Using a scale as a way to "see how you're doing" keeps you focused externally. Even if you've let go of all other diet mentality and dieting tools, stepping on the scale will continue to pull you outside of your body. Weighing yourself undermines the process of eating intuitively. It causes you to lose sight of, and makes it harder to listen to, your internal signals of what, when, and how much to eat. Also, being hung up on the number on the scale can lead to obsessing about food and your body and can be linked to lower self-esteem, negative body image, repeated weight loss and gain, and disordered eating. Weighing can detract from other health goals, too. When you spend so much time focused on the number on the scale, you have less time to change behaviors that can help your health (and may even attempt behaviors that are harmful to your health).

Still unsure about tossing the scale? Try taking a break from it for one month to find out what happens. Notice how you feel and how you behave. I know; it's scary. You'll feel like you're letting go of control, and, in a way, you are because you're letting go of allowing a number on the scale to dictate how you feel and how you behave. One of my clients tried this recently and shared, "Leaving this morning without weighing myself felt so freeing! It honestly never occurred to me that giving myself a break from the number on the scale would have such a positive impact on my day." Remember, your weight is not an indicator of your worth, your value, your health, or your progress.

Move Away from Binary Thinking

Humans dislike ambiguity. The unknown can be anxiety-provoking. So we tend to simplify things into two mutually exclusive categories: good/bad, either/or, right/wrong. This type of binary thinking makes us feel safe. Diet culture plays right into binary thinking. The implication of "If you do this, everything will be okay" is part of the reason dieting behaviors feel safe, and moving away from them can feel scary. However, life doesn't happen in the binary, and talking about food and bodies and reducing ourselves to such inflexible, black-and-white terms limits us from growing and changing.

Language is powerful. The ways you talk about food (and bodies) affect your thoughts, emotions, and behaviors. Using binary terms like good/bad, healthy/unhealthy, guilt-free/indulgent, or clean/toxic causes a split between body and mind. Rather than listening to your internal signals of hunger, satisfaction, and fullness, you end up reacting to the language and labels placed on food. For example, one of my clients noticed that when they ate something they considered "bad" or "junk," they'd immediately feel like the day was blown. This caused them to think "screw it," ignore their body's feelings, and mindlessly eat whatever other "bad" foods they had around—because tomorrow they'd "start over."

Eating foods that you've labeled as "bad" or "unhealthy" can also cause increased feelings of guilt (hello, food police!) and shame. Words like this assign a moral value to food, so eating a "bad" food then affects a person's self-worth, making them feel as though they are a "bad" person, creating more shame and possibly leading to self-punishing behaviors (often using food).

Likewise, describing food as "good" or "healthy" is also a harmful type of binary thinking. When someone thinks of a food as "good," they usually assume it's better for them (known as the *health halo* effect), which often leads to eating more of the food, regardless of how hungry the person is or whether they like the food. Similar to words like *bad* or *unhealthy, good* and *healthy* also pull us outside of our body cues. For example, my client Roxanne would frequently binge-eat several protein bars or a few pints of one of the so-called "healthy" ice creams. She wasn't physically hungry, but because she was dieting, she never felt satisfied. So she turned to these foods she thought were "good" and ended up bingeing on them (because they also were not satisfying).

Binary thinking is an all-or-nothing thing that sets you up for success or failure. The scale goes down a few pounds; you're "good." It creeps up; you're "bad." When it's always one or the other, there is no space to engage, reflect, learn, or grow. Instead, if you can suspend judgment and sit with any uneasiness or anxiety that arises, a third element emerges: the gray area. I know, I know; everyone *hates* the gray area. But it is here where meaningful learning, growing, and changing occurs. Living in the gray means each life experience (and eating experience) is an opportunity to learn and experiment rather than to pass or fail. Moving away from the binary enables you to explore and dig deeper, uncovering your beliefs about food and bodies. The gray area allows for nuance and flexibility to emerge. Using neutral language levels the playing field and takes morality and shame out of the decision, which enables you to make decisions based on your internal cues rather than your external environment. This space in the in-between brings together your mind *and* body, allowing you to explore and find a more balanced, inclusive relationship both to food and with yourself.

Observe what happens when you use dichotomous, black-and-white language. Become aware of judgments like, "I was good today up until dinner," or, "Today was so bad." Call this out as an unhelpful diet mentality and shift your language. Try to use more neutral, nonjudgmental terms. More helpful words to describe food include *nourishing, delicious, comforting, fueling, fun, colorful,* or *satisfying.* Or you may say, "I ate a lot of desserts this week, but I enjoyed them, and I also had other foods." Remember, the day doesn't magically reset at midnight (that's another type of binary thinking). Remind yourself that all foods provide nutrients. Some foods have fewer ingredients; some have more. Some are less processed; some are more. Those qualities don't make them "good" or "bad"; it just makes them *food.* Taking the morality out of food allows you to separate your food choices from your self-worth and gives you space to learn, grow, and move in a more meaningful direction.

Language Matters

Make a list of all of the words that you use to describe or think about food. Which of these words have judgment attached? How do these terms affect you? What effect does it have on your behaviors? On your thoughts? Do you feel guiltier when you eat foods that you refer to as "bad" or "unhealthy"? As you become more aware of how these words affect you, start to practice shifting your language to neutral terms.

Create an Anti-Diet Bubble

Remember, diet culture is *everywhere*. The mainstream approach to food and bodies encourages dieting and disordered eating while perpetuating fatphobia and weight stigma. Although you will never be able to avoid diet culture completely, you can take steps to move away from it in certain aspects of your life. Evaluate the types of media that you consume each day, including social media, books or magazines, televisions shows, movies, and podcasts. What types of messages do they promote? Filter out diet-culture messages and opt out of diet culture as much as you can. For example, you may start by

- Unfollowing anyone on social media that promotes dieting or weight loss
- Getting rid of any diet or weight-loss books and magazines
- Thinking critically about the television shows and movies that you watch and how they reinforce characteristics of diet culture

You can also opt out of diet conversations or body-bashing sessions. When these topics come up in conversation, avoid contributing to the conversation. Change the subject if you can. If those topics feel particularly triggering, excuse yourself and go to the restroom for a breather. This is also a place where you can set an explicit boundary around what topics you will and will not talk about or tolerate; I'll talk more about boundary setting in Chapter 16.

When you've opted out of diet culture as much as you can, then create an "anti-diet bubble" for yourself. Surround yourself with supportive, inclusive messages in the form of books, podcasts, blogs, social media accounts, and more. I'll talk more about diversifying your media sources and finding community later in Chapters 12 and 13. You can also find some of my favorite anti-diet resources in Appendix B. These messages will provide support and community as you deprogram and unlearn all of the arbitrary rules that diet culture has taught you.

After reading this chapter and taking inventory of all the ways diet culture and diet mentality show up, you've probably begun to notice it in places you never did before. As many people in the anti-diet community say, once you "see" it, it's almost impossible ever to "unsee" it. For many folks, this new knowledge can feel liberating. I've had so many people say to me, "I never knew that there was another way to operate outside of dieting and trying to lose weight or change my body." The realization that there is nothing wrong with their bodies and that their "failures" to lose weight had nothing to do with a lack of willpower or control can feel incredibly freeing.

This new path may also feel scary. Some people, when they learn about diet culture and the alternatives that exist, wish in part that they *could* unsee it. For some folks who live in marginalized bodies, this alternative path can feel like walking away from acceptance and the idea that they will one day achieve a body that will be accepted by society. For others, to whom dieting is all, or most, of what they have ever known, giving up the structure and rules can feel terrifying. I get that; I've been there, too.

If you're still feeling unsure or nervous about giving up the diet mentality, know that the feeling is normal. This journey is a process, and it takes time. Letting go of something you've used for a while, even if it hasn't always worked how you wanted it to, can be tough. Making the change can also be difficult if you're still surrounded by people who are wrapped up in diet culture. Trying to heal your relationship to food and your body in a world where diet culture and fatphobia are ingrained into every institution is exhausting. If you relate to any of these issues, I encourage you to notice what fears might be coming up for you right now. In the next chapter, I'll share how you can continue to dig deeper and explore more about how and why your thoughts, beliefs, and behaviors about food and bodies first began.

CHAPTER 5

Exploring Your History with Food and Your Body

Janella, a twenty-five-year-old living in New York City, couldn't figure out why she kept overeating. "I feel like I'm addicted to sugar," she told me when we first met. "So I try to tell myself that I can't have any sugar and cut it out completely. It works for a little while, but the moment I add any sugary foods back into my diet, I end up bingeing. Then I totally beat myself up about it." Janella was clearly stuck in a cycle of restriction, followed by bingeing and extreme guilt. In our first session together, I asked her what food was like in her house when she was growing up. Without hesitating, she replied, "Complicated." Looking back, she realizes that both of her parents were out of touch with their bodies. Her earliest memories involve watching her mom track her food and then sneak food from the kitchen at night. "Each time my mom would eat dessert, or any type of sweet, my dad would make comments about it, like 'Are you sure you should be eating that?'"

Meanwhile, her dad was always trying to "get in shape" and hopped around from diet to diet. "Almost every diet he tried didn't allow sweets, which meant that we couldn't keep any in the house. I seldom had access to these types of foods, and I remember visiting friends' houses and going wild eating the sweets that they had available." Janella also recalls her dad eating very little throughout the day and then beating himself up at night when he would eat a huge amount at dinner. "I don't have any memories of my parents talking about enjoying their food; food was only associated with guilty feelings. I always heard them say, 'I'm so bad for eating this.' There was so much judgment."

Listening to Janella describe the food environment in the house where she grew up, it was clear to me (as it may be to you, too) why, according to her, her main "problem" was with sugar. It had been something that was restricted, and therefore scarce, for about as long as she could remember. Not only that, but she grew up learning that sugar was "bad," something that shouldn't be eaten and—if it was consumed—was cause for guilt, shame, and judgment. It's no wonder that now, as an adult, she struggles with cycles of restriction and bingeing, with a huge side of guilt and shame.

It's a natural human impulse to want to "fix" our problems. When it comes to food, people often try to "fix" their eating behaviors by dieting to try to stop the "bad" behavior and replace it with a "good" or "healthy" behavior. But by trying to immediately change your behavior without doing any work to dissect and understand where this behavior came from, all you end up doing is putting a Band-Aid on things. Before you work to shift your behaviors—even if you're attempting to do so through a non-diet lens—it's crucial to bring awareness to and gain an understanding of where your thoughts, beliefs, and behaviors are coming from.

Examining Your Beliefs

I hate my stomach pooch because I hate my stomach pooch.

I can't stand my cellulite; it looks so gross.

Carbohydrates are awful for you; it's not okay to have them at every meal.

Despite how familiar these statements sound (perhaps you've uttered at least one of them before, too?), no one pops out of the womb holding these beliefs. So, where did these ideas come from? Who told you a flat stomach was the epitome of attractiveness? (Side note: Babies and small children would beg to differ; squishy bellies are the stuff napping dreams are made of. Or so I've been told.) Where did you get the message that carbohydrates are bad for you? Who told you that you shouldn't have cellulite? What assumptions are behind this belief? And who's benefiting from you holding these beliefs, disliking your body, and dieting to try to change it?

In Chapter 1, I shared some of the historical roots of diet culture and beauty ideals. Now it's time to do some investigating of your own. Let's unpack all of the things you've been told about your body and begin having a better understanding of your history with food. I want you to start to think critically about where you learned and absorbed these messages. What has informed your beliefs and feelings about your body, other people's bodies, food, eating, and weight?

Family Narratives

When you were growing up, what was your family's attitude toward food? When I was asked a similar question during an interview for the podcast *Food Psych,* my mind went to early childhood, where my memories related to food were generally pretty happy. My mom cooked dinner most nights. On nights she worked, my dad would cook for my brother and me (though my mom loves to tell the story about the time my dad called her at work to ask her how to make grilled cheese, and she said, "Ask Alissa; she knows"— I was five years old). I also have great memories of Sunday breakfast. From a young age, I would cook crêpes for my whole family. When I was little, I wanted to be a waitress when I grew up, so I would make the meal, take everyone's order, then plate the food and bring it to the table. There was always a lot of food around, and nothing was really restricted. I don't remember the health impacts of food coming up, but I was a picky eater, so I do have a vivid memory of an all-out fight at dinner when I refused to take even one bite of tomato. My mom wouldn't let me get up from the table until I did, I refused, and a stand-off ensued. I remained at the table for hours, bawling my eyes out. Sometime around 10:00 p.m., I finally took a bite of the tomato and promptly ran to the kitchen sink and "threw up" (ha, showed you, Mom!).

Although I was lucky to have mostly positive associations with food as a child, not everyone can say the same—like Janella, whom I introduced earlier. She had almost no positive childhood memories involving food. Or my client Codie, who had a family that constantly "pushed" food onto her, so she felt a lot of pressure to eat and finish a meal while also receiving negative comments about the size of her body.

What comes up for you when you think about what food was like in your house as a child? Many factors can affect your relationship to food, including what and how your parents or caregivers ate, what the food environment was like, and how food and body size was discussed.

Parental Eating Behaviors

Your parents' eating behaviors and beliefs about food (and how those beliefs showed up in your household) shape the relationship you have to food. At the beginning of this chapter, I shared the story of Janella, whose parents dieted on and off throughout her child and teen years. Children who grow up in a household with adults who frequently diet, like Janella did, are more likely to have disordered eating behaviors, including higher rates of binge-eating.[1] If you grew up with parents who were preoccupied with their weight and often dieted, you may have learned that being thin was very important—in general, but also specifically to your parents.

Even if your parents did not explicitly diet, how they spoke about food, how they served food, and what foods they kept around the house play into the behaviors and attitudes you have as an adult. When Maura, now thirty-nine, was growing up, her parents never kept much food at home. Her mom would buy just what she needed to make meals; if anyone got hungry between meals, there were never any snacks to eat. "I used to binge-eat as a kid, and I've always blamed myself and my lack of control," Maura shared with me. "But I've come to realize that the fact that food was so scarce in our house probably had something to do with my binge tendencies. There was real food restriction that was outside of my control, and if I was hungry between meals, there was often nothing for me to eat. No wonder I then began bingeing whenever I did have access to food."

Food and Identity

Even positive feedback about eating can have an unintended harmful effect. When Maura ate "good" foods, her parents rewarded her with lots of praise. She began to attach herself to the label of "someone who eats healthy food," and she knew that a surefire way to get her parents—and society's—approval was to eat healthy. "I always tried to keep up the appearance of eating healthy, because if I was *eating* healthy then I was healthy, and if I was healthy then I was worthy."

I can relate: In high school, when I started to diet and eat what I believed was "healthier," I got a lot of praise and attention from my classmates and my teachers. Recently, when cleaning out my parents' basement, I came across a senior year biology assignment in which I had to track everything I ate in a day and complete a nutrient analysis. Looking at this assignment now, it was clear that I was severely undereating. My "day's worth" of food was barely enough to meet half my needs. Yet right up top was a comment from my teacher, "Wow, you eat so healthy—I need to pick up some of your habits!" Throughout college, as I majored in nutrition and exercise science, my identity was closely intertwined with eating healthy and exercising like a ridiculous amount. If I wasn't able to keep up appearances, then I wasn't a "good" nutrition student.

Unfortunately, I was not alone: There is a huge body of research to support a higher rate of eating disorders and disordered eating in nutrition students compared to other non-nutrition majors. A study published in 2015 found that nutrition students had more rigid, restrictive eating patterns and a higher rate of binge-eating (which makes sense because we know that restriction leads to bingeing).[2] Another study surveyed college nutrition students from fourteen different countries and found that 77 percent felt that eating disorders were an issue among their peers.[3]

When the food you eat and the body you have becomes so intertwined with your identity, any "slip up" can send you into a downward spiral because it's not just about the food, but who you are as a person. I'll explore these shame narratives more shortly.

The Family Food Environment

Any food rules that were in place when you were a child can have a lasting impact. A common one is the "clean plate club." Perhaps you weren't allowed to leave the table until your plate was clear. ("There are starving children in other countries!") Or you had to eat all your dinner to have dessert. If you continue to have a tough time leaving food on your plate, even when you feel full, this policy from your childhood could be part of the reason. (It could also be a leftover side effect of dieting.)

The environment at mealtime also plays a role in your eating behaviors. Maybe you had several siblings, and getting enough to eat at dinner was a case of every person for themselves. "I had two older brothers, and dinners were always served family style, so it was a race to get enough food before my brothers would eat it all," Janella told me. "Even if I got the food on my plate, certain family members would eat off my plate, so it still didn't feel like enough. I used to hide food in my room under my mattress so that I would have something to eat if I didn't feel like I got enough at dinner."

You may experience similar feelings of scarcity if you grew up in a food-insecure household. If there were times when there wasn't enough to eat or you didn't know when your next meal would be coming, then you may have developed some coping mechanisms related to food. Situations like these, where food either felt scarce or actually *was* scarce, can affect how you eat—even decades later. Your childhood experiences with food and mealtimes, and the way your parents or caregivers spoke about food, shape how you learn to view food, which affects your eating behaviors and relationship to food. Take some time to explore and reflect upon what food was like in your home when you were growing up.

Reflection Questions _____

What memories come to mind for you when you think about food and childhood? Are there happy memories? Any anxieties or fears? Who prepared your food? Were there ever times when food was scarce? Was food ever used as a reward? Did your caregiver(s) ever use food to express love or comfort? Were mealtimes ever stressful? Were there rules about how much you had to eat before you could leave the table? Did you ever have a fear that other family members would finish the food before you got a chance to eat more? Did you ever feel like you needed to sneak or hide food?

Body Size Discussions

You weren't born holding the belief that fat is bad and thin is better, but, depending on the household you were raised in, you may have begun to learn that message very early. Around age two to three, children first start to develop a sense of their bodies as "this is mine." By age five to six, young girls already show a desire for thinness as they begin to internalize the messages that they hear. Whether these messages are directed toward the child specifically or just said in front of a child doesn't seem to make too much of a difference. From a young age, kids learn that certain bodies have more value than others and begin to compare their bodies to others, assigning them as "better" or "worse."

"I remember being six years old, watching my mom stand in front of the bathroom mirror and pick her body apart. She was always making critical comments about her body," Janella told me. "I look very similar to my mom—we have the exact same body type. While she never directly commented on my size, I internalized the beliefs she had about her body and directed them at myself. When I did lose weight and got praised for how 'good' I was doing, it only served to reinforce these beliefs." There is research to support this: One study found that girls whose mothers dieted and made self-critical comments had lower self-esteem, lower body satisfaction, and more disordered eating behaviors.[4]

People who grow up in households where body size is a topic of conversation are taught, directly or indirectly, that being thin is better and more valuable than being fat. Maura was always a "chubby kid," as she puts it, and she remembers watching her dad go on and off various diets for much of her childhood. When she was twelve years old, her parents put her on her first diet. That led to a twenty-five-year struggle as Maura vacillated between restricting to get her weight down and bingeing the second the diet ended. Even now, as a thirty-nine-year-old who has made peace with her body, Maura still has moments when she worries what her family will say to her. "They always made it so clear that weight gain was a bad thing, and there is still part of me that fears their judgment. Even though I know it's generally coming from a place of concern, it still feels awful."

Research studies have found that almost 40 percent of parents have encouraged their children to diet.[5] The reasons for this vary and include concerns about their child's health, worry about their child being teased, and cultural or social norms. Parents often are motivated by not wanting to see their children suffer as they did as children. Adults whose parents dieted or who were weight-shamed can pass down the consequences to their own children. Parents have been found to provide weight-related feedback to their children during adolescence, regardless of whether the child was "overweight." In fact, 34 percent of parents reported having conversations about weight with their "nonoverweight" adolescents; this is compared to 61 percent of parents with "overweight" adolescents.[6]

As Janella shared with me, "From an early age, my parents used to say to my siblings and me, 'Weight will always be a thing for our family; we have to watch it.' Everything was centered around what you ate and how much you ate and if it would make you fat. My grandmother was always evaluating and commenting on what people were eating, like 'Do you really need to eat that?'" So Janella's mom—the one who was constantly dieting and trying to lose weight—grew up with a mother who was always critical of her body and what she was eating. Janella recalls her grandmother being close to dying and still not wanting to gain weight. "Even though my mom wasn't directly critical of my body, the way that she spoke about her own body and the way that she constantly dieted trickled down to me," said Janella. "I know that she 'struggled' with her weight and just didn't want to see me do the same, but watching her diet and criticize her body set off a decades-long struggle with food and my body."

We call this *intergenerational dieting* trauma—a focus on diet and weight causes trauma in past generations that then affects how people within a family view food and their bodies. If no one in the family heals from dieting, parent's will continue passing this diet and weight focus down to further generations.[7] Even when parents are coming from a place of trying to help and protect their children, the negative side effects of intergenerational dieting trauma persist. Children and adolescents of parents who provide weight-related feedback are more likely to diet, more likely to use unhealthy behaviors to try to control their weight, engage in more binge-eating, and have a higher BMI compared to children whose parents did not provide weight-related feedback.[8] In this case, it doesn't matter what the child's weight was; regardless of whether the person had been a "normal" weight child or an "overweight" child, any weight-related feedback caused similar issues. Weight-focused talk has also been found to cause depression and low self-esteem in children. As I discussed in Chapter 3, weight-related feedback—whether from a healthcare provider or a well-meaning parent—is not a helpful motivator for behavior change, and it causes negative physical and mental side effects down the road.

Reflection Questions ——————————————

Did any of your family or caregivers restrict their food choices? Did you understand why? Was your body size discussed in relation to your food choices? What about other people's body sizes? Did a parent or caregiver ever encourage you to diet? How did your family, parents, and caregivers discuss food? Were the health impacts of food a common discussion?

Adolescence and Puberty

How do your memories around food and your body change as you age? Throughout childhood and into my early teen years, I never really thought about what I was eating. That was until high school, when puberty coincided with my decision to stop playing basketball, and I started to gain weight. The weight gain prompted me to go on my first diet, and I joined Weight Watchers with my mom. It was there that I learned about how different foods had different "points" values, and I diligently tracked what I ate in a little paper journal. This experience was my indoctrination into dieting: No longer was food just "food." It was now zero points, low points, or high points, which made the difference between a "good" weekly weigh-in or a "bad" one.

Unfortunately, I am not alone. A survey of U.S. high school students found that 60 percent of women were attempting to lose weight.[9] Meanwhile, a 2018 report from Australia found that 54 percent of fourteen- to fifteen-year-old girls said they were afraid of gaining weight, and two-thirds of them said they would be upset if they gained 2 to 4 pounds.[10]

Although I didn't know it at the time, most people will naturally gain 40 to 50 pounds during puberty as their body prepares for menstruation.[11] Seriously, where was that statistic when we were teenagers?! Healthcare providers and parents need to do a much better job communicating that weight gain is both normal and expected during adolescence. If teenagers are worried about gaining 2 to 4 pounds, then they have no idea what their bodies are supposed to do, and it is no wonder that puberty—and its associated weight gain—causes so many of them to begin dieting.

The average age that people begin menstruating is age thirteen. If you look at the CDC's weight-for-age growth charts before and after age thirteen, there is—on average—a 10-pound-per-year weight gain over the course of about four years. This is the equivalent of approximately 40 to 50 pounds of weight gain during puberty.

Reflection Questions ─────────────────────

How do your memories related to food change as you age? What about memories of your body? How do things differ between childhood, adolescence, and then into your late teens and early twenties? Recall any body-related or food-related memories at each stage of life that stand out. These memories may be positive, negative, or neutral.

Media Messages

Although your parents', caregivers', or family's relationship to food and body size have likely affected your relationship with those things, the blame for any of your disordered eating behaviors or body image struggles does not belong with them. They were a product of the same diet culture that you grew up in and likely did not know any better. So let's broaden the scope and look outside the family unit: The messages presented by the media—either directly or indirectly—continue to reinforce the idea that appearance matters and that thin is best. Just look at children's movies and fairy tales: Kids learn at an early age that princesses—and any other story protagonist—are slim and beautiful, whereas the evil villain characters—or the antagonists—tend to be portrayed as ugly or fat, like the stepsisters in *Cinderella* or Ursula in *The Little Mermaid*. Not only do young children get the message that beauty matters and that there is a beauty ideal to live up to, but they also are taught that appearance is relevant and what you get out of life depends on what you look like. The beautiful, thin princess ends up with the guy and lives happily ever after, whereas the ugly, fat character loses out.

While things have somewhat improved since I was a kid in the 1980s, even the more diverse children's shows and movies feature traditionally beautiful leads. I loved the story arc behind Disney's *Moana* (which I only agreed to watch once a friend assured me that it wasn't another "get the guy and live happily ever after" movie), and it was refreshing to see a non-white culture and characters represented in a Disney movie. However, the central character is still a slim, traditionally beautiful young woman. For many young children, Disney princesses are among their first role models outside of their parents. This becomes problematic because girls are not just being told to watch the movies or choosing to dress up like them; they are being given the idea that they need to be like them. "Disney princesses are seen as the epitome of beauty, and even as a young girl, I quickly learnt that meant I wasn't beautiful," body positivity advocate Michelle Elman told the *Independent* in 2017.[12] These messages directly or indirectly affect a little kid's idea of who they are and who they want to be. And when messages are by and large portraying a narrow, rigid idea of what is "beautiful"—and therefore acceptable, desirable, and valuable—girls are taught to fit into this ideal rather than be who they really are.

In the top family films, men outnumber women two to one and have more leading roles, supporting roles, screen time, and speaking time.[13] Women are three times more likely to be portrayed in sexually revealing clothing and veritably objectified compared to the men. Also, teen girl characters are shown in revealing clothing at higher rates (61 percent) than the women whose characters are in their twenties (44 percent). Similar themes are seen with race and ethnicity, with white characters outnumbering characters of color three to one in leading roles. In terms of body size, only 8 percent of characters are fat.[14] Plus, many of the fat characters that do exist are portrayed in a negative light. These characters are more likely to be depicted as lazy, slow, stupid, clumsy, or poorly dressed. This representation matters because the stories told in TV and movies send messages about who has value in our society and who doesn't. These messages continue to permeate the media that we consume after childhood and throughout adulthood.

Social Comparison Theory

The desire to learn about one's self through comparison to others is a universal human characteristic. It is thought that it may have come from an evolutionary need to measure one's strength against competitors, which back in the day became a matter of survival. There is even neuroscience to support this: The brain's reward center will light up not only when a person performs well but also when they perform better than other people. The tendency to compare oneself to others is not new; however, today's digital landscape and 24/7 access to media only serve to heighten it. We now have many more opportunities to compare ourselves to others than we had in the past, and we're no longer making comparisons to just a handful of people in a neighboring cave. We are now able to compare ourselves to people who we will never know or meet.

Although some comparisons can be healthy and helpful, research shows that people who compare themselves to others more frequently tend to have lower self-esteem, are more self-conscious, and have more depressive tendencies. Constant comparison also leads to negative feelings such as inadequacy, guilt, and dissatisfaction, as well as to behaviors like dieting and disordered eating.

Uniform Beauty Standards

The current media and social media landscape tend to portray just one very similar female beauty ideal: white or light-skinned, young, a thin waist and flat stomach but always voluptuous curves in the "right places" (i.e., boobs and butt), and smooth, flawless skin. We see this ideal even though 67 percent of women in the United States are size 14 or larger, more than 50 percent are aged 35 or older, and 40 percent are not white. All told, less than 5 percent of the people in this world naturally have what is on display as the "perfect body."

Social media has made unattainable beauty ideals be even more pervasive and constantly in our face. It has caused us to become accustomed to extremely rigid and uniform beauty standards. Even among people who are considered "traditionally beautiful," Photoshop and filtering apps are so pervasive that almost every image we see in the media is altered in some way. The majority of the photos you see on social media, on television, in magazines, or on billboards have been edited. The proliferation of "face tune" apps has made it so that anyone can alter their appearance with just a few clicks on the phone. On top of this, Botox, fillers, and other injectables are so common, with many celebrities and influencers starting as early as age eighteen to twenty, that even if an image *is* unaltered, a "real" woman doesn't stand a chance. Between Photoshop, Facetune, and Botox, being "beautiful" is seen as real, normal, and attainable, even if the standards that these images uphold are anything but. Yet we still hold ourselves to that standard. Although I've carefully curated who I follow on Instagram, on the rare occasion that I go down a celebrity or influencer rabbit hole, I will feel bad about myself, even though I know full well that the images have been altered. How screwed up is that?!

Even more problematic are the messages that we see in the media of how women who *don't* live up to this beauty standard are treated. Celebrities who gain weight, have cellulite, or—God forbid—step out of the house without makeup are splashed across magazine covers and media sites as their appearance is dissected and often ridiculed. This negative attention demonstrates to women that not only is their appearance and body size important but that the way they look determines how they are treated, whether they are successful, and whether they can find love. This further cements the narrative that starts seeping into our brains as kids: that you have to be thin and beautiful to find your happily ever after. The root of the problem isn't necessarily the unrealistic beauty ideals, although those are unhelpful, but the fact that a woman is continuously taught that her value is dependent on her ability to meet those ideals.

Media Influence Assessment

Grab any women's magazine, and flip through it as you answer the following questions:

- What do the majority of the people in the magazine look like? Describe them.
- Do they look like most people that you know?
- How many of the images do you think are edited in some way?
- Did you find that you were comparing yourself to these images, either consciously or subconsciously?
- How do you feel after looking at these images?

Companies and Consumerism

When I was in the fifth grade, several of the girls in my class started to develop breasts. They then had the attention of the entire grade, girls and boys alike. Meanwhile, I was still flat as a board, desperately hoping that my chest would grow. (I finally gave up on this hope the year I turned thirty and decided just to accept my tiny boobs.) I convinced my mom to let me get a training bra because so many of my friends had them, and I wanted to fit in. The fact that a training bra is even a thing is evidence of the effect that companies have on us. Before the 1950s, most young girls would wear thin camisoles or undershirts until they were able to fit into an adult bra. Companies saw an opportunity to profit: If they could create a lead up to a bra and persuade prepubescent girls and their parents that their nonexistent breasts needed support, the companies could cash in. Enter the training bra. Its popularity was helped along by doctors of the 1950s who declared that bras were needed to stop breasts from sagging and prevent stretched blood vessels and poor circulation—all of which was believed to be a problem if a woman wanted to be able to nurse children in the future (and all of which has since been disproven).[15] One of the physicians who warned that bras were needed to be able to successfully nurse future children also commented that sagging breasts were "not so attractive." A training bra was therefore supposed to help women progress toward successful motherhood *and* have a sexually appealing body. There's our oppressive, patriarchal society for you again.

Companies continue to profit from women's self-loathing and desire to fit in. The ideas that you have about all the ways your body is wrong and needs to be "fixed" did not come from within yourself. As I detailed in Chapter 1, beauty ideals were helped along and often created by companies and advertisers who make money selling a "solution" to fix women's body problems. If we didn't believe that gray hair, cellulite, or wrinkles were a problem, would we spend so much money purchasing products to try to change these things? And if we didn't believe that belly rolls or jiggly thighs were an issue, would we spend our money signing up for diet programs or buying low-calorie meals and shakes? Remember: The dieting industry makes more than $70 billion per year from selling the idea that fat is bad and our bodies need to be changed. If everyone chooses to be comfortable in their own skin, the diet industry goes out of business.

Reflection Questions

Get curious about all the things you believe about your body. Who gave you those ideas? Where did you hear those messages? Who is benefiting from all the ways you think you don't measure up? Who makes money from you feeling inadequate? Who is profiting from you believing you need to change yourself?

Socialization

All humans begin the process of socialization at birth, which varies depending on your biological sex. You are assigned a sex at birth (usually male or female, though some people are intersex) based on multiple factors including your genitals, hormones, and chromosomes. Biological or assigned sex is often used interchangeably with gender—i.e., a biological male is a boy, whereas a biological female is a girl. In reality, sex and gender are two distinct concepts. Sex is based on biology and anatomy, and gender is based upon society's expectations and standards of how biological males and biological females are "supposed" to act. Meanwhile, gender identity is how a person feels and interprets their own identity outside of societal expectations. Some people have an assigned sex and gender identity that is the same (cisgender), whereas other people have a gender identity that does not match the sex they were assigned at birth (transgender). Gender identity is a spectrum with many identities between cisgender and transgender.

Although there are biological differences between the sexes, socialization exaggerates these differences based on a person's assigned sex and assumed gender in a way that people have little to no control over. Socialization is defined as "a continuing process whereby an individual acquires a personal identity and learns the norms, values, behavior, and social skills appropriate to his or her social position."[16] This process of socialization varies greatly between the sexes and happens as a result of the people around us, including family, peers, and friends, as well as cultural and social norms and the media that perpetuates these gender norms. These people and systems influence how children are taught to behave so that they can be accepted by society.

Gender roles encompass the ways we are expected to dress, act, speak, and conduct ourselves based upon our assigned sex. For girls and women in the U.S., a much greater emphasis is placed on appearance, including the size of their bodies, how they look, and what they wear. Girls and women also internalize expectations on how they are "supposed" to act. Our culture socializes girls to be nice, kind, and nurturing. Boys and men, on the other hand, are socialized to be strong, assertive, and tough. Although these stereotypes on their own may not be harmful, they have been used across society as a tool of oppression, which becomes personally damaging on both the individual and the collective levels. Gender socialization contributes to inequalities in education, employment, income, and empowerment.

Socialization of gender roles starts at birth. One study found that parents described their newborn daughters as "less strong" and "more delicate," even though there was no difference in the infant's weight or length.[17] What starts at birth only intensifies as girls age. Little girls are more apt to receive compliments that are appearance-focused, such as, "You look so pretty," or, "Look how cute you are!" whereas boys are more likely to receive praise for their abilities, such as, "You run so fast," or, "You are so strong!"

With one glance at the selection in a children's clothing store, you can easily see the differences between assigned genders. The girls' section is typically full of racks of dresses and tights that are pink or purple, frilly, sequined, and "pretty." I've always enjoyed buying clothes for friends who have little girls because I thought it was more "fun" to pick out this type of outfit rather than the clothing in the boys' section. Although girls' clothing may be adorable and cute, they are more often than not also tight and uncomfortable. Meanwhile, most boys' clothes are built for function, with stretchy fabrics, deep pockets, and reinforced knees and elbows. Girls' clothing sends the message that a girl's function is to *look* nice; boys' clothing is made for them to *do* things.

At face value, the compliments a child receives and the clothes they wear might not seem like a problem (my niece *is* really damn cute!), but what this divide does is teach girls from a young age that the most important thing about them is how they look—especially how they look *to other people*. It teaches them that a girl's main form of currency is her appearance and that how she looks is more important than how she thinks or what she can do. Yes, girls' clothing can be cute and fun, but it also creates a standard from very early on that girls need to spend energy and time looking good while boys can just be.

Clothing also is a way in which society polices girls' bodies. From a young age, we are told to close our legs and cover ourselves up. We hear, "Don't wear that; you're sending the wrong message," or, "What will people think?" Girls are taught to be ashamed of their bodies and hide themselves lest someone think the "wrong" thing about them. These messages teach both young girls and boys that women are objects to be looked at and judged. (For more on this, check out the work of Lexie and Lindsay Kite and their nonprofit organization, Beauty Redefined, at morethanabody.org.)

Even when children aren't directly told or made to perform specific gender norms, they still implicitly learn about gender through social patterns and behaviors that they observe. For example, a friend's twin son and daughter had been raised to share toys and clothes since birth. At age two, they were given a princess dress-up outfit, and their parents allowed the son (as well as the daughter) to wear the dress whenever he wanted. Yet by age four, he refused to put on the dress, telling them it was "for girls." No one had ever directly told him that princess dresses were for girls, yet he had picked up on this gender norm quickly.

Socialization goes beyond appearance. In her now-viral TED talk, "We Should All Be Feminists," Chimamanda Ngozi Adichie states, "We teach girls to shrink themselves, to make themselves smaller. We say to girls, 'You can have ambition, but not too much. You should aim to be successful, but not too successful.'" Over and over again, girls and young women are taught—either directly or indirectly—that they can only take up so much space.

When I was growing up, I was told that I could be and do whatever I wanted. I was an outspoken, assertive kid. From early on, instead of nurturing that, my assertiveness was deemed "bossy" and was determined to be something that needed to be changed. My first grade report card told my parents that I needed to be more "agreeable." This judgment was made because girls are trained to be quiet, nice, and submissive, and when we break these gender norms, we receive feedback that we need to change. Funny, isn't it, how women who speak out and take charge are labeled "bossy," a word with a negative connotation and consequences, whereas men who do the same are labeled "assertive" and "leadership material." Although women are twice as likely to be called bossy at work, men act bossy just as often as women.[19]

Not every person internalizes these socialized gender roles, but those who do end up applying these expectations to themselves, which creates a harmful feedback loop. Little girls who internalize society's desire for women to look attractive and be nice tend to grow up to be women who shrink and silence themselves—who think not only about what they look like or what they're going to say, but what *other people* will think about how they look or what they say. They grow into women whose sense of self is tightly wound up with what their bodies look like and what others think of them. This gets in the way of absolutely everything and affects our ability to be our whole selves. It blocks us from being fully present and participating in our lives. It impacts our relationships, the jobs that we take, the salaries we make, and the world as a whole.

Gender socialization hurts boys as well. Any vulnerability or weakness is automatically shut down, which leads to a power imbalance where men feel like they have to be strong and tough, and women have to be submissive and weak. "Be a man," they're told, yet what is considered "masculine" is such a narrow definition that men end up hiding their true selves as well.

For transgender and nonbinary children and adults, who don't adhere to society's mainstream gender binary of "male" or "female," the forces of socialization are even tougher to navigate and manage. Transgender people experience much higher levels of discrimination, stigma, and oppression, which in turn affect their physical and mental health. As many as 70 to 80 percent of transgender people experience mental health problems such as depression, anxiety, and eating disorders, and more than 40 percent of transgender people have attempted suicide. Many trans and nonbinary people are subject to gender policing and harassment. This can happen because they "fail" to embody their assigned gender "correctly" *or* because others think they are not "doing" their gender identity the "right way."

Many of the socialized gender examples I shared here are most common in white, middle-class society, but these are not necessarily the norm. Gender expectations and socialization norms can vary greatly between cultures. I was raised in a white, middle-class social environment, so my lived experience reflects this. At the end of the day, each individual has had their own experience with socialization. Your experience is important because it affects how you feel, think, act, and present yourself to the world. Unlearning what you have been taught about gender—yours and other people's—will free you from the weight of society's expectations and allow you to discover who you are rather than who you think you are supposed to be.

Reflection Questions

Growing up, what were you taught about how you were "supposed to" behave, dress, or look? What toys did you play with as a kid? What messages did those toys communicate? When was the first time you realized you held a certain gender identity? Have you ever felt like you couldn't do something you wanted to do because of your gender? Write about the first time that you learned something was "for girls" or "for boys." How did that make you feel? What is the hardest part of being who you are in a society with a gender binary and without gender equality?

Exploring Shame Narratives

Chesa, a forty-three-year-old from California, grew up in a big Filipino family. "The joke was always that if you gain weight, you will always know because your family will tell you," she says. While Chesa's family never directly shamed her food choices, they were quick to point out whenever someone had gained weight. "I always worried about whether or not my mother would notice if I gained weight. If she told me I looked good, then I knew I was okay." But when her mother failed to comment on how Chesa looked, she would start to spiral. "I'd just go into a complete shame cycle," she says. "Thoughts like *I am so awful, What is my problem?* and *I'm never going to be good enough* were my constant companions."

What Chesa is describing here is shame. Shame and guilt are often lumped together, but they are distinctly different. Whereas guilt is a focus on behavior—e.g., "I did something bad"—shame is a focus on self—e.g., "I am bad." Shame is that inner dialogue that pops in to tell you that you're not good enough or pretty enough or smart enough. It's the nagging voice that, in the face of failure (real, potential, or imagined), says things like *Who do you think you are trying to do this?* or *You'll never be able to do it.* Shame is that deep-seated belief that something is wrong with you. Often shame can manifest as behaviors such as people-pleasing, perfectionism, self-blame, avoidance of certain situations or people, or shutting down.

It's important to explore and work through shame because it directly affects your ability to learn, grow, and change. Shame shuts you down, keeps you stuck, and prevents you from taking care of yourself. It's impossible to treat something well if you don't think it is worthy or good enough. Shame only serves to disconnect you from your body. But when you can start to understand your shame, see it for what it is, and figure out where it came from, you can then work through it.

The Development of Shame

Shame is the underlying feeling that something is fundamentally wrong with you and that, because of this, you don't deserve acceptance, belonging, or love. As Brené Brown, a well-known shame researcher, writes in her book *I Thought It Was Just Me,* "Women often experience shame when they are entangled in a web of layered, conflicting and competing social-community expectations. These expectations dictate: who we should be, what we should be, how we should be."[20] Shame narratives about food and our bodies develop as a result of family comments, socialization, cultural or media messages, and experiences of trauma, bullying, neglect, or abuse. What may seem like an offhand comment, when heard in the context of our fatphobic, racist, diet culture, can be something that stays with a person for years.

When Victoria was a little girl, her dad would affectionately call her "pumpkin head." "He used to say, 'You have a pumpkin head just like me!'" she recalls. "So, I thought it was a good thing." That was until Victoria was ten years old, and her aunt made an offhand comment about Victoria's round head. "I asked my aunt what she meant by that, and she said that I had a very round head and big cheeks," Victoria said. "That word 'big' stuck with me—I already knew at that time that 'big' was not a good thing. I started to question my dad's nickname for me—was it really good to be called a pumpkin head?"

Heard in the context of a fatphobic culture, "You have a big head," is no longer a neutral comment. Victoria, on the cusp of puberty, began associating the word "big" with the rest of her body. "I heard the word 'big' and immediately attached it to being fat...and I knew that fat wasn't a good thing. Everybody wanted to be the pretty girl, and the pretty girls were all rail-thin and tiny. I began to feel ashamed about my body." Victoria recounts how she proceeded to spend years sucking in her cheeks to try to make her face look skinny and dieting to try to get her body to do the same. "I wanted to be liked; I wanted to not stick out—and I believed that in order to do that, I had to be smaller."

What began as an off-the-cuff comment to a ten-year-old girl turned into a decades-long shame narrative. I see this happen often, where feelings of shame about a person's food behaviors or body size or shape turn into a story or belief about themselves and their value in the world. At some point in our lives, most of us will internalize a false belief that something is wrong with us. Often it begins, as Victoria's did, around the beginning stages of puberty. Changing bodies, coupled with the increased desire to want to fit in, and an acute awareness of how society values certain (thin) bodies over other (fat) ones, create a recipe for shame narratives to start and thrive. Many children and adolescents are directly told that they need to change their appearance to "fit in" or "be better." Others may not have been criticized directly, but if they lived in a household where adults made negative comments about fat bodies, they may have internalized the message that their body wasn't good enough as it was.

Exactly

Once you attach to this core shame story, it can be hard to let go of it. Some people may use these stories as a way to hide from or put off dealing with other emotions, blaming any perceived food or body "failures" on themselves instead. Or it could be that their shame story helps them to feel in control—if something is their fault, then maybe they can do something about it by changing themselves. Like Shanna, who for years believed that it was *her* lack of willpower that kept her from losing weight and that there was something wrong with *her* for being unable to stick to any diet. "I'm so bad at dieting—if only I didn't love ice cream so much," was a frequent refrain in her mind. She felt a lot of shame, but it also made her feel like she had control over her body and the reactions of others: If she could just have more willpower, she'd be able to "fix" herself, and therefore be accepted.

Changing your body may seem like the answer. How many times have you said some version of, "If only I could be thinner/stronger/more in shape, then I'd feel much better"? For Shanna, focusing on trying to change herself also allowed her not to have to deal with the deeper, harder-to-process feelings that she was experiencing. But the reality is that focusing on the external rather than the internal most often leads to spending life in a state of "if only." And, as many people experience, if you do get to your "if only," it is never the answer to the deeper-rooted problem or pain. Your external appearance may be different, but you still haven't healed the internal shame stories.

The Negative Effects of Shame

Shame causes us to feel disconnected, unworthy, and less capable of positive change and growth. The story becomes *This is just who I am,* which can leave you stuck and unable to connect with your authentic self or have meaningful relationships with others. As psychologist Gershen Kaufman writes, "Shame is a wound felt from the inside, dividing us both from ourselves and from one another."[21]

Shame is associated with increased rates of eating disorders, depression, anxiety, bullying, addiction, and suicide. Shame causes people to withdraw and hide, and it prevents them from being vulnerable with others. The ability to be vulnerable is the gateway to connection, both with ourselves and with others. Shame is just one more way that diet culture blocks your ability to be fully present, open, satisfied, joyful, and connected. Plus, when you have thoughts of *I don't matter,* or *I'm not good enough,* there is no space to relate to your body differently and no space for positive self-care.

When it comes to your relationship to food and your body, shame gets in the way of being able to tune in to what's really going on and blocks your ability to give your body what it needs. When Chesa came to see me, she was caught in a cycle of gaining a few pounds, which would cause immense shame and negative self-talk, and then she would seek comfort in food. She'd immediately have regret and panic, then join a weight-loss program to try to "regain control," which just made everything much worse. "I had deep-rooted feelings of shame, panic, and anxiety with eating," she explains. "It wasn't until I realized that dieting was a reaction to an underlying shame and took steps to name that shame and heal from the stories I had developed that I finally got out of this cycle." The feelings of shame led Chesa to try to "rein in" her eating and be "in control." By reacting to the shame with dieting, she was never able to bring her shame to light and explore where it came from. Dieting covered up her shame temporarily, but it never allowed her to get to the root cause, which is where the healing can begin.

Healing from Shame

Brené Brown says that for shame to survive and thrive, it needs three things: secrecy, silence, and judgment. Shame thrives in darkness; it's only when we bring it to the light that we can begin to heal it. The following steps can help you to work through your shame narratives:

1. Bring awareness to your shame.
2. Start unpacking where these stories or beliefs came from.
3. Talk about it with others.
4. Directly challenge the stories you've been telling yourself.
5. Develop a self-compassionate voice.[22]

Bring Awareness

The first step is to bring awareness to and name your shame. What is it that you feeling (or being made to feel) shame about? For example, Chesa felt ashamed every time she looked in the mirror and saw the size of her body. She also felt ashamed that she could never stick to a diet or lose weight and that she couldn't be around certain foods without bingeing on them. Her shame stories centered on the belief that she would never be good enough or pretty enough for her family or for society to accept her fully.

Start Unpacking

Once you've brought your shame narratives to light, it's time to explore where these beliefs came from. It's common to feel as though the thoughts you have about yourself are true, yet they only exist because of the experiences you've had. Your thoughts do not exist in a silo; they are molded by society and cultural influences. It's only when you step away from the assumption that everything your brain states is true and start to question when, where, and why these thoughts started that you can begin to untangle your true self from your deeply held beliefs and thought patterns. In other words, any shame you may have is something you've been *made* to feel thanks to the society and culture you live in. Consider the following questions:

- What is your first memory of feeling shame?
- What happened? How did you feel?
- When you feel shame, how do you react?
- How does shame impact your life?

Talk About It with Others

Shame flourishes in secrecy, so by opening up to people close to you and sharing your stories, you can begin to stop shame in its tracks. The key here is to open up to people who can really listen and whom you trust. When shame is met with empathy and understanding, there is no place for it to grow. The ability to hear someone else say "me too" and validate your experience takes the wind right out of shame's sails. You are not alone in this experience; every human being experiences shame. *Note: If you don't have someone in your life that can be this person for you, or even if you do, a trained therapist can be very helpful.*

Directly Challenge Your Shame Stories

Not only does shame need secrecy and darkness to flourish but it also thrives with judgment. Moving through your shame narratives requires openness and curiosity as you ask your judgment to step back. To unlearn the beliefs you hold about yourself, you need to open up to the possibility that you've been wrong about your body and that you *are* good enough, lovable enough, worthy enough as you are right now. Begin to challenge the shame stories you've been telling yourself. Are there facts to support the belief that you are not enough? Or is this something that someone has told you over time? You may *feel* like you're not enough or *feel* like you're unworthy of love, but that feeling doesn't mean that you *are* these things.

Develop a Self-Compassionate Voice

Shame does not breed growth or change. You need self-compassion to do those things. Work to develop a self-compassionate, kind voice, and start to change the narrative. When you recognize that the shame voice is popping up, call it out for what it is: something that is unhelpful and potentially harmful. Replace it with a more helpful statement, like *I am enough, I am not alone, This is part of the human experience,* or *My worth is not dependent on how I look.* I'll talk more about self-compassion in Chapter 11, but for now, remind yourself that no one is perfect and that making a mistake does not make you a bad person. Try to forgive yourself so that you can move forward.

The process of untangling your deeply held beliefs does not happen overnight. It is something that takes weeks or months to begin to understand, and you often need years to detach from it fully. But recognizing and naming your shame will enable you to start finding your way back to yourself.

The Stories You're Telling Yourself _____

Write out any beliefs about yourself that cause you to feel shame, especially concerning your body and food experiences. What are some of the go-to things that you shame yourself for? The following prompts may help:

- I feel shame because I am _____.
- I feel shame because I am not _____ enough.
- I feel shame about how _____ I am.
- I feel shame because I think that I will never _____.

Note: If you have experienced trauma or are feeling unsafe, it may not be safe to process your shame alone. Please seek out a licensed therapist to help.

Moving from Fixing to Allowing

Hopefully, you have begun to see that not only has trying to "fix" yourself not helped you to be healthier—mentally or physically—but it has also served to cause more stress, shame, and disconnection with your body and with others. It's okay if you're still nervous or scared about giving up dieting and the pursuit of weight loss. This fear makes a lot of sense: It's what you've been taught to believe through years of social and cultural messages, and it may be all you have experience doing. Giving up something that you've relied on for many years is scary. However, on the other side is something so much greater. What if you can take all that energy and put it into something that you actually *want* to do and *enjoy* doing rather than trying to live up to socially constructed ideals? Let's start that journey by learning how to sit with your thoughts, feelings, and experiences as you begin to shift from *fixing to allowing*.

PART 2

Allowing

CHAPTER 6

Cultivating Awareness and Mindfulness

Kamala, a thirty-eight-year-old marketing executive in New York City, always wanted something sweet after eating a meal. These cravings usually came in the mid-afternoon, while she was at work, and in the evening, after she'd had dinner. She had tried for years to "get a handle" on her cravings, doing everything from cutting out sugar completely to "allowing herself" a small portion each time. Diet culture had taught her that "too much" sugar (whatever that meant) was bad, and those daily desserts were not part of a "healthy diet." (See all the internalized diet mentality here?)

Most recently, Kamala had been trying to eat more mindfully in the hope that she would eat less dessert. "I allow myself to eat something sweet but make sure I am eating with no distractions, so I am fully present and able to enjoy it," she told me. Yet, more often than not, the cravings still felt overwhelming, and she would end up eating until she was uncomfortably full. Then Kamala would experience the inevitable internal boxing match where she'd verbally beat herself up for ingesting so much sugar. When Kamala came to me, she was frustrated. "I just feel like I have no control or willpower," she shared, "I know sugar isn't necessarily bad, but the need for dessert after every meal feels like a compulsion. And it can't be healthy, right?"

Kamala, like many people, dove right into mindful eating, thinking that if she could *just be more mindful* at meals, maybe she wouldn't feel so driven to eat dessert all the time. She was making a common mistake: jumping straight into attempting mindfulness around food and *using it as a dieting tool.* When mindful eating becomes a way to try to "eat less"—whether consciously or subconsciously—it then is a type of diet mentality that will keep you in the dieting cycle. That said, mindful eating can be a helpful tool in the process of healing your relationship to food. But before you apply mindfulness to food, you first must work to cultivate mindfulness skills within yourself so you can learn how to sit with your thoughts, feelings, and experiences (rather than trying to "fix" them).

What Is Mindfulness?

At its simplest, mindfulness is the act of paying attention to something on purpose. We can expand this definition and say that mindfulness is about bringing your *awareness* into the present moment, where you can *purposefully notice* your experiences in a *nonjudgmental* way.[1] Mindfulness allows you to be in the present rather than the past or the future. The present moment includes external experiences, like things that you see or hear, as well as internal experiences like your thoughts, feelings, or body sensations. Mindfulness is the process of being aware and *observing* yourself with openness, flexibility, and curiosity. Instead of getting caught up in your thoughts and intellectualizing things, you take a step back, shift your attention in a deliberate, intentional way and instead observe what is happening in that moment.

It's common to have some misconceptions about mindfulness. For example, when I first learned about mindfulness and was trying to incorporate it into my day, my thoughts would go something like this:

Okay, just focus, focus, focus, focus. Don't think of anything else.
NO, don't think about that. What are you doing? You're so bad at this.
Okay, focus, focus, focus.
Ugh, why do these thoughts keep coming up! I just want to focus.

I was used to using discipline and willpower to make myself do things, so naturally, I tried to approach mindfulness the same way. What I did not realize at the time is that mindfulness is not about *forcing* yourself to focus, and it doesn't entail trying to control or manipulate your thoughts and feelings. Mindfulness is not something that you try to do "perfectly," which means it's not something you can fail at (good news!). Rather than focusing on the *outcome* of what is going to happen, mindfulness focuses on the *process*.

For example, when Kamala was practicing mindful eating, she was doing so with the hope that the *outcome* would change (i.e., that she'd eat less sugar or dessert) instead of focusing on the *process* of making external and internal observations as she ate. As Fiona Sutherland, a non-diet dietitian and yoga teacher from Melbourne, Australia, said in a training I attended, "Mindfulness is a sense of 'being with' rather than 'doing to.'" When practicing mindfulness, you're not trying to coerce yourself to do something; instead, you're allowing yourself the space to notice and observe what is going on—whether that is externally around you or internally within your brain.

Another common misunderstanding of mindfulness is this idea that you need to stop your thoughts or make your mind blank. This is what I was trying to do when I was yelling (internally) "focus, focus, focus," and then beating myself up when thoughts would intrude. Because you're a human being with a complex brain, stopping thoughts or making your mind completely blank is pretty much impossible. Instead, it's about observing your thoughts without attaching to them. Years ago, a friend shared the analogy of imagining all your thoughts as clouds in the sky. It works like this:

Picture each thought as a cloud; try to notice the cloud but let it drift by.

Observe the cloud and be aware of it, but don't attach to it or try to jump onto it.

Just let the clouds, and the thoughts, go by one by one.

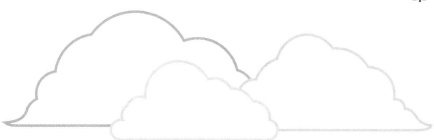

The clouds will always be there, somewhere. The goal is not to have a completely clear blue sky or for the skies to be calm all of the time. But if you can observe the cloud as just a cloud, and let it pass on by, calm skies will return.

Why Mindfulness Is Essential

Both internal events (such as thoughts, feelings, or body sensations) and external events (like visiting the doctor, trying on clothes, or seeing a magazine cover) can provoke negative or upsetting thoughts and feelings. These thoughts and feelings may cause you to try to "fix" them or numb and avoid them by engaging in harmful actions and behaviors. When it comes to healing your relationship to food and your body, mindfulness allows you to

- **Identify** the specific experiences, thoughts, and feelings that cause you to feel pain
- Allow for space to **observe** your experiences as they are happening
- Create a "pause" to **respond** to your experience rather than pushing it away (numbing and avoiding) or reacting to it (fixing)

Through the process of practicing mindfulness, you begin to build more awareness of the different internal and external cues that can cause unhelpful thoughts and feelings. Mindfulness can also help you notice the different behaviors that you engage in and be able to have a better understanding of whether they are helpful or not so helpful. Once you have that awareness, you are then able to take a "pause" to observe what is going on and then consciously choose how you are going to *respond* rather than just *react* to the cue.

Typical chain of events:

Experience > Reaction

Mindfulness chain of events:

Experience > Notice > Pause > Get Curious > Respond

For example, my client Susan had decided to try on her summer clothes from the previous year. One of her favorite pairs of pants was really tight, and she immediately had all sorts of negative thoughts and feelings bubble up. "I felt awful in that moment," she told me later. "I felt sadness, regret, and fear. My mind immediately went to, 'My body is the problem,' and 'Well, I just can't trust my body.' This spiraled into body-checking all weekend, and I stood in front of the mirror picking apart my body. I began second-guessing all the progress I had made."

In the past, an experience like this would send Susan straight toward dieting. She'd react to the uncomfortable sensation of her clothes being tight and want to "fix" it. This time around, she used her mindfulness skills, like this:

Experience: A pair of pants that feel snug.

Notice: I'm feeling really scared, sad, and upset that my pants are so tight. It's bringing up my fear of gaining weight, being judged, and not being loved.

Pause: Okay, let me just pause for a second and consider my options.

Get Curious: When I think about it, these pants have always been on the tight side and were pretty uncomfortable last year too. I think this is affecting me more than normal because I'm already on edge after spending some stressful days with my in-laws. Things have felt out of control around the house; I'm probably projecting some of that onto my body.

Respond: I have many other pairs of pants that are just as cute and are more comfortable. I'm going to toss these into the donation pile; it's okay to get rid of them. I don't want to let them spoil how good I've been feeling and all the progress I have made.

Susan didn't miraculously feel better. For the rest of the day, she still felt sad and a little low. But she allowed herself to experience these feelings and explore where they came from without trying to avoid them by fixing or by numbing. In doing so, she was able to move through the feelings. Not only did that shorten the amount of time she felt bad but she started to build her skills and resilience so that the next time she had an experience like this, it didn't affect her as much.

When you can bring your thoughts to the surface, you can identify what assumptions are behind that thought, which allows you to uncover your core beliefs. I learned a helpful technique for doing this from Brianna Campos, LPC:

$$\text{Automatic thought} \longrightarrow \text{Assumption(s)} \longrightarrow \text{Core belief(s)}$$

For example:

Automatic thought: "I can't stand my cellulite."
Why is this so bad?

Assumption(s) behind that thought: "Cellulite is gross and unattractive."
What does this say about me?

Core belief(s): "No one will find me attractive; I'm unlovable."

Another way you can break this experience down is to notice your automatic thoughts and then pause to think of some alternative thoughts that don't scapegoat your body. For instance, when a pair of pants feels tight, your first thought may be, "My body is the problem; I need to lose weight." You can then pause to come up with an alternative thought: "My body is changing, and these pants no longer fit, so I need to get new pants." Whereas the automatic thought blames or pathologizes your body, the alternative thought explores a different reality.

Both internal and external experiences or events may provoke automatic reactions. Internal events include any thoughts, feelings, emotions, or body sensations that cause you to go into a negative spiral of thoughts, feelings, or behaviors:

- **Thoughts:** Body criticisms, food police voices, comparisons to another person, shoulds and shouldn'ts
- **Feelings and emotions:** Shame, anger, anxiety, stress, sadness
- **Body sensations:** Bloating, nausea, fatigue, headaches, muscle tension, stomach pain

External events are those that originate outside of yourself, including
- Looking in the mirror
- Weighing yourself
- Trying on clothes or getting dressed
- Seeing a photo of yourself
- Reading a social media post
- Comments from another person about your appearance
- Comments from someone about what you're eating
- Conversations about diet or weight
- Subtle or not-so-subtle media messages

Mindfulness helps you recognize these internal and external experiences as a cue to pause. This pause gives you the space to notice when you are tempted to react to a negative experience by trying to "fix" your body and instead respond to the experience. This responsiveness allows you to *be with* whatever experience you're having, explore what is really going on, and respond to it rather than pushing it away or distracting yourself from it by trying to make a "fix."

When you can view your experiences as experiences—without attaching to them or avoiding them—then you can *respond* rather than *react*. This goes for experiences that may be painful or uncomfortable or unwanted, as well as those that are pleasant and enjoyable.

Separating Yourself from Your Thoughts and Beliefs

Here's something that blew my mind the first time I heard it: Just because you have a thought *does not mean that it is true.* Mind. Blown. You have thousands of thoughts every day. Some are true, and some are not true. Some of the thoughts are helpful, and some are not so helpful. Problems don't arise from the thought itself, but problems can happen because of your *reaction* to that thought—specifically from the thoughts and feelings that you have *about* that thought. When you attach or fuse yourself to a thought and view it as being true and worth listening to, the thought—and your reaction to it—can overshadow the real truth and can stand in the way of doing what is most meaningful and important. It could even cause you to partake in unhelpful and even harmful behaviors. Here's an example that came up during a client session:

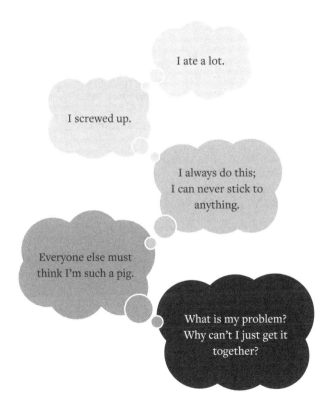

In this example, a fairly neutral thought led to a cascade of thoughts and feelings, including guilt, self-judgment, and shame. If you can instead use mindfulness, it enables you to notice your thoughts as just thoughts. They're not necessarily true or untrue but are instead either helpful or unhelpful.

When you are aware of your thoughts as they are happening and can call them out for what they are, then you can "pause" before having an automatic reaction to the thought. Over time, the more you can practice this, these unhelpful (or untrue) thoughts will no longer dominate your experience or affect your behaviors as much.

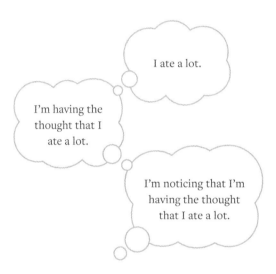

The Brain's Negativity Bias

Do you ever notice how one negative comment will stay with you for years, whereas you easily forget multiple positive comments? You can blame the brain's negativity bias. The human brain is wired to watch out for danger and promptly respond. It's designed to be able to notice danger quickly, look for similar past experiences, and build a story that imprints on your mind. Evolutionarily, this process was beneficial—humans' survival depended on how well they could notice and dodge danger. This bias toward negative thoughts and experiences remains today, even though, more often than not, it is not helpful and can cause a lot of pain and suffering.

Although you can't automatically stop your brain's tendency toward negativity, you can strengthen your mindfulness skills. The human brain adapts constantly, and research has found that mindfulness practices can actually change your brain (neuroplasticity is your friend!). That means that you can train your brain not to attach to negative thoughts automatically so that those thoughts have less effect on and influence over you. Let's look at some practical ways that you can go about retraining your brain.

Trauma-Informed Note _____

In the next section, I'm going to walk through several different ways that you can connect with your body, which can include noticing different body sensations like your breath or how your body feels.

For some people, especially those who have experienced any sort of trauma (including dieting) or those who live in a body that is oppressed in our society (such as BIPOC, fat, queer, or trans folks, or folks with a disability), noticing and feeling in the body may not feel safe.

If this is the case, please be thoughtful about practicing any of the exercises I suggest. If anything does not feel okay, such as closing your eyes, or causes any kind of anxiety, you can modify as you see fit. Stop the exercise if anything doesn't feel good or safe and consider bringing this into a therapy session with a skilled practitioner.

Four Steps to Cultivate Mindfulness

The first step to practice mindfulness is to notice and bring awareness to your experience. From there, you'll practice shifting your awareness and creating a "pause" between your experience and your reaction. Then you'll engage in curiosity as you ask some questions to dig deeper into your experience and your thoughts, feelings, and beliefs about that experience; then you'll decide how you want to respond. Let's dive in.

Step 1: Noticing

To build skills in "pausing" between your experience and your response, you first need to have an awareness of your thoughts, feelings, and beliefs. Cultivating this awareness must happen before you try to make any changes because if you aren't aware of how you speak to yourself and the specific words or phrases that you use to criticize or shame yourself, then you end up reacting instead of responding. Before you begin exploring your thoughts and feelings, try a simple mindfulness exercise to practice bringing your attention to different senses. Reminder: If any of these exercises bring up anxiety or don't feel good, you can stop.

Mindfulness Exercise: Exploring the Room _____

All you need for this exercise is somewhere to sit. Ideally, you'll be in a room or place where you can be by yourself.

1. Find a comfortable place to sit.
2. Look around you: What do you see? Name those things in your head.
3. If it feels comfortable, close your eyes. What do you hear? Name those things in your head.
4. With your eyes still closed, notice what you smell. Name those things in your head.
5. Notice your naming of the things you see, hear, and smell. For example, "I see a red water bottle" $\longrightarrow$ "I noticed that I had the thought that I saw a red water bottle."
6. Notice any thoughts or feelings that arose when you named what you could see and hear. For example, perhaps seeing the red water bottle made you think: "I haven't had much water today. I should get a glass of water after this; I'm probably getting dehydrated."

This mindfulness activity is one that you can practice doing at any time. Although it may not seem like traditional meditation, that's exactly what you are doing. Meditation is simply focusing your thoughts and attention on one particular thing. In this case, you were focusing on what you could see and hear in the space around you. The ability to connect with the present moment and notice what is going on is a skill that can be honed through practice and repetition. The more you bring your awareness to the here and now, the easier it will become.

Bringing Awareness to Your Thoughts

Now that you've had some practice bringing awareness to the space around you, it's time to shift that noticing skill to your thoughts, feelings, and body sensations. When it comes to internal and external experiences related to food and bodies, here are a few common things that may arise:

- **Rules** about how you should act, what you should eat, how you should look, and so on. *Words that may signal a rule*: always, never, right, wrong, should, shouldn't, have to, must.
- **Judgments** about your body, yourself, the food you're eating or not eating, your thoughts, your feelings, other people, and so on. These are usually negative. *Words that may signal a judgment*: best, worst, better, worse, great, terrible, disgusting, awful, deserve, not enough.
- **Past and future thoughts**, including worrying, fantasizing, blaming, predicting the worst, reliving past experiences, catastrophizing, regretting, ruminating on circular thoughts, or blaming. *Phrases that may signal a past/future thought*: if only, I can't wait until, what if X happens, I can't believe I, why did it happen, I should have.
- **Self-labeling,** including self-judgmental thoughts and limiting beliefs about who you are or what you can do. These thoughts may hold you back from doing certain things or going after certain opportunities. *Phrases that may signal self-labeling*: I am not ____ enough, I don't deserve it, I'm too _____, I can't trust myself, I'm just going to fail, why bother.

I asked Kamala to allow herself to eat dessert whenever she wanted it as she practiced noticing her thoughts. Later, she reported on her thoughts, which included

- I shouldn't be eating dessert; I already had sweets earlier today.
- I have no willpower or self-control.
- I can't believe I'm eating so much sugar.
- This is so unhealthy.

I'll come back to Kamala shortly. For now, take a few minutes to complete the Identifying Your Thoughts activity. The ability to notice your thoughts takes some practice, so don't get discouraged if it feels challenging at first. Over time, as you build the skill, it will get easier and easier to bring awareness to any thoughts you are having (and to notice when you are getting carried away by them).

Identifying Your Thoughts _____

Thinking about the common types of thoughts that I just described, write down any thoughts you have about food or your body. For example, *I shouldn't eat too many carbs* or *I look so disgusting*. Get specific, writing down the words and phrases that often go through your brain. It might help to think of a recent negative internal or external experience you had.

After you have a list of words or phrases, answer the following questions:

- How often do these thoughts pop up?
- When are they more likely or less likely to occur?
- When you have this thought, what other thoughts, feelings, emotions, judgments, or body sensations do you feel?
- Write down anything else that you notice when you have this thought.

Dropping Anchor

Sometimes, paying attention to your thoughts and feelings may feel uncomfortable and even painful. You may feel the urge to push these thoughts away; or you may feel yourself spiraling down into more and more negative thoughts and feelings, which can feel very overwhelming. When you notice this happening (again—using your awareness!), it can help to use a technique known as *dropping anchor*.

Envision your swirling thoughts, feelings, emotions, and memories like a strong storm that you are trying to sail through. It can feel overwhelming to be tossed around, unable to gain any control in the storm. Dropping anchor allows you to feel more grounded.

The purpose is not to distract from or escape your thoughts; rather it's about allowing yourself to *be with* your thoughts in the present moment. It doesn't make the storm go away, but it allows you stay steady and not get carried away by your thoughts.

Mindfulness Exercise: Dropping Anchor —

Try out this exercise whenever a thought, feeling, or experience occurs that feels overwhelming, uncomfortable, or painful.[2]

1. Notice that there is something causing discomfort, pain, or suffering.
2. Put your feet on the ground and press them hard into the floor.
3. Bring your palms together until they touch and press your fingertips together.
4. Notice and find your breath. If possible, take two or three deep breaths in through your nose, and out of your mouth.
5. Notice that there is something uncomfortable or painful that you are struggling with, and also notice how your body is in the chair.
6. Keeping your palms together and your feet on the floor, start to move your elbows and your shoulders around in small circles, then larger ones.

After dropping anchor, do you notice any difference? Are you less caught up in the storm of thoughts and feelings?

Step 2: Shifting Attention

After you notice the thoughts that you are having, it is time to insert the "pause." This is where you can bring even more awareness to how you speak to yourself, what feelings or body sensations you experience, and where your mind goes once you have that initial thought. For example, Kamala practiced taking a step back and pausing once she noticed her thoughts. "When I eat dessert or sweets, I have the thought that I have no willpower or self-control," she told me. I asked her what happens when she starts to have these thoughts, and she shared that she starts beating herself up with a lot of negative self-judgment. At this point, she doesn't even really taste what she is eating because she feels so guilty about it.

This shifting of attention from the thought that Kamala had to the act of observing her thoughts (and her reaction to the thoughts) is what allows for actual neurobiological shifts to occur. That's right: Your brain will start to change as a result of redirecting your attention. It can feel difficult in the moment, but practicing will help you to be better able to tolerate and handle discomfort.

Practice Shifting Attention _____

In Step 1, you began to notice the thoughts that pop into your brain. Now try to practice shifting the attention, creating the "pause" to allow some space between the experience you're having and your response. The next time you experience an internal or external event that prompts a negative thought, answer the following questions:

- What is (or was) your mind telling you?
- Do you notice what your mind is doing? Think of the example from earlier in this chapter: "I ate a lot." ⟶ "I'm having the thought that I ate a lot." ⟶ "I'm noticing that I'm having the thought that I ate a lot."
- What happens when you get caught up in these thoughts?
- What do you do next, or where does your mind go, after you've gotten attached to or pulled into these thoughts?
- What could you do differently the next time this thought shows up?

Step 3: Engage in Curiosity

At this point, you have noticed your thoughts and shifted attention by inserting a "pause." Within that pause, it's time to practice cultivating curiosity about your experience, thoughts, and feelings. As I shared earlier in this chapter, an initial thought often is followed by a (usually negative) judgment. If you instead engage in curiosity, you have the opportunity to approach what's going on in your mind with openness, interest, and compassion.

Curiosity means that you observe your thoughts, *pay attention* to where your mind goes, and *ask questions* to understand what is happening. What you are *not* doing is evaluating or assigning a judgment of good or bad, should or shouldn't. Instead, you're taking a step back to make space for curiosity and exploration. When engaging in curiosity, try to listen and notice. Pay attention to what you're feeling. Notice any physical sensations in your body. Get curious: Where are these feelings coming from? Why might you be feeling the way you are? What may have happened that caused these thoughts or feelings? Try to get a better understanding of where your thoughts came from and what beliefs you may hold that have led to them.

When Kamala began to ask herself questions about what was really going on in the moment, she realized that she was exhausted. "No wonder I want something sweet in the afternoon," she told me. "I'm so tired, and my body is looking for energy to get through the last few hours of my workday."

Get Curious

After you've noticed your thoughts (*I'm having the thought that... and I'm noticing that I'm having the thought that...*) and created some space to "pause," it's time to get curious. Ask yourself the following questions:

- What other thoughts, feelings, emotions, or memories arise in response to this thought?
- What do you notice in your body? Are any physical sensations occurring? If so, where?
- What thoughts are causing these feelings?
- Where did these thoughts come from?
- What beliefs or assumptions do you have that led to these thoughts?
- Where did these beliefs come from? Where did you learn them?
- How have these beliefs affected you?

Step 4: Respond

If you usually react to an experience by disconnecting and pushing it away, or by attaching to it and spiraling into negative, judgmental thoughts, this four-step mindfulness process gives you space to respond. For many of my clients, certain experiences, whether internal thoughts or external events, cause them to want to diet and/or exercise to "fix" their bodies (or cope by eating or bingeing because "eff it"). This is a *reaction*. With mindfulness, after you've taken a step back and created a "pause" to explore, you instead can decide how you want to *respond* to the experience that you're having.

At this point, Kamala had brought awareness to her thoughts, created a "pause," and realized that she was craving sweets because she was tired and wanted energy. By noticing, shifting her awareness, and engaging in curiosity, Kamala was able to shift her response. "Understanding what is going on allows me to have more compassion for myself. Sugar DOES give me an energy boost, so it makes sense that I'm craving it!" Mindfulness didn't mean that she stopped eating dessert, but it allowed her to do so without the side of guilt and shame. She could eat dessert, get an energy boost, and then move on with her afternoon feeling content and satisfied.

When responding, it is helpful to use self-compassion. We'll talk more about self-compassion in Chapter 11, but a great place to start is "What would I say to a friend right now?" or "How would I treat a friend who was in this position?" Try to respond to yourself with that same compassion. For example, when I asked Susan what she would say to a friend who had the experience of putting on a pair of pants that no longer fit, her answer was, "I'd tell them that bodies are not supposed to stay the same and that it is okay if you need to buy a different size of pants." Then these words became some of the self-compassionate self-talk she used toward herself in that moment.

As you practice responding to your experiences with self-compassion, you begin to rebuild a positive, trusting relationship with your body. Honing these skills is hard work. But with continued practice, you will start to notice more shifts and more tolerance in your ability to "sit with" your experiences, responding rather than reacting. Remember the neurobiology: When you redirect your mind, create space to explore, and engage in curiosity, you can literally begin to change your brain.

Reflection Questions ─────────────────────────

How might your life be different if these thoughts about food and your body were still there, but they didn't affect you in the same way?

What would it be like if the thoughts were still there, but you were able to move through them and not let them stop you from living your life?

───

Building Mindfulness Skills

Mindfulness is a skill, and it takes practice. It is not something to try to get "perfect" or to do "right." Remember, mindfulness is not about stopping your thoughts or emptying your mind. Rather it's about consistently noticing when your thoughts are swirling, or self-judgment is happening and then using that moment to take a pause and employ curiosity.

There are many different ways that you can build your mindfulness skills. Meditation is a "formal" way, but, in reality, "informal" mindfulness practice is available to you at any moment of the day. Similar to learning how to drive a car or play an instrument, mindfulness takes consistent practice. Let's explore some of the formal and informal ways that you can do this.

Formal Practice: Meditation

Tell me the truth: Was your first thought when I mentioned meditation something along the lines of *I'm bad at meditating*; *I've tried in the past, but I had such a hard time sitting quietly*; or *I think I'm someone who just cannot meditate*? If yes, I've said those exact words, too.

So here's the good news: *It is not about being good at meditating.* Phew, the pressure is off! Meditating is also not about quieting your mind or making your thoughts go away. Rather, it's about *noticing* thoughts and *shifting* your awareness. The simple act of noticing and shifting awareness is what builds up your mindfulness skills. In fact, if you were to make your mind go blank, your mindfulness skills would not improve because the deliberate process of shifting your attention is what creates the changes in your brain.

156

What Is Meditation?

There are many different descriptions and definitions of mediation. However, I'm sharing here the definition from Mindful.org, which encompasses several things that I believe are important on your journey of food and body peace:

> *Meditation is exploring. It's not a fixed destination... Mindfulness meditation asks us to suspend judgment and unleash our natural curiosity about the workings of the mind, approaching our experience with warmth and kindness, to ourselves and others.*[3]

Exploring. Curiosity. Suspending judgment. All things that allow you to get more in touch with *your* body and with who *you* are and what *you* want. It asks you to get curious about how your mind came to believe certain things or make certain assumptions, which allows you to get to the truth of what is important to you rather than listening to others or society: *You get to decide what is right for you.*

Meditation involves training your mind to build up your awareness skills. There are many different styles of meditation, all of which can help you connect to yourself, get to know your thoughts, lower your stress levels, improve your focus, and ultimately be kinder to yourself and others. I'm going to focus here on mindfulness meditation because it's a skill that can help you improve your relationship to food, with your body, and with yourself (and that's why you're here, right?!).

How Do I Start Meditating?

If you are new to meditation, there are many fantastic guided meditations available for beginners. A guided meditation is one in which you listen to a recording where someone walks you through the different aspects of the meditation. Even if you have some experience meditating, guided meditations can be a useful part of your meditation practice. Some of my favorite (free) guided beginner meditations include

- Headspace app: Meditation for Beginners, ten-day series
- Mindful.org: Meditation 101, three-part audio-guided series
- Calm app: 7 Days of Calm, beginner's meditation series

Meditation Techniques _____

The following are a few meditation techniques that you can use to practice meditation on your own. Find a comfortable, quiet place to sit and set a timer. If you're just beginning, it may be helpful to pick a short time frame, like five or ten minutes. (Insight Timer is a free meditation timing app that I love.) You can either close your eyes or leave them open, whichever feels best for you.

1. **Focus on your breath.** Try counting "one" for every in-breath and "two" for every out-breath. When your mind wanders (which it will), just return your focus to your breath and start counting again. Remember: it is the act of noticing and redirecting your attention that builds the skill.

2. **Do a body scan.** Starting at the top of your head and moving downward, bring your attention to each part of your body and check in: How is it feeling? What sensations do you notice? How intense are the sensations, on a scale of 1 to 10? Move down your body slowly, checking in with each part in the same way.

3. **Progressive relaxation.** Similar to the body scan, you are going to start at the top of your head. This time, when you bring your attention to each body part, try to relax it. It can sometimes help to tighten the muscle and then relax it to have a better sense of what relaxation feels like. Continue from the top of your head down to your toes. This exercise is a great one whenever you feel a lot of tension or (my favorite) as you're lying in bed trying to fall asleep.

4. **Senses meditation.** This one is similar to the "Exploring the Room" activity from earlier in this chapter. Sitting quietly, first bring your attention to what you see, trying to notice without judgment. Then bring your attention to what you can hear and then to what you can smell. Finally, bring your attention to what you can feel in your body. You can do this anywhere at any time. Try it at different moments of your day—both indoors and outdoors.

5. **Music meditation.** I'm not sure everyone would consider this type of meditation "formal," but it's quickly become one of my favorite ways to meditate. I like to think that I "discovered" this type of meditation myself, though it's certainly possible (or probable) that someone else has written about it before. In any case, here is how I like to do what I call "music meditation": Sit or lie down somewhere quiet and comfortable, then put on one of your favorite songs (I find that instrumental songs work great for this, but any song you enjoy will work). If it feels comfortable, close your eyes. Bring your attention to the music, and pick out one of the instruments or sounds that you hear. Continue to follow that specific sound as it flows through the song. If that sound ends, choose another one. Try to focus on just one aspect of the

song at a time. A few of my favorite albums to do music meditation with are Slow Meadow *Happy Occident*, Alaskan Tapes *Views from Sixteen Stories*, and Ludovico Einaudi *Seven Days Walking*. (Before you think I know a ton about music, I don't; the credit goes to my partner who introduced me to all three of these.) All of these albums are mainly instrumental and feature several different "layers" of sound, making it fun to pick different parts to pay attention to each time you listen.

Informal Practice

Although having some type of formal meditation practice helps increase your mindfulness skills, you can practice mindfulness at any moment of the day. Most recently, I've been doing an "informal" mindfulness practice several times a week as I walk through a park near my apartment. I stop underneath a different tree each time and look up. I stand there for a few minutes, taking in this new perspective. I've been walking through this park for years, but it wasn't until I started paying more attention that I really noticed the many different plants (and animals) in that park. For example, I recently noticed that several of the trees have leaves that are green on top but silver underneath. It's amazing what you can notice with a simple shift in perspective. (I credit my photographer friend Diego for teaching me to "look up.")

Here are a few other "informal" mindfulness practices you can try:

- As you walk down the street, bring your attention to what is going on around you. What do you see? What do you hear? What do you smell? What else do you notice?
- During a conversation with a friend, notice when you are planning your response in your head rather than listening fully. Bring your full attention back to what that person is saying.
- During your day, take two or three minutes to pause and check in with yourself. How are you feeling? How does your body feel? What do you notice?

Gratitude

Another type of informal mindfulness work is practicing gratitude. As I mentioned earlier, by nature, humans tend to focus on the negative and neglect to think about the positive things going on. Cultivating an intentional gratitude routine can be a helpful tool to practice pausing, shifting your awareness, gaining perspective, and counteracting the brain's inherent negativity bias. Bonus: Research has shown that reflecting on what you are grateful for each day can help you be happier and feel better about yourself.

You can practice gratitude at any moment of the day, but I find it most helpful to take a minute or two at the end (or the beginning) of each day to write down a few things for which I am grateful in that moment. Even if you think you *know* what you are grateful for, writing it down can be a powerful way to see it spelled out in print and is especially useful for the days when you are feeling down.

Gratitude Practice

Grab a blank notebook or piece of paper or jot it down in your phone. For one week, spend two minutes each night (or each morning) writing down five things that you are grateful for that day. It doesn't always have to be something deep; it can be as simple as, "I sat in the sun for five minutes at lunch today," or "I got to talk to my niece on the phone." It's okay if you're grateful for the same things each day (the latte from my local coffee shop ends up on my list several times a week). It is the conscious and intentional practice of reflecting and writing down what you're grateful for that helps.

Mindfulness in Food and Body Image Work

The constant chatter in your brain about food and your body—much of it (or all of it) informed by diet culture—can't be turned off completely. This internal programming will always be there, talking and judging. But you *can* lower the volume a bit and, in doing so, refuse to let the chatter dictate your life choices. Mindfulness allows you to become aware of your thoughts and respond to them rather than reacting by doing what they say. Plus, as I'll talk about in later chapters, you can reprogram your brain by reading and consuming diet-culture-free content (like this book!). So, although the diet culture programming may never completely go away, mindfulness allows you the space to make a decision that is more in line with what you and your body need. Mindfulness also allows you to be with your body, your thoughts, your feelings, and your experiences. It is in this "being with" and "sitting with" place that growth and change happen. In the next few chapters, you will learn how to use these mindfulness skills to connect to your body's inner wisdom, move away from dieting, and begin to heal your relationship to food.

CHAPTER 7

If Not Dieting, Then What?

It's right about now that you may be thinking, *Well, if I'm not dieting, then what do I do instead?* In this chapter, I'll introduce you to an alternative approach known as *intuitive eating*. I'll also encourage you to explore the reasons *why* healing your relationship to food and with your body is important to you—and that's something you'll return to frequently during this process. Plus, I'll share a foundational element that must happen first before you can dive into intuitive eating.

You Were Born an Intuitive Eater

Many adults struggle to feel their body's signals of hunger and fullness and decipher what those signals are trying to tell them. But this disconnect was not always present. We are all born with the instinct to know when we are hungry and how much we need to eat. It is programmed into our brains from birth; we come into the world knowing how to feel hunger and use that cue to drive us toward food and eating. Just watch any baby, and you will see this instinctive eating at play. When babies feel hungry, they will cry until fed. Once they start feeding, they will eat until full and then refuse any more. This cycle then repeats itself every few hours. Babies naturally know how to honor their hunger cues; the drive to eat is instinctive.

Humans aren't born holding judgments of what foods are "good" or "bad," what the "proper portion" is, or how much food is "too much." If you look at any toddler who has adequate access to a variety of food, you can see this at play. I witnessed this firsthand with my twin niece and nephew when they were around two years old. They loved all kinds of foods, and they loved to eat, but what and how much they ate varied greatly from day to day. Some days, even if I fed them one of their favorite foods, they'd take just a few bites before confidently proclaiming, "All done!" and hopping up to go play. Then, without fail, the next day or two, they would be bottomless pits—I couldn't feed them enough! And that makes sense because, despite what diet culture tells us, our bodies do not need the same amount of food every single day.

I could see how my niece and nephew used their internal cues to guide them in what and how much to eat. They didn't look at their plate and think, "This looks like too many carbs," or "I already had bread today, so I really shouldn't eat pasta." Instead, provided they were offered a variety of food, they ate what their bodies needed. Some days, they finished all their pasta and didn't touch their vegetables. Other days, the opposite occurred, and they'd go to town on the veggies while barely touching the pasta or pizza on the plate. They'd eat what they wanted and happily enjoy it without guilt or apology.

Research supports what I observed with the twins. Infants and young children, barring any kind of health issue and assuming adequate access to a variety of food, will innately balance their food and nutrient intake from week to week. Although their food intake will vary meal to meal, and often day to day, over the course of a week, children will eat what they need when left to their own devices (and provided with enough access to food).[1]

As we get older, outside factors begin to get in the way of this deep connection to our inner body wisdom. Any situation in which you experience food deprivation will make it difficult to listen to your natural hunger, fullness, and satisfaction cues. Whether this deprivation is caused by poverty, where there is a very real chance that you won't have enough food, a medical condition that causes trauma and disrupts your connection to your body (I'll address both these factors in more detail later in this chapter), or via diet culture, the outcome is the same. In these circumstances, food—and our relationship to it—is no longer simple and pleasurable; it becomes complicated and often problematic.

Diet culture is a big factor in deprivation for many people. As I mentioned in Chapter 4, diet culture weasels its way into our brains from a very young age. Most of my clients can recall being as young as four or five years old and having an adult limit their food because they were eating "too much" or because sugar was "bad." Well-meaning parents or caregivers may have set rules and restrictions related to food dictating what, when, and how much you were allowed to eat. You may have been taught to finish everything on your plate or learned that dessert is a reward that can only be eaten after eating vegetables (and can be taken away if you misbehave). Over time, you were taught that your body—and your appetite—can't be trusted. That *you* can't be trusted.

The chasm between your body wisdom and your brain knowledge widens until any decision about food becomes something that is made only (or mostly) using external factors. You stop honoring your feelings of hunger. Hunger and fullness become sensations that feel scary rather than safe. If food is pleasurable, it often comes with a huge helping of guilt. The innate confidence that you know what you need and can be trusted to eat it gets eroded. When you repeatedly ignore your body's inner wisdom in favor of listening to outside information, a disconnect occurs. The good news is that no matter how long you've been ignoring your intuition, that wisdom is still in you, and you can find your way back to it.

Getting Back to Intuitive Eating

You were born a natural, intuitive eater, and you can get back to this "default" mode. Although this way of eating has been around since the beginning of time, intuitive eating as a framework was created by two registered dietitians, Evelyn Tribole and Elyse Resch. The first edition of their book *Intuitive Eating* was published in 1995 (the book is now on the fourth edition). Since then, the intuitive eating framework has been extensively researched. To date, more than 125 studies have shown the benefits of intuitive eating.[2] These studies have found that intuitive eating, as measured by a validated assessment scale,[3] is associated with

- ◆ Higher self-esteem
- ◆ Better body image

- More body appreciation and acceptance
- Higher optimism and well-being
- Proactive coping skills
- More enjoyment of food
- Higher HDL ("good") cholesterol levels
- Lower rates of binge eating
- Lower triglyceride levels
- Improved blood pressure
- Lower rates of disordered eating and eating disorders

Tribole and Resch's intuitive eating framework is a non-diet, self-care approach to nutrition, health, and well-being that helps people make decisions based upon their body's inner wisdom instead of external rules or restrictions. Rather than using outside sources—such as counting calories or points, measuring portions, or following certain eating or food rules—to determine what, when, and how much to eat, you turn inward and listen to, and trust, your body's cues to guide you.

The foundation for intuitive eating is this ability to bring attention to your body and notice, feel, and understand all of the different physical sensations that arise. This skill is known as *interoceptive awareness*, and it's one of the reasons why intuitive eating can be so powerful. By connecting to your body, you can not only understand what you need food-wise but also what it is that you *truly* feel and want. Intuitive eating starts with food, but in the end, it ends up being life-changing in many ways. Trusting your body around food then transfers over to other areas of your life: you learn to trust your intuition when it comes to decision-making, boundary-setting, and all sorts of life choices; you learn to be flexible; you stop people-pleasing behaviors; you develop more awareness and overall appreciation with life.

That said, some people—such as those in low-income communities who lack access to food and other essential social services or marginalized folks who experience systemic oppression and microaggressions on a daily basis (I'll talk more about this shortly)—find that parts of intuitive eating feel inaccessible at times. Intuitive eating also can become problematic when it is applied as a rigid set of "rules" that must be followed sequentially and precisely as the book dictates. In reality, the principles of intuitive eating are just one tool that can be used in your anti-diet, anti-oppression toolbox. Certain parts of it may feel more helpful; other parts not so much. As Heather Caplan, a dietitian and the host of the RD Real Talk podcast, says in one of her podcast episodes, "Many of the principles of intuitive eating can be applicable to every human being in some way, shape, or form. However, this is only true when we see intuitive eating as a foundation. Not a set of rules that apply in the same way to the same people across the board."[4]

Intuitive Eating Versus Diet Mentality

As I outlined in Chapter 4, diet mentality involves thoughts or feelings about food that cause you to eat based on external factors. Diet mentality is rigid, is dictated by rules or restrictions, often ignores physical eating cues, and is judgmental; it's also usually accompanied by feelings of guilt or shame. Emphasis is often put on weight and body size. In contrast, intuitive eating involves listening to your body and, once you're reconnected to your body cues, using your body *and* your brain knowledge to decide what, when, and how much to eat.

Intuitive eating is

- Flexible
- Based upon internal body cues
- An emphasis on satisfaction and health
- Focused on curiosity instead of judgment
- Eating a wide variety of foods with no guilt or shame

When making decisions about what to eat, diet mentality takes the form of "What *should* I have for dinner?" or "What *can* I have for dinner?"

The same decisions, when made using your inner body awareness, can be

- "What *sounds good* to me right now?"
- "What do I *want* to have for dinner?"
- "What am I *hungry* for?"
- "What foods would *feel good* to eat?"
- "What kind of taste am I in the *mood* for?"
- "What would *satisfy* me right now?"

Intuitive eating is about *caring* for your body by eating foods that are pleasurable, satisfying, and sound good at that moment, rather than trying to *control* your body with rules or restrictions.

Intuitive Eating Compared to Mindful Eating

Before I started my training in intuitive eating, I used the terms *mindful eating* and *intuitive eating* interchangeably. Although there are some overlaps, the two concepts are different. The Center for Mindful Eating defines mindful eating as "allowing yourself to become aware of the positive and nurturing opportunities that are available through food selection and preparation by respecting your own inner wisdom" and "using all your senses in choosing to eat food that is both satisfying to you and nourishing to your body and becoming aware of physical hunger and satiety cues to guide your decisions to begin and end eating."[5]

It's evident from this definition that intuitive eating encompasses the principles of mindful eating. However, intuitive eating goes a step further by also addressing the importance of rejecting the dieting mentality, respecting your body (regardless of your weight or shape), coping with emotions, and using gentle movement and nutrition without judgment. I like to imagine the intuitive eating framework as an umbrella, and mindful eating is one spoke that helps to support the umbrella. Mindful eating—that is, paying attention to what and how you're eating—can be a helpful tool as you work toward listening to your body. As I mentioned in Chapter 5, mindfulness skills allow you to notice, pause, and explore your thoughts, feelings, and experiences. Using mindfulness skills during a meal or eating experience can be helpful.

The problem I see is that many people turn the idea of mindful eating into something black and white (binary thinking strikes again!). It becomes something that must be done "perfectly," where eating must take place with absolutely no distractions (or else it is "mindless," which is "bad"). For most people, this interpretation of mindful eating is entirely unrealistic, not to mention inflexible. This approach vilifies "mindless eating," and partaking in any type of distracted eating can set people up for feelings of guilt, shame, and failure.

Approaching mindful versus mindless eating using binary thinking leaves no room for nuance, flexibility, or exploration. For example, my client Chantal had a habit of mindlessly eating popcorn in bed every night, to the point that she would feel uncomfortably full and have difficulty sleeping. In the past, she had tried a variety of ways to "fix" the problem, including eating more mindfully, trying different foods, or attempting not to eat in bed. These solutions would work for a little bit, but inevitably her "habit" would start again. And it's no wonder: All of these attempts to "fix" were just diet mentality in disguise. Similar to Kamala in Chapter 5, Chantal was using mindful eating to try to eat less of the popcorn. Her inability to do so was causing negative self-shaming and self-judgment. "As soon as I finish the popcorn, my immediate thought is, 'What the eff is wrong with you? Why are you doing this to yourself? You know that this is why you can't lose weight,'" Chantal explained.

When Chantal came to see me, she was feeling tremendously frustrated by what she felt was a lack of willpower and inability to change. She was surprised then when I told her that I didn't want her to stop eating the popcorn. Clearly, this "mindless" eating had some benefit; otherwise, she wouldn't continue to do it. Instead of trying to "fix" the problem by eating more mindfully (which carries with it an undercurrent of diet culture), I asked Chantal to try to set aside her guilt and self-judgment and explore the parts of the eating experience that she felt were helpful.

During our conversation, Chantal recalled that popcorn was something she had associated with comfort ever since childhood. Her mother always made her popcorn whenever Chantal had a tough day. Popcorn also signified many happy times from childhood, like when her mother would take her to a baseball game. "Whenever we were able to go to a baseball game and eat popcorn, it meant all was well in the world," Chantal told me. Well, no wonder she was having such a hard time "stopping mindless eating." Not only was she operating from a place of diet mentality but also popcorn had been a powerful coping mechanism for much of Chantal's life. Plus, she realized that feeling guilty about eating immediately after finishing meant that any small amount of pleasure she may have gotten was gone right away.

Rather than try to use mindful eating to "fix" a problem, I find that it's most helpful to use mindfulness techniques to unpack, explore, and get curious about what is happening. Try not to approach it with the assumption that mindful eating will help you eat less because this will just keep you in the dieting cycle. Instead, notice, pause, and check in with yourself. In this way, mindful eating can be a useful tool to help you reconnect with your body and get back to a place of eating more intuitively.

The Ten Principles of Intuitive Eating

The intuitive eating framework, as described by Tribole and Resch, consists of ten principles that work together to help you to break out of the dieting cycle. The process involves learning to tune in to your body's physical sensations of hunger, fullness, and satisfaction as you remove any barriers that disrupt your ability to be attuned to these sensations. Intuitive eating honors both physical *and* mental health to get you back to a place where eating can again be simple, pleasurable, and satisfying.

The 10 Principles of Intuitive Eating

1. Reject the Diet Mentality
2. Honor Your Hunger
3. Make Peace with Food
4. Challenge the Food Police
5. Discover the Satisfaction Factor
6. Feel Your Fullness
7. Cope with Your Emotions with Kindness
8. Respect Your Body
9. Movement—Feel the Difference
10. Honor Your Health with Gentle Nutrition

Source: www.intuitiveeating.org

The first principle—*Reject the Diet Mentality*—is the foundation on which all the other intuitive eating principles rest. In Chapter 4, I explained how insidious diet culture is and how it causes you to internalize the unhelpful thoughts, feelings, rules, and restrictions related to food known as *diet mentality*. This principle is first for a reason: to move away from dieting, you need to be aware of how the diet mentality shows up in your life *and* the ways it undermines your connection to your body.

Rejecting the diet mentality isn't a one-and-done affair that happens overnight. It is a process you'll work on throughout your journey (and probably in some fashion for the rest of your life). Although you may have already figured out some ways diet mentality is harmful, there may be times when dieting—or gaining "control" over your eating or your body—will feel tempting. Understanding the reasons *why* you want to heal your relationship to food (and your body and yourself) will help you when the process gets tough.

Finding Your "Why"

If you're reading this book, my guess is that there is at least a small part of you that is tired of spending so much time worrying about food and your body. If this is true, connect with that part of yourself and answer these questions:

1. Why is it important to you to heal your relationship to food and your body? Write down all the things that come to mind.

2. Go back through your list and, one item at a time, put the items through the "if/then" test to get to the root of your "why." For example, if one of the whys you wrote down was, "so I'll have more confidence," you'd then ask, "If I had more confidence then what?" Do the if/then exercise at least four times for each of your original "whys" to distill your main reason(s) for doing this work.

3. Make a final list that includes all of the reasons why it's important for you to move away from dieting and make peace with food and your body. Keep this list somewhere so you can remind yourself of your "why" whenever you're going through a rough patch in this process.

Using Process Thinking

It's easy to fall into the diet mentality with intuitive eating and treat it like a set of ten "check boxes" to get through and follow to a T, but this isn't how it works. Intuitive eating is not a simple, linear process. It's not something that you work your way through step by step (as much as my perfectionist's brain would like it to be!) with "becoming an intuitive eater" as the finish line. In fact (please don't hate me for saying this), there is no finish line. There is also no "right way" to "do" intuitive eating. Although this can feel scary, I also think it is a *good* thing because if there is no arbitrary end goal, and if there is no "right way," that also means there's no wrong way and no way for you to "fail." The principles of intuitive eating are not a set of rules to follow; instead, they are a series of tools you can use to reconnect to your body signals and relearn how to eat outside the constraints of dieting.

In this way, intuitive eating is the exact opposite of dieting. While dieting or following some external plan or rules feels easy at first, it gets harder and harder to follow, and eventually, there is nothing to do but "fail." Intuitive eating is the opposite: It is harder at the beginning, but over time it gets easier and easier as you become more in tune with your body and build back trust with your body. Instead of focusing on the end goal or the destination, healing your relationship to food is about being present in the *process,* which is not a linear, neat path but a messy, back-and-forth, few-steps-forward-few-steps-back journey. Depending on where you are in your journey, certain parts of the intuitive eating process may feel more useful than others. (Though if you're inclined to start with "feel your fullness"—don't; I'll explain more in Chapter 8.)

Every eating experience is an opportunity to learn more about yourself and your body. In this way, intuitive eating is an example of the cliché, "It's a journey, not a destination." There is a lot of nuance and a ton of gray area. I'll talk about that more in later chapters, but for now, continue to remind yourself that *every eating experience is a learning experience.*

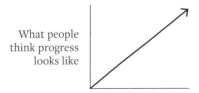
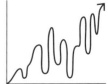

What people think progress looks like

What progress actually looks like

A Note About Weight

Intuitive eating is *not* an intentional weight-loss method. It also does not promise to lower your set point weight range. While earlier editions of *Intuitive Eating* contained some weight-centric language, the authors have shared their evolution and have since made it clear that intuitive eating is a weight-inclusive approach. Intuitive eating is fully aligned with the Health at Every Size® paradigm, meaning it does not promote *intentional* weight loss. Unfortunately, as intuitive eating becomes more mainstream, diet culture has begun to co-opt it. Calorie-tracking apps and "wellness" gurus now claim to "heal your relationship with food" and encourage you to "stop dieting," even though the methods they promote rely on external mechanisms that control what and how much you eat. And that is, in fact, dieting.

The danger in blending intuitive eating with any form of intentional weight loss or putting the emphasis on lowering or getting to your set point is that it keeps you focused on an external number. Weight, rather than your inner body signals, continues to be the measurement of how you are "doing." This external weight focus can impede your ability to listen to and trust your body cues. It sends conflicting messages that can be confusing and undermine the intuitive eating process. A client of mine discovered this firsthand when she decided to weigh herself after several weeks of an inner body focus. Before stepping on the scale, she was feeling great; she was noticing her body signals and eating foods that felt satisfying, and her guilt around food was way down. Then she got on the scale, saw a higher number than she hoped to see, and immediately started second-guessing all of her body signals.

Understandably, there may be part of you that still wants to lose weight. After all, as I've discussed in previous chapters, our society puts thin people on a pedestal. And in many ways, it *is* easier to be a thin person in our society. But actively pursuing weight loss keeps you in the dieting cycle or bouncing back and forth on the deprivation-binge pendulum. You will continue to obsess about or feel out of control with food. It will continue to take up so much brain space and time. I am a full believer in body autonomy, and you have to do what feels best for you. But if pursuing weight loss is holding you back from growth in other areas of your life, you have to ask yourself, "Is it worth it?"

Anxieties about weight and body size may pop up as you go through this process, and that's very normal. Struggling to accept your body in a white supremacist, patriarchal society is not your fault. In a culture that oppresses marginalized bodies, you've been conditioned to feel body shame. Folks in fat bodies can do all of the internal work, but at the end of the day, they still have to deal with living in a world that actively tries to oppress them. Add any other marginalized identities—Black, disabled, queer, trans—and it becomes even harder to just "accept" your body. This struggle speaks to how body image is a cultural flaw, not a character flaw.

Although fatphobic beliefs about weight or body size and worth may still be embedded in your brain, you can actively challenge and start to move away from them as you go through the intuitive eating process. Some people find it helpful to put weight on the back burner during the early stages of intuitive eating as they work to reconnect to their body cues. For others, actively challenging beliefs about weight and body size go hand in hand with learning to listen to and trust their body signals. It can be helpful (and often necessary) to revisit your "why" daily to remind yourself of the reasons you are doing this work. It is also helpful to review your history with dieting to reconfirm all of the reasons it didn't work in the past or potentially caused you harm. Go back to the foundational work around rejecting the diet mentality, revisit your "why," and remember the following:

- Weight and body size don't determine your worth as a human being.
- Your health is not dictated by your weight or where you fall on the BMI chart.
- A focus on weight and body size can prevent you from improving true physical, mental, and emotional health.
- Diet culture, and the idea that thinner is better, is a by-product of racism, classism, and sexism and serves to keep women distracted (and keep others, mainly white men, in power).

First Things First: Eating Enough

Before you dive into attempting to reconnect with your internal body cues, you must eat *enough* food to support your body. If you're not eating enough, then your hunger and fullness cues are not going to be reliable indicators of when, what, and how much your body needs.

This is especially true in people with anorexia, whose bodies are in a constant starved state, but this is also often the case in chronic dieters. A very thin body is *not* a prerequisite for anorexia, which affects people of all sizes. Even if you are at a higher weight, you could still be chronically underfeeding yourself and in a starvation state.

The longer you eat based upon external cues, harbor diet mentality, and restrict your food intake, the more your hunger and fullness cues atrophy and become harder to sense. These body signals can return, but you first need to be eating adequately and consistently.

Here's another problem with eating too little. Your brain (and your body) don't have enough energy to focus, and your brain tries to get your attention and continues to seek out food. This is your body's survival response. If it isn't getting enough nutrients, it will direct all your energy toward finding food, which is a large part of the reason why, whenever you're dieting or restricting your food intake, you find yourself thinking about food all of the time. This food obsession is one sign that you are probably not eating enough.

Other signs you need to eat more include the following:

- You get frequent cravings.
- You're often tired and irritable.
- You have large energy swings during the day.
- You're not sleeping well.
- You get full easily.
- You have a hard time knowing when you are hungry.

What Is "Enough"?

You may be thinking there's no way you need to eat more because you already "overeat" or binge. However, in my own experience with food and as I've worked with hundreds of clients, I've found that most people do not allow themselves to eat enough. Bingeing is often a sign that you are *not* getting enough food, no matter what size you are.

Diet culture has completely skewed our perception of what "enough" is—to the point that most people have no idea how much their body actually needs. Diet culture has also indoctrinated us to believe that we must make up for any instance of "overeating" by restricting our food intake, which keeps us in the binge-restrict-binge-restrict pendulum I described in Chapter 2. When I say eat "enough," I'm referring to overall calories as well as carbohydrates. These two things are what I find lacking in most people's—especially chronic dieter's—diets.

Calories

Enough calories are necessary so that your body isn't triggered into thinking that you're starving. It's only once you are eating enough calories to meet your body's needs that you can quell your body's starvation response and get out of feast or famine mode. Calories are a measure of energy, so when we talk about eating a certain number of calories, we're really talking about how much energy you're getting. When you look at it this way, restricting calories means restricting energy. Low-calorie meals and snacks are not going to provide much energy.

The majority of calories you need each day—about 70 percent—are required just to keep your organs functioning properly: your heart beating, your lungs expanding, and your gastrointestinal system digesting food. That means even if all you do is lie in bed all day long, you still require a minimum number of calories to survive.

Although I don't like to talk about calories because the numbers can often pull you out of your body (and it's your body that knows how much you need), I think it's important to note that most adult women need a minimum of 1,600 to 1,800 calories *just for their bodies to function* (this doesn't include any type of movement or activity).[6] While we're on the topic of numbers, let me note that 1,200 to 1,400 calories is the range that the *average toddler needs.* I don't think I need to tell you that adult women *are not* toddlers. Yet it is this range of numbers that I often hear women clinging to, somewhat arbitrarily, when it comes to "deciding" what they should eat each day. That 1,200- to 1,400-calorie range is also what most "meal plans" in popular magazines recommend, or the result you get when you plug your information into an app and say you want to "lose weight." If you've been trying to stick to a low level of calories like this, it's no wonder you're unable to sustain it long term: Your body needs more.

Bottom line: Calories are energy. Calories are fuel. And you need a bare minimum just to stay alive (and much more than that to thrive).

Carbohydrates

Aside from making sure you get adequate calories, you must also be eating enough carbohydrates. Carbohydrates have gotten an awful rap over the last few decades as they've been diet culture's scapegoat of choice. The fact is that carbohydrates are our bodies' best source of energy.

Carbohydrate Metabolism

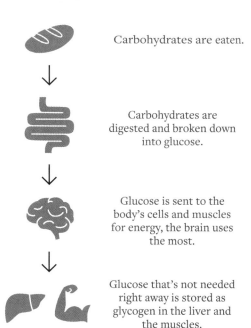

Carbohydrates are eaten.

Carbohydrates are digested and broken down into glucose.

Glucose is sent to the body's cells and muscles for energy, the brain uses the most.

Glucose that's not needed right away is stored as glycogen in the liver and the muscles.

When you eat something like bread, pasta, rice, crackers, or fruit, the carbohydrates in the food are broken down into glucose through the digestive process. Glucose then provides fuel and energy for your body. Small amounts of glucose are stored in your muscles and liver but, depending on your activity level, there is only enough to provide the energy your body needs for about three to eight hours. After that, you need to eat some type of carbohydrate to provide enough energy for your body and your brain to function. This is also why it's important to eat consistently throughout the day.

Here's another reason carbohydrates are so important: Your brain, nervous system, and red blood cells require glucose to function. In fact, your brain needs the equivalent of about 3 cups of pasta per day to function optimally.* (This is *just* your brain—not including all the rest of your body parts.) While the body can adapt somewhat and convert protein (from muscle) and stored fat into energy, these fueling mechanisms are nowhere near as efficient and can cause muscle tissue to break down. If you've ever tried to restrict carbohydrates, this inefficient conversion is why you may have felt tired, low on energy, and foggy-brained. Your brain and your body need enough carbohydrates to function properly.

---

*Based upon the Institute of Medicine's finding that 130 grams of carbohydrate per day is the amount required to provide the brain with an adequate supply of glucose.[7]

How to Eat Enough

If you aren't eating adequately and consistently throughout the day, any hunger and fullness cues that you feel may not be reliable indicators of when to eat and when to stop. Intuitive eating emphasizes flexibility, but if you aren't eating enough to begin with, it can help to have some structure.

Start with feeding your body at consistent intervals or times during the day. A general rule of thumb is to eat three meals per day, plus several snacks. Most people feel best when they eat every three to five hours. If you don't currently feel hunger cues, it may help to come up with an eating schedule, such as the following example:

- Breakfast between 8:00 and 8:30 a.m.
- Snack between 10:00 and 10:30 a.m.
- Lunch between 12:30 and 1:00 p.m.
- Snack between 3:00 and 3:30 p.m.
- Dinner between 6:30 and 7:00 p.m.
- Snack between 8:30 and 9:00 p.m.

Eating at regular intervals will help you have enough energy for your brain to function, for you to think properly, and for you to get in touch with your feelings of hunger. Meals and snacks should include plenty of carbohydrates, along with protein and fat. Although "enough" will be somewhat different for each person, a good sign that you have eaten a sufficient amount is if you can go several hours without thinking or obsessing about food. *Thinking* about food is often a sign that your body needs food and is physically hungry. I'll talk more about this shortly.

If you're unsure whether you're eating enough, or if increasing the amount of food you eat feels scary or causes you anxiety, this is a great time to meet with a weight-inclusive dietitian who specializes in disordered eating. You can visit intuitiveeating.org or HAEScommunity.org to find someone in your area.

> Note: If you are struggling with an eating disorder, or think you might be, you can find support, resources, and treatment options at www.nationaleatingdisorders.org/help-support/contact-helpline.

Are You Eating "Enough"?

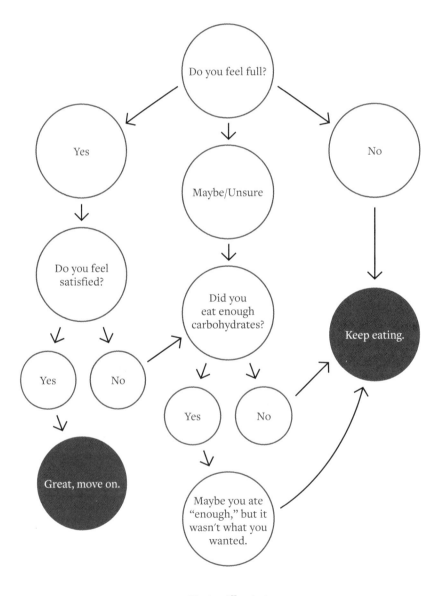

What If There Really Isn't Enough?

People living with financial instability may deal with *involuntary* food restriction. When you can't buy enough food to be able to eat until you're full, can't buy the food that sounds good to you, or have to choose between paying your rent or buying food, intuitive eating becomes much more complicated. Poverty and food insecurity can lead to disordered eating in much the same way as dieting. Being unable to buy enough food to feed yourself can set off the deprivation-binge cycle. If your body feels restricted and deprived, even if the restriction is not self-imposed, then it makes sense that when more food is available, you may eat large quantities. It is challenging to stop at "comfortable" fullness when you don't know the next time you'll have that kind of meal. Several studies have shown that people with food insecurity have higher levels of binge-eating, restrictive eating, stress, and bulimia compared to people who never experience food insecurity.[8]

Eating exactly what you want, whenever you want, and having pleasurable eating experiences are all a function of privilege. In other words, being able to eat intuitively is a privileged experience. To be fully at peace with food, you have to have food security and know that you can access *enough* food. Maslow's Hierarchy of Needs, which I mentioned in Chapter 3, describes how our basic physiological needs have to be met before we can attend to needs at higher levels. These basic needs include a safe place to live, enough sleep, and enough food to eat. So, if you don't have reliable access to consistent, adequate amounts of food, it can be challenging to have a positive relationship to food. Dietitian Ellyn Satter also created a hierarchy called Satter's Hierarchy of Food Needs, which has "enough food" as the foundation of the pyramid, followed by acceptable food, reliable access to food, "good tasting" food, "novel" food (meaning a wide variety), and finally "instrumental" food (the level where you may take a food's nutrition into consideration) at the peak.[9]

Survival is your body's main priority. Until you have access to enough food, and a variety of foods that you like to eat, then the more nuanced parts of intuitive eating are not so helpful. But the beauty of intuitive eating is that it is not all about food and body cues, and it does allow for you to address other areas of health including chronic stress, emotions, eating to support chronic diseases or athletic performance, and more.

If you are dealing with food insecurity and still want to move away from diet culture, the resources available as of the writing of this book are unfortunately limited. The following suggestions are by no means an all-inclusive list, but they're a few considerations to keep in mind as you work to practice intuitive eating:

- Try to find ways to increase your access to consistent, reliable food so that you can *honor your hunger* as much as possible. Look into services or programs in your area that provide inexpensive, low- or no-cost foods like SNAP (Supplemental Nutrition Assistance Program), food pantries, soup kitchens, community gardens, or other local resources.
- If you're already limited in the food you can eat for financial reasons, labeling even more foods as "off-limits" due to diet mentality can cause even more stress. Some of the *reject the diet mentality* concepts that I shared in Chapter 4 can be helpful here.
- Work on thinking of food and speaking about food in more neutral terms. Although you may not be able to physically eat whatever you want, permitting yourself to eat whatever is available, without guilt, will help release some of the mental restriction that you may hold. (Read more on this later in Chapter 9.)
- When you find yourself being judgmental or self-critical, try using self-compassion. Self-judgment causes stress, which is not helpful or beneficial when you're trying to take care of yourself. I'll discuss ways to practice self-compassion in Chapter 11.
- If you find yourself frequently eating more than what feels good because you're not sure when you'll get the chance to eat again, this can be a place to pause and check in. Are you reacting to a fear of *potential* scarcity or real, legit, you-know-you-won't-be-able-to-eat-for-a-really-long-time scarcity? You have permission to eat no matter what, but this can be a great place to start getting curious and exploring.

Even if you have plenty of access to food now, if you've ever dealt with food insecurity, your body may still feel the effects. Food insecurity, or having your food restricted in any way during childhood, is a form of trauma that can cause challenges and anxiety related to food well into adulthood. If you are struggling with this, your reactions make perfect sense. Focus on continuing to show abundance with food, both physically and mentally (which I'll talk more about in Chapter 9), while exploring more of the thoughts, feelings, and emotions that arise for you related to food.

Your Brain Wants to Keep You Safe

Most people think of trauma as huge, life-changing events, such as abuse, neglect, or assault, or experiences like growing up with an alcoholic, having a parent with severe mental illness, or dealing with the death of a loved one. In reality, trauma is anything that we've lived through or experienced that remains unprocessed and unresolved. Aside from these types of "macro" traumas (sometimes referred to as "capital T trauma"), there are also many forms of "micro" traumas, which are experiences or events that may seem insignificant but are still emotionally damaging. I put the word "micro" in quotes because these experiences may have felt small at the moment they happened, but they can have life-changing consequences. The effects of these "micro" traumas can accumulate over time and can have profound effects on your relationship to food, your body, and your physical and mental health.

These "micro" traumas can include periods when your emotional needs were not being met; when you felt disconnected in some way from a partner, loved one, or group; or when someone close to you suddenly abandoned you (the dating term *ghosting* comes to mind). If you were unable to depend on your parents or caregivers, were not allowed to express your emotions, or were frequently belittled, bullied, or shamed, you experienced trauma.

Another common type of trauma involves *microaggressions*, which are frequently experienced by people who hold marginalized identities. Microaggressions come in the form of subtle comments, questions, insults, behaviors, or put-downs that demonstrate bias based upon race, ethnicity, body size, gender, socioeconomic status, or ability. Often the person making the comment has no idea that they're doing something harmful, which makes it slightly different than *overt* racism, sexism, homophobia, classism, or ableism (all of which can be a form of trauma, too).

Here are some examples of microaggressions:

- Commenting on how fit someone is "for a fat person"
- Telling a Black person that they sound "so educated"
- Going to the doctor and being told to lose weight, even if what you're there for has nothing to do with your body size
- Assuming a person's sexuality based upon their gender presentation and appearance

- Assuming that a fat person eats "unhealthy" and doesn't exercise just because of their body size
- Receiving looks of pity or disgust when a person mentions they live in the "poor" part of town
- Commenting to someone with a disability that you could "never deal with that"
- Misgendering someone by using incorrect pronouns or not intervening when you hear someone being misgendered
- A doctor being surprised that a person's labs and blood pressure are normal "because their BMI is so high"
- Assuming someone with a disability "suffers" or resents their experience
- Being complimented on losing weight and then being ignored when your body gets bigger

Dieting is also a form of trauma. Chronically restricting your food intake, ignoring your body's hunger signals, and feeling deprived can set off a trauma response in your body. In the aftermath of dieting, many people experience serious mental or physical consequences (or both) even if they are no longer restricting. For example, many of the people I work with describe feeling anxious around food, being overcome with cravings, feeling worried about what others think of what they're eating or how their body looks, and living in terror of holidays or social events where they'll be around large varieties of food.

Dieting may also occur in *response* to a trauma, such as being told your body is too big, wrong, not okay, or a problem that needs to be solved. Engaging in dieting, as I described in Chapter 1, can be a form of coping from trauma and may serve to distract from the deeper wounds this trauma has caused.

No matter what kind of trauma you've experienced, if you don't fully work through that trauma, it will likely continue to affect your experience with your food, your body, and yourself.

Trauma Affects Your Brain and Body

Research has found that trauma causes physiological changes in both your brain and your body. Our brains are designed to keep us safe in part by identifying and reacting to any perceived threat. After experiencing a trauma, whether "macro" or "micro," your brain becomes hypervigilant to threats and develops tools to help you feel safe. These tools may help in the moment, but over time, they can come at the expense of being present in your body and day-to-day life.

When your brain perceives danger, real or not, your body will automatically react with one of four responses: fight, flight, freeze, or fawn. Although we all react to stress or danger in this way, people who've experienced any type of trauma often overuse one or more of these responses (not necessarily consciously or purposefully) to the point it disconnects them from their experiences.

For example, many of my clients' fawn responses show up in the form of people-pleasing, frequent apologizing (regardless of whether something is their fault), or seeking and relying on external validation. They often struggle to set boundaries and revert to telling people what they want to hear and putting others' needs before their own. Although this behavior may come across as being nice or considerate, in truth, it is a learned behavior that they are (usually subconsciously) using to feel safe, and they've often developed it in response to some large or small trauma.

While the trauma may have occurred years in the past, your brain and body have encoded that trauma and continue to remain on high alert for any perceived danger. When it comes to your relationship to food, past traumas (including dieting) can cause a significant disconnect between you and your body to the point where it may not feel safe to be "in" your body.

How to Break the Cycle

Start by identifying any unhelpful patterns, coping tools, or behaviors that you find yourself using, including behaviors or tools that you use to avoid, numb, or distract yourself from uncomfortable feelings or experiences. Notice these patterns and think about where they may have started. To address food experiences and body experiences, it may help to return to the reflection questions in Chapter 5.

Exploring Coping Responses ————————————————

What patterns do you notice in how you respond to stressful situations? Where may these coping tools have originated? How may they have been helpful in the past? Are they still helpful today? If not, how are these responses causing a disconnect between you and your body?

———————————————————————————————

Healing from trauma of any kind requires unpacking and processing your past experiences. If you've experienced any type of major or complex trauma, working with a trauma-informed therapist can help you shift your deeply ingrained brain and body response. For "micro" traumas, a trained therapist or dietitian can also help explore your experiences and how they may be affecting your relationship to food and your body. You may also try other coping tools, like journaling or talking with a trusted friend. In Chapter 10, I share some other practical ways in which you can start building a set of helpful coping skills. No matter what, be patient with yourself: healing from any form of trauma takes time, experimentation, and practice.

———————————————————————————————

To find a professional in your area who specializes in trauma-informed therapy, visit https://www.psychologytoday.com/us/therapists/trauma-and-ptsd.

———————————————————————————————

Reconnecting with Yourself

Dieting, like any other form of trauma, causes you to become disconnected from your body. The more you listen to external voices or messages telling you what, when, and how to eat, the tougher it becomes to connect with your body cues. In Chapter 5, I explained how to use mindfulness to bring awareness to and start to explore your thoughts and feelings. In the next chapter, I'll be sharing how you can use those same skills to become more attuned to your body sensations and reconnect with your inner wisdom.

CHAPTER 8

How to Honor Your Inner Wisdom

After many years of dieting or ignoring your internal body cues in favor of external rules, restrictions, "shoulds" or "shouldn'ts," the idea of listening to what your body is telling you may seem challenging. Many of the people I work with tell me that they have no idea what "slight" hunger feels like; they typically only notice the more extreme "starving" forms of hunger. Others say that they never really feel full or satisfied (which, as I'll talk about shortly, is very different from fullness). Other folks find that they do feel their hunger and fullness cues but have trouble honoring them.

Not only does diet culture disconnect you from your body cues but it also teaches you that your body is not to be trusted. "But if I don't have any rules, I'll just eat donuts and cookies all day" is a common concern. If you think that, you're not alone. But trust me when I tell you this: The reason that you are craving donuts and cookies so much *is because diet culture has told you that you can't have them*. Remember what I shared in Chapter 2: Any form of restriction will end up triggering *more* eating. So diet culture gets to have its cake and (metaphorically) eat it, too. By teaching you that you can't trust your body, diet culture causes you to feel *more* out of control, which means you're more likely to turn back to diet culture to help "fix" your "problem." In reality, it was diet culture that was at fault all along—*not you*—and something cannot be both the poison *and* the antidote. So it's time to start moving away from external constraints and turn inward to connect with your body's inner wisdom.

You were born with the innate ability to trust your body. Your body intuitively *knows* what it is that you need. Although that trust may have been eroded through years of ignoring your body's wants and needs, you can rebuild it. Body trust is established by fostering a sense of reliability, consistency, and connection with your body. (The Body Trust® paradigm was developed by and is a registered trademark of Dana Sturtevant, a dietitian, and Hilary Kinavey, a licensed professional counselor, through their company Be Nourished.[1]) You are in a relationship with your body, and trust with your body is fostered the same way you foster external relationships with other people. In those relationships, you may build trust with another person by showing up, being supportive and kind, being a person they can rely on, and being responsive to what they share with you. It's just like that with your body—a two-way street where your body is sending you information and you are interpreting and honoring that information. In practice, body trust includes the following aspects:

- Becoming in-tune with your body's subtle and not-so-subtle cues
- Honoring your hunger by consistently eating enough
- Eating satisfying foods
- Giving yourself unconditional permission to eat
- Allowing yourself to feel pleasure from food, without a side of guilt
- Respecting and taking care of your body

In this chapter, I'll share how to begin to reconnect with your body cues, including feelings of hunger, fullness, and satisfaction. I'll cover the other pieces of regenerating trust in your body signals, including unconditional permission to eat, lessening guilt, and respecting your body, in the next few chapters.

Hunger Is a Biological Cue

For something necessary for life, hunger gets a pretty bad rap. When's the last time you heard someone say, "I'm so excited that I feel hungry"? It's much more likely that you heard, or thought to yourself, "Ugh, I can't believe I'm hungry again." Hunger is often believed to be something to be feared or suppressed. Magazine articles, diet plans, and entire books are dedicated to how to "control" hunger. In reality, hunger is a life-giving, and lifesaving, interoceptive cue from your body. *Interoception* is the ability to feel your body's physical sensations, including those of hunger, satiety, thirst, or temperature. Being able to notice and feel these physical sensations and body cues is necessary for survival.

Let's compare hunger to another interoceptive body cue: the urge to pee. When's the last time you had to pee and thought to yourself, "Damn, I just peed an hour ago. I shouldn't have to pee again." Or, "My next pee-break is in two hours. I can wait until then to pee." Or imagine that instead of simply peeing, you try to chew gum or do something to distract yourself from the urge to urinate. Sounds ridiculous, right? Yet we do this to ourselves with feelings of hunger all of the time. I can't tell you how often I hear people say, "I got hungry this morning, but I had already had breakfast, so I just waited until lunch to eat," or "I was starving by 5:00 p.m., but dinner was at 7:00, so I just waited."

Feeling hungry—just like feeling the urge to urinate—is a normal, lifesaving biological cue. Think of these biological cues as a sign that your body is speaking to you and asking you to listen and take care of it. Just as you respond to other signals your body gives you (like going to the bathroom when you need to pee), you need to respond to hunger in the same way: by eating. If you ignore your hunger cues, your body responds with increasing signals to try to get you to eat. Your mouth salivates. Your stomach growls. Your brain can think of nothing but food.

Learning to feel, trust, and *honor* your hunger cues is a foundational part of the intuitive eating journey and will help you to improve your interoceptive awareness. Studies have found that people who practice intuitive eating have better interoceptive awareness skills,[2] which makes sense given that the foundational elements of intuitive eating—honoring your hunger, respecting your fullness, discovering the satisfaction factor—all require the ability to feel the body's physical sensations.

As you build (or rebuild) your interoceptive skills and are more aware of what is going on in your body, you will begin to rebuild body trust. On the other hand, if you aren't eating when you're hungry (whether you're trying not to eat "too much," you're too busy, or you just aren't paying attention to body cues) then a disconnect occurs, and your body starts to distrust you. Your body needs to know that it will consistently have access to food. Otherwise, your body is biologically wired to respond to any deprivation (real or mental) with cravings and binges.

Your body has a complex system, regulated by hormones, that gauges your energy (i.e., calorie) needs and signals you to eat to maintain homeostasis (and keep you alive). Your body's energy needs vary greatly from day to day and are affected by variables such as stress, activity level, amount of sleep, menstrual cycles, and your meals and snacks both that day as well as several days prior. In other words, your body doesn't need the same number of calories every day. Some days you'll need more, and some days you'll need less. If you're tuned in to your hunger cues, you'll notice that your hunger levels will *also* vary greatly from day to day. One of the first things I noticed when I started tuning back into my body was that one week of the month my appetite was much higher than "normal." Then I realized that I also had about one week a month in which my appetite was lower than "normal." This fluctuation is very common in folks who menstruate because our hormone levels fluctuate throughout the month and can greatly affect our energy needs (and thereby our feelings of hunger).

Earlier in the book, I mentioned that babies and small children naturally balance out their calorie and nutrient intake from week to week (assuming they're provided with enough food), and we adults can do that, too. We just need two things: enough access to food (which I spoke about in Chapter 7) and the ability to recognize—and honor—our body's feelings of hunger.

Reconnecting with Hunger

Hunger can be felt and experienced in a variety of ways. It is a subjective feeling and can differ from person to person. Contrary to popular belief, hunger is not only felt in the stomach. For some people, a growling stomach is one of the last signs of hunger they feel, which comes on only at the point at which they are completely ravenous (and ideally you are able to eat before it gets to that point). Here are some ways in which you may sense hunger:

- **Energy:** Tired, low-energy, sluggish
- **Head:** Trouble concentrating, headache, dizzy, unable to focus, feeling light-headed
- **Mood:** Irritable, on edge, cranky (the classic "hanger"), uninterested
- **Stomach:** Growling or rumbling, slight pain (i.e., a hunger "pang"), empty feeling, a gnawing feeling

One tool that can be helpful to practice getting in tune with your hunger cues is the hunger-fullness scale, which rates your level of hunger on a scale from 1 to 10. A 5 is neutral—when you are not necessarily hungry, but you're also not full. Working down the scale, a 4 indicates the early feelings of hunger; you could eat and are even ready to eat, but you don't feel a lot of urgency. Next is a 3, which is when you feel very hungry and are looking forward to eating; you feel some urgency at this point. A step below that is 2, which is where you may begin to feel irritable, have a headache, and feel ravenous. At the low end of the scale you have 1, which is a painful, primal feeling of hunger. At this level, you may feel dizzy, shaky, or nauseated because you are so hungry.

Hunger-Fullness Scale[3]

1 Painfully hungry—Dizzy, nauseous, physically ill.

2 Extremely hungry—Ravenous, gnawing emptiness in stomach, headache, moody, anxious to eat.

3 Very Hungry—Stomach growling, low energy, some urgency.

4 Hungry—Ready to eat, stomach slightly empty feeling, not much urgency.

5 Neutral—Neither hungry nor full

6 Mild fullness—Feeling some early sensations of fullness, but can still eat and not yet satisfied.

7 Comfortably full—Feeling content and satisfied.

8 A little too full—Slightly uncomfortable

9 Very full—Really uncomfortable, feel stuffed, may have some belly distention.

10 Painfully full—Physically ill, may feel sick or nauseous.

These numbers, as I've just described them, may not best suit your experience or sensations of hunger. For example, one of my clients starts to get a headache as an early sign of hunger, which puts her around a 4 on the scale. Another client never experiences an "empty" or growling stomach feeling, even when she's at a 1 or 2. As you practice tuning in to your body and bringing awareness to your hunger cues, it may be helpful to personalize the hunger-fullness scale based on your hunger cues. Make note of what feelings and sensations seem to correlate with the ravenous/starving low end of the scale and which ones seem to signal earlier signs of hunger.

As I shared in the previous chapter, if you have been chronically dieting, restricting, or are in recovery from an eating disorder, it may be too soon to start using the hunger scale. The priority for you, as discussed in Chapter 7, is to eat consistent meals and be eating enough calories and carbohydrates.

For most people, eating experiences feel best when eating occurs somewhere between a 3 and 4 on the scale. While this may not always be possible, eating before you hit that extreme or painful hunger point has several benefits. For one, eating soon after your first signs of hunger helps to build back trust with your body. Remember, hunger is a biological signal, and the more you ignore it or try to push through without eating, the more your body distrusts that you are going to feed it when it cues you to. Ignoring hunger, or frequently waiting until you are ravenous before eating, can cause increased cravings and increased hunger cues. Your body doesn't know whether you are going to feed it, and to do its job to keep you alive, it compensates by sending more and more signals to get you to eat.

Waiting to eat until you are extremely hungry can feel really uncomfortable. You may feel so much urgency to eat at that point that your eating habits become more quick and chaotic, which is typically not a satisfying way to eat. Not only are you more apt to eat until you feel uncomfortably full, but you may also experience bloating, gas, and indigestion. A cycle I frequently see is a person waiting much too long to eat, then when they finally do sit down to have something, they eat quickly and end up at the "very full" end of the hunger-fullness scale. This overly stuffed feeling causes them to feel guilty, and they vow not to eat so much next time. This person's thought of, "I won't overeat this time," is interpreted by their body as, "Starvation is coming; better increase signals to make sure they eat enough to stay alive." By ignoring their hunger cues, or just not being aware of the more subtle signs of hunger, and by having guilty or food police–type thoughts, this person stays stuck in the diet cycle. If you are someone who rarely feels hunger until you hit a 2, or even 1, on the scale and feel "totally ravenous," then it can help to practice noticing the earlier, sometimes more subtle sensations of hunger.

When you honor your inner wisdom, you are *present-focused*. You are noticing and becoming more attuned to how your body feels *in that moment* and honoring that feeling. If you find yourself saving up for meals or choosing (or avoiding) certain foods based on what you might eat later, you are *future-focused*. It is impossible to know what your body will need later on or how you will feel when you get there. When you base *current* eating decisions on what you think *might* happen in the future, it will prevent you from being able to reconnect with your body cues fully. Bring yourself back into the present moment, check in with your body, and challenge yourself to honor your body's desires.

If using the 1 to 10 hunger-fullness scale feels overwhelming, or you notice that it triggers any diet mentality thoughts, simply start by identifying whether your stomach feels comfortable, uncomfortable, or neutral. If you try to use the scale, remember you're not striving for perfection (repeat to yourself: find the gray area). Sometimes you don't know what your body is feeling, and that is okay! Just the simple act of tuning in to see if it feels comfortable or not is often enough.

Practice Tuning in to Hunger Cues _____

For the next few days, try using your mindfulness skills to bring attention to your body before meals and snacks. Reflect on the following questions:

- How do you feel hunger during the day?
- Where in your body do you feel the sensations of hunger?
- What do the different levels of hunger feel like?
- How does it feel in your body when you are really hungry?
- Are you able to notice any of the more subtle, earlier signs of hunger?
- Were there times when you felt hungry, but didn't eat? Why?

You may have noticed that I've introduced the hunger-fullness scale, but I haven't brought up anything related to fullness. *I'm doing this intentionally.* You may be tempted to jump ahead to the fullness piece because you think that honoring your hunger cues isn't your issue and stopping when full is. (I hear this all the time.) Trust me when I say, "Wait." If you are not honoring every hunger signal (by eating), then you're going to find it next to impossible to stop when you feel full, which is why honoring your hunger needs to come *before* feeling your fullness. Otherwise, and I say this with love and compassion, you'll just be turning intuitive eating into a diet.

It Is Not the "Hunger-Fullness Diet"

If you've been in the habit of following rules for how you deal with food, your brain will likely try to turn intuitive eating into a diet. The "Hunger-Fullness Diet" happens when people turn hunger and fullness into rules to follow. Here are some examples:

- Only allowing yourself to eat when you are physically hungry and berating yourself if you eat something in the absence of physical signs of hunger. "I can't believe I ate that cupcake. I wasn't even hungry."

- Trying so hard to stop eating when you feel "comfortably full" and feeling guilty if you eat past that point. "I totally messed up. I knew I felt full at dinner but then I kept on eating."
- Attempting to "do" intuitive eating "right"—and worrying that you're not.

Diet culture teaches us that we can't trust ourselves and that we must follow external rules to stay "in control," so it makes sense if your brain attempts to do the same with hunger and fullness. If you are still in a part of your journey where you do not trust your body, it's common to latch onto rules like "only eat when hungry" and "stop when you feel full."

However, this is diet mentality talking. Intuitive eating is not all or nothing, and it's not black and white; it's about finding the gray. When you refer to yourself as "good" for eating one way and "bad" for eating another, this is black-and-white diet-mentality thinking. If you find yourself feeling like you "screwed up," you're using all-or-nothing diet-mentality thinking, which will inevitably trigger bingeing and cause you to feel out of control around food.

Intuitive eating does not say that you can eat *only* when you are hungry because that type of guideline would require applying rigid, diet-mentality thinking. It's okay to eat when you're not physically hungry because more than one type of hunger exists. (I'll talk more about that in the next section.) For example, when a restaurant brings out dessert menus, I'm rarely still *physically* hungry. But if something on the menu looks good or sounds good, or I'm just in the mood for dessert, I will order it (and eat it). This is one form of intuitive eating.

Likewise, intuitive eating does not mean that you *must* stop eating when you're comfortably full. That idea is also diet mentality. You can be tuned in to your body's hunger and fullness cues and still eat past the point of comfortable fullness, which is okay (and completely normal!). If you say, "I will eat only when I'm hungry, and I'll always stop when I'm full," you're setting yourself up for failure. Instead, try to notice any rigid pattern of thinking and call it out as diet mentality. Use self-compassion and remind yourself that there is no such thing as "perfect" eating. You're involved in a learning process with the goal of exploring your body's sensations and cues. Exploration, experimenting, and curiosity are the goals—not perfection.

Get Off the Hunger-Fullness Diet ————————

- Try giving yourself permission to eat when you're not hungry; then pay attention, get curious, and notice what that eating experience was like. How did your body feel before eating, and how it does it feel after? What was driving this eating?
- Try giving yourself permission to eat past the point of fullness. The next time this happens, pay attention and reflect. Did you notice when you were getting full? What thoughts were going through your head? What was this eating experience like? What might have been driving you to keep eating?

Types of Hunger

As I just shared, if you are trying to eat only when you are physically hungry, this is a form of diet mentality. Physical hunger is a type of hunger that stems from your body's need for energy (in the form of food). But there are other common, and just as valid, types of hunger that can drive eating. These other forms of hunger, as described originally in the book *Intuitive Eating*, include

- Practical hunger
- Taste hunger
- Emotional hunger

All three types of hunger are legitimate reasons to eat, but knowing which type of hunger you are feeling can help you decide what food(s) will be most satisfying in that moment. For example, I may be experiencing taste hunger for chips, but I also know that it's been several hours since breakfast, so I will probably be feeling physical hunger soon. I take that knowledge, and eat something that includes chips, along with other filling foods that satisfy my need for a meal, too.

Practical Hunger

When honoring your inner wisdom, you will use both brain and body knowledge. With practical (or planned) hunger, brain knowledge comes into play. Practical hunger can take a couple of forms:

- You know you may not be able to eat although you are physically hungry—for instance, you have a job in which you have set meal breaks (hi to all my teachers out there!) or you are going somewhere that eating isn't feasible, like a play or musical performance.
- Certain factors—like stress, anxiety, or exercise—are suppressing your hunger, so you don't feel physically hungry, but you know you need to eat.

Practical hunger may mean that you use your brain knowledge over, or in addition to, your body knowledge. For instance, your job and work schedule might mean that your only chance to eat is early in the morning before work; otherwise, you won't get anything until lunch. Although you may not feel hungry that early in the morning, you sure as heck need to eat to get through until lunch. Or say you're heading out to see an evening movie. You may not be physically hungry before you leave the house, but you know you'll be out during dinner, so you choose to eat at home ahead of time.

Stress, anxiety, and even certain types of exercise can mask hunger cues and necessitate using brain knowledge to decide when to eat. Stress activates the sympathetic nervous system as part of the fight-or-flight response, and blood is diverted away from the stomach and gastrointestinal tract. This can cause you not to feel hungry; you may even feel nauseated or have an upset stomach. But not eating, especially if it's been several hours since your last meal, will only make your body's stress response worse, so, in this case, it is smart to eat even if you are not physically hungry because it is what your body really needs.

A similar response happens in your body after exercise. One of my clients is a prime example: She often exercises in the morning before breakfast and doesn't feel at all hungry afterward. She learned that if she doesn't eat right away, she ends up nauseated and totally ravenous a couple of hours later. Although she's not always hungry immediately following her workout, she chooses to eat something anyway to stave off the hunger that she knows will come.

Note: Practical hunger that's also future-focused hunger is different from what I mentioned earlier in this chapter because it comes from a place of self-care and abundance rather than from a place of fear and restriction.

Taste Hunger

Taste hunger is just what it sounds like: eating because something sounds good, looks good, smells good, or tastes good. When I visited Paris, I experienced a lot of taste hunger (a whole week's worth in fact!). The food in Paris is, in my opinion, unmatched, especially for my favorites: bread, croissants, and cheese. During my week visiting the city, I spent my days hopping around from one boulangerie to the next. I'm pretty sure I didn't feel any physical hunger that entire time, but I sure did eat, and it was So. Good.

You may also run into taste hunger when a certain occasion calls for eating—for example, when someone is having a birthday, you want to celebrate with them, but you just had lunch and aren't that hungry. Sure, you could turn down the cake if you want, but you could also eat it with them in celebration.

Emotional Hunger

Ah, emotional hunger: perhaps the most maligned form of hunger of them all. You may have read the stories—or at least the headlines—before: "Gain Control of Emotional Eating" and "Conquer Emotional Eating." We're constantly told that emotional eating—eating to soothe, suppress, or distract from negative emotions, including stress, boredom, sadness, anger, excitement, or celebrate positive emotions like happiness—is a problem, and, we need to stop doing it to be healthy or have a good relationship to food.

But that is all plain wrong. Consider this: Eating *is* emotional. Food is not just nutrition and fuel for our bodies; it is part of our history, our culture, our families. Food is something that is meant to be enjoyed for the taste and pleasure it brings us, not for the vitamins, minerals, or fiber it provides. Cooking, baking, and eating are all ways in which we connect with others and care for ourselves and for the people we love. Emotional eating is vilified, but what's the alternative—emotionless eating?

Emotional hunger—or feeling a drive to eat due to emotions like stress, anxiety, boredom, or sadness—is a valid reason to eat. Food affects the way we feel, which means it is a totally natural thing to use as a coping mechanism. I'm not just talking about "healthy" foods here; I'm including any food that helps you to feel better. My go-to emotional eating foods are chocolate chip cookies and chocolate peanut butter cups.

If you aren't convinced that emotional eating isn't so bad, consider this: trying to stop it only makes things worse. If you feel guilty and ashamed any time you eat for reasons other than physical hunger, it can be worse for your body than the eating itself. Shame creates a stress response and causes physical side effects that can affect your digestion and sleep, increase inflammation, and more. Plus, you'll likely stay trapped in the vicious emotional eating cycle: You feel guilty and ashamed for emotional eating, so you continue to eat emotionally. Wouldn't it be better to accept emotional eating for what it is—a coping mechanism—and move on once it's served its purpose?

All that said, emotional eating *could* be a problem if eating is your only coping mechanism or you are constantly using food to numb yourself from feeling and processing your emotions. In Chapter 10, I'll share more about cultivating multiple coping skills and discuss how to use food in a way where it can actually help you to feel better.

Hunger Is a Normal Response to Restriction

After dieting or restricting, it is normal to feel an insatiable hunger once you begin eating enough. Your body is healing from restriction, and it requires a lot of energy to shift out of starvation mode. You will likely feel really hungry. Evelyn Tribole, one of the co-founders of intuitive eating, likens it to what you feel after you've held your breath. "If you hold your breath for a long time and finally take your first panicked inhale, no one calls it 'loss of control breathing' or 'binge breathing,'" she said recently in an Instagram post. "It's a natural compensatory response to air deprivation. We need that perspective for eating."[4]

It's normal to eat quickly and eat past the point of fullness if you haven't had enough to eat, just like it's normal to gulp in several huge breaths after you've been submerged under a wave. This is your body working to ensure your survival by providing you with oxygen and food. Your body is not broken, and neither are you. It may feel uncomfortable, but try to sit with that discomfort, feel it, and experience it to get to the other side. Eventually, as you continue to consistently feed your body sufficiently and use self-compassion to reduce restrictive thoughts, the discomfort will dissipate, and your hunger cues will balance out.

If You're Not Satisfied, You're Not Done

Contrary to popular belief, physical feelings of fullness are *not* what turn off our drive to eat. Satisfaction is involved, as well. *Merriam-Webster Dictionary* defines satisfaction as: "fulfillment of a need or want; a source or means of enjoyment."[5] For your body to feel truly fulfilled by a meal or snack, you have to eat something that you find satisfying and enjoyable.

There is a difference between feeling physically full and feeling satisfied. My favorite explanation of this comes from Rachael Hartley, a weight-inclusive registered dietitian in Colombia, South Carolina, and the author of *Gentle Nutrition*. She says, "Fullness is a *physical* sensation of satiety, while satisfaction is the *mental* sensation of satiety."[6] For example, if I eat a huge bowl of raw vegetables, my stomach feels physically full, but I am in no way satisfied.

If you are not satisfied with what you are eating, you will probably continue to feel the urge to keep eating, even if you are physically full. One of my clients calls this "the search." I used to experience this all the time. I'd eat dinner and feel full, but then I'd spend the next several hours going back and forth to the kitchen to graze on all sorts of foods. A little chocolate here, a handful of crackers there. This pattern would usually continue until I went to bed. I know now that this happened because I wasn't satisfied with my dinner: I was restricting, so not only was I not eating enough, but I often was not including foods that I really enjoyed. Once I stopped restricting, ate enough, and included satisfying foods at dinner, this drive to keep eating decreased.

Food is meant to provide pleasure. Yet, in much of the Western world, we are taught that we have to choose between enjoyment and health when it comes to eating. If something tastes good, then it must be bad for us. And if we're going to eat healthy, we must "give up" all of our favorite foods. Although pleasure hasn't disappeared from food, it has become closely intertwined with negative emotions like guilt, fear, shame, and judgment. We've come to see food as the enemy, which is a major problem.

Pleasure, satisfaction, and enjoyment are important components of a healthy diet. The Japanese even include "pleasure" within their dietary guidelines as one of the goals of healthy eating.[7] Research has found that when you enjoy the food that you eat, you absorb *more* nutrients. You also digest your food better and are better able to honor your body's feelings of hunger and fullness. When you don't get the pleasure that you are seeking, your brain interprets that missed experience as hunger, so you continue to eat more and more in an attempt to feel satisfied.

At the same time, negative emotions related to eating like guilt, fear, and shame have real consequences for your health and well-being. When you feel bad about what you've eaten, your body's stress response is triggered, which partially shuts down digestion and can lead to insulin spikes, fat storage, and gut issues like bloating, constipation, or diarrhea. That's right: Stress can *cause* gut issues—no matter what food you are eating. The end result is that if you're choosing foods you think you *should* eat rather than the foods you *want* to eat, you are unlikely to have a very satisfying eating experience and more apt to feel guilty, stressed, and/or experience gastrointestinal side effects from indigestion.

The Problem with "Air Foods"

Rice cakes. Plain popcorn. Celery sticks. High-fiber crackers. Raw veggies. "Healthy" ice cream. These very different foods have one thing in common: They fill your stomach but contain very few calories. I refer to these types of foods as *air foods*. They're common on diets because eating them can make you feel like you're eating a lot without consuming many calories (or as one of those "healthy" ice cream brands proclaims, "Eat until you see the bottom!"). Although eating a high volume of food with less calories may sound like a good thing, it's really not.

As I've mentioned, feeling full is not the same thing as being satisfied. The foods I mentioned above do a great job at physically filling up and stretching our stomachs. You can only eat so many broccoli florets or high-fiber crackers before you feel full (or get constipated). But while these foods may take care of the *physical* part of satiety, they are severely lacking when it comes to the *mental* aspect of satiety.

Take that "healthy" ice cream. Does it taste as good as real ice cream? What about the texture or the mouth feel? You can eat a whole pint of it for fewer calories than real ice cream, but if the flavor or the texture isn't satisfying, then you'll eventually end up wanting more food (or real ice cream). This is definitely what happens to me: I've tried half a dozen varieties of "healthy" ice creams, and they are never satisfying. I can eat and eat and eat them without ever getting that satiated feeling. Hand me a pint of Talenti gelato, though, and I can eat some, feel completely satisfied, and move on (especially if it's the Sea Salt Caramel flavor). Sure, there are nights where I still eat most of a pint, but the difference is that a) I feel fully satiated after eating and b) eating the entire pint occurs less frequently because the gelato tastes so much better compared to the "healthified" stuff (and because I keep it in my house all the time—more on that soon).

The other problem with these "air foods" is that you are—in essence—trying to trick your body into eating less, which never works in the long run. Your body is smart, and trying to manipulate yourself into eating less than your body needs will only set off the restriction-binge cycle. Take, for example, the common nutrition advice to "eat your salad or vegetable first." As one client of mine shared, "I've always had this rule that I need to eat my vegetable first. But then I watched my daughter eat, and realized that she always eats the part of her meal that she likes first." So this woman decided to follow her daughter's lead. She discovered that when she did so, she felt way more satisfied with the meal—in part because physically filling your stomach is only one part of your body's appetite regulation equation.

What Makes a Satisfying Meal?

If you're like many of my clients, you may have no idea where to start when it comes to finding foods that are satisfying to you. Or you may be noticing that the first foods that come to mind are things like sweets or carbs (have you been keeping those foods off-limits?). It's normal to have a hard time figuring out what foods are most satisfying. It takes a lot of experimentation and a big dose of self-compassion. With some practice, though, you can start to figure out what foods give you the most pleasure and enjoyment.

In general, a satisfying meal includes several components:

- A mix of carbohydrates, fat, and protein
- A food (or foods) that you enjoy
- Your food environment

A Mix of Macronutrients

Although carbohydrates, fat, and protein may be filling or satisfying individually, when you eat them together, you get more bang for your buck. These three macronutrients work in different ways to help signal fullness. Carbohydrates raise your blood sugar, which causes the release of hormones such as insulin, amylin, and GLP-1, all of which signal your body to stop eating. Protein and fat trigger the release of other hormones, like cholecystokinin or CCK, which triggers satiety in your brain.

Common Sources of Carbohydrate, Protein, and Fat

Carbohydrate	Protein	Fat
Grains such as bread, cereal, crackers, oatmeal, pasta, rice	Chicken and turkey	Animal fats, including fat in butter, cheese, dairy products, eggs, and meats
Fruit	Dairy products such as cheese, cottage cheese, milk, and yogurt	Avocado
Starchy vegetables like corn, potatoes, and yucca	Eggs	Condiments such as mayo and salad dressing
Milk and yogurt	Fish	Nuts and seeds (including nut or seed butter)
	Meats	Oils such as avocado, algae, canola, coconut, olive, peanut, and sesame
	Nuts and seeds (including nut or seed butter)	Olives
	Pulses such as beans, chickpeas, dried peas, and lentils	
	Soy products such as edamame, tempeh, and tofu	

Although there will certainly be instances where you eat a meal with one or two of these macronutrients and still feel satisfied, a general rule of thumb is that all three make a more satisfying—and filling—meal. When you're picking something to eat, verify whether it has some type of carbohydrate, protein, and fat. One of my clients often had a salad for lunch, but her diet mentality meant that it usually fell short in fat and carbohydrate. She decided to add a big scoop of cooked grains and bump up the fat by adding avocado and mixing in more dressing. When she did so, she ended up being much more satisfied and full after she ate. Another client was skipping carbs at most meals, so she added them and found she was much more satisfied (and didn't graze as much at night).

Foods You Enjoy

The second part of satisfaction is *pleasure*. For a food to be satisfying and pleasurable, it needs to look good, smell good, and taste good—to you. Instead of choosing foods that you think you "should" eat, choose foods that you enjoy eating. Take into consideration not just taste, but also texture, aroma, appearance, and culturally relevant foods. Maybe you find that you like creamy foods better than crunchy foods, or that hot foods are more satisfying than cold, or that you like to have multiple tastes and textures all at once to be most satisfied. One client of mine discovered that she needed to have some element of "crunch"; otherwise, she felt unsatisfied.

Your Food Environment

A third component of satisfaction is your food environment. I'm not just talking about setting the table and lighting a candle (though I discovered recently that this makes my meals much more satisfying), but any inviting food environment that feels pleasurable. This can include who prepared the meal for you, who you prepared it with, who you ate the meal with, where you ate the meal, or the experience you had while you ate it. Here are some qualities that might contribute to a satisfying food environment:

- A meal prepared for you by a friend or loved one
- Cooking with a friend or family member and making fun memories
- Getting your kids involved in the meal preparation
- A fresh bouquet of flowers on the table

- ◆ Eating outdoors in the sunshine
- ◆ Going out to eat and having a relaxing meal (and no dishes!)
- ◆ Listening to your favorite music
- ◆ Being surprised and gifted with a meal or dessert
- ◆ Enjoying good conversation and laughs

You may feel satisfied with just one or two of these three components—like a food that you love in the company of people you love. What satisfies you can change from week to week and even day to day, so start to experiment and notice how your body feels after different meals.

Finding Foods That Satisfy You _____

1. **Make a list of all the foods you enjoy eating.** Taste is one factor of enjoyment, but it's also about texture, temperature, smell, or happy memories. Chips and salsa won't be that enjoyable if you're really in the mood for a warm, filling meal. A few foods on my list include fresh pasta in Little Italy, the texture of creamy gelato, the smell (and taste) of a just-baked New York City bagel, and breakfast crêpes that I grew up making with my family.
2. **Before each meal, ask yourself, "What do I really want to eat right now?" If you're not sure, that's okay.** Pick something, eat it, and then note how full and satisfied (or hungry and unsatisfied) you feel after eating that meal. You may find it helpful to keep a journal so that you can start to notice patterns.

Fullness

"My problem is I just can't stop eating when I'm full"—I hear this all the time. Here's the thing: The reason you may eat past the point of "comfortable" fullness has pretty much nothing to do with noticing and feeling your fullness. Yes, some people are out of touch with what "comfortable" fullness feels like, but just being able to tell what various types fullness cues feel like is usually not what *actually* makes people stop eating.

Trying to force yourself to "stop when full" never works long term. It always ends up backfiring because it causes a sense of scarcity in the body and can bring up restrictive thoughts or feelings. I find that most people will get to a point where they naturally feel "done" eating—not because they are forcing themselves to stop, but because their body stops wanting food. To get to the point where you naturally notice and honor your fullness signals, you need to

- Be aware of your hunger cues.
- Eat every time you feel hungry.
- Allow yourself permission to eat whatever you want.

If you aren't able to notice your hunger cues and eat every time you feel hungry, then it is going to be really hard to stop eating once you feel full. Your body doesn't trust that you'll eat the next time you're hungry, so you'll feel the urge to continue eating even once you notice a "comfortable" fullness feeling. On top of that, diet culture and chronic dieting often cause us to feel like we "have" to eat at mealtimes—when it is allowed—which means that leaving food behind can be difficult. This is why, before tackling "how to stop when I'm full," you first have to build back body trust by honoring your hunger and giving yourself unconditional permission to eat (which I'll talk more about in the next chapter). Only then can you focus on feeling your fullness.

Components of a Filling Meal

In general, a filling meal will include all three macronutrients: carbohydrate, protein, and fat. It may also include some fiber, which slows down digestion and can keep you full for longer. Similar to what I shared earlier about a satisfying meal, a filling meal includes several different foods that all will work to signal your brain to decrease hunger hormones and increase fullness cues.

Certain foods will fill you up for a longer period, and others will keep you full for a shorter time. Neither one is "good" or "bad"; it's just information. You can file that information away and use it—as part of your brain knowledge—along with your body knowledge to help make food decisions down the road.

A client of mine, Jasmine, craved dessert all of the time and would beat herself up for eating past her fullness cues. She had relegated sweets to the "bad" category, so she was only "allowing" herself to have dessert a certain number of times each week. When we started working together, one of the first things we did was remove the dessert restriction. Jasmine also made an effort to notice her hunger cues and eat more consistently throughout the day whenever she felt hungry.

After several weeks of doing this, Jasmine shared, "Before, my favorite thing to eat would be dessert. I would crave it all the time, especially when I got home from work and after dinner. Now that I'm allowing myself to have dessert whenever I want, I've realized that the meals that are most filling and satisfying are those that are full meals that are more substantial. I've been craving meals that have some type of meat or protein, a starchy carb, and vegetables. I still want dessert, but I feel so much more full and satiated during the day when I eat a 'full' meal."

Finding "Comfortable" Fullness

Here's a little secret: When you are tuned in to your hunger signals, eating satisfying and filling foods whenever you feel hungry, letting go of physical restriction, and reframing restrictive thoughts, then you don't really need to pay much attention to fullness. You may be thinking something to the effect of, "Yeahhhh...no way." But trust me; when you're doing all of these things, what you're really doing is building back body trust. So your body begins to trust that you'll allow it whatever it wants the next time it sends a hunger cue. When you build back that trust, you'll start to naturally notice that you will hit a point when you feel "done" eating.

Although it can help to play around with your feelings of fullness and examine what those sensations feel like in your body, try not to force the "stop when comfortably full" thing. This tends to backfire because it causes a feeling of scarcity and can trigger the rebellious part of you to say, "Eff it. I'm going to do what I want," and keep eating. When you feel ready to practice noticing different levels of fullness, the hunger-fullness scale on page 189 can be a helpful tool. The sensation of fullness varies from person to person, so play around with what "comfortable" versus "slightly overfull" versus "really uncomfortable" feel like to you.

Are You Truly Eating Enough?

Don't mistake feeling "neutral" as being full. This confusion occurs often, especially in chronic dieters or people who've been restricting their food intake. They end up stopping at "neutral" instead of eating until full. Here are some signs you may be doing this:

- You never feel fully satisfied.
- You often get hungry soon—within one to two hours—after eating.
- You end up grazing throughout much of the day instead of eating meals.

Although needing to eat every few hours doesn't necessarily mean you aren't eating until fullness, this need could be a sign that you're stopping closer to "neutral." Notice where you may have sneaky diet mentality rules popping up, like one client who said, "I should have a lunch that keeps me full enough to not want to eat all afternoon." That *should* is a red flag; it's diet mentality. There's nothing wrong with you if you want to eat between meals, and if your meals are more than several hours apart, then it might feel most supportive to have some snacks. But if you find yourself unable to go more than an hour or two without thinking about food, you may not be eating enough. (Remember: Thinking about food can be a sign of physical hunger.)

This is a great place to experiment: What happens if you push a bit past what you *think* "comfortable" fullness is? How does that feel? Do you feel more satiated? Are you able to go several hours before thinking about food? When do you start to get hungry again? Again, there is no right or wrong and no "messing up." Experiment, get curious, and notice what you feel in your body.

Some Bloating Is Normal

If you're not used to eating enough, then "comfortable" fullness may feel a bit uncomfortable, but that doesn't mean you've eaten "too much." It means that your body may legitimately need much more food than your feeling of "comfortable" (or "acceptable") fullness suggests. You may need to get used to what *fullness* actually feels like. For example, occasional bloating and gas is totally normal and is not necessarily a sign that you've eaten "too much." This is your body just doing its thing, and unless it's happening on a regular basis or becomes painful, it's probably not something to worry about (though when in doubt, check with your doctor).

For people who've been restricting or engaging in other disordered eating behaviors, some level of delayed stomach emptying is very common. This means that you may feel heartburn, bloating, or gas, or you may notice that you get full quickly. Most of the time, this is a normal and expected part of the process. Over time, as you eat more, have a larger variety of food, and work on reducing anxiety or stress (which can cause gastrointestinal issues), these symptoms do typically resolve.

Often, any bloating or stomach discomfort is met with the recommendation to eliminate foods or eat less. Elimination diets—like gluten-free, dairy-free, or low-FODMAP diets—have become popular for "healing" gastrointestinal symptoms but can, in fact, mask disordered eating, which is a much more likely cause of digestive issues. Up to 98 percent of people with eating disorders have gastrointestinal issues, and as many as 44 percent of people with gastrointestinal disorders also have disordered eating behaviors.[8] I've had several clients with doctors who told them to "try" a low-FODMAP diet without doing much else to investigate what may have been causing their gastrointestinal issues. The low-FODMAP diet is a very restrictive elimination diet that removes certain classes of carbohydrates. While some people have success using it to identify intolerances, if the doctor doesn't screen the person for disordered eating (which I find doesn't happen most of the time), cutting out all these foods can mask or exacerbate underlying eating problems. Also, the elimination part of the low-FODMAP diet is meant to be only short term. With many people either self-diagnosing or following the advice of a healthcare provider without fully reintegrating foods, the diet can have a lot of negative consequences.

This isn't to say that food couldn't be the cause of some people's gastrointestinal symptoms, but if you have any history of dieting or restricting your food intake, then eliminating foods could actually cause your symptoms to worsen in the long run. It's much more likely that the symptoms are a result of the restriction, stress, anxiety, and/or a diet that includes too many high-fiber, raw, "clean" foods (because these will most *definitely* cause bloating and gas). In some cases, even *anticipating* that you will feel bad after eating something can cause gastrointestinal symptoms. A 2013 study found that gluten especially has a strong "nocebo effect"—meaning people who *thought* that gluten was making them sick ended up with actual symptoms, even when they never ingested any gluten.[9]

Cutting out foods or food groups should never be the default response. Often the symptoms can be reduced or eliminated through minimizing restriction, dealing with stress (and other feelings), and finding helpful coping mechanisms.

Not Every Meal Can Be Satisfying (And That's Okay)

I often find that people approach the concept of satisfaction in much the same way as the "hunger-fullness diet," where eating an unsatisfying meal means they are doing things "wrong." In reality, not every single eating experience is going to be 100 percent satisfying, and that is okay! It's unrealistic to expect you'll always be able to eat exactly what you want to eat. Having that expectation creates a lot of pressure, meaning you may find yourself back in that diet mentality of trying to do things "perfectly."

Although you can ideally consider what sounds good for each meal, sometimes food just needs to be fuel in response to a hunger cue. Recently, I went on a road trip, driving for hours through a rural area where the only option was gas station food. Several hours in, I really wanted a "full" meal, but that wasn't possible. So I satiated my hunger as best I could with the food from the gas station, picking some of the snacks that sounded best in the moment. I ate enough to feel full, though I still wasn't satisfied. But it was fine, and it got me through until I got to a bigger town, where I immediately swung into a fast-food drive-through to get some more "meal" food.

There may be other times when, for reasons outside your control, you're unable to satisfy your hunger fully, such as when you feel completely exhausted, which some people find makes it really hard to be satisfied by food (potentially because what your body really needs is sleep). Or if you menstruate, you may find that during certain times of the month, nothing seems to satisfy your hunger. It is okay if you don't always feel satisfied. In these cases, try to do the best you can by picking what sounds good and opting for some combination of carbs, protein, and fat if possible, so that you'll hopefully feel some semblance of fullness. You can also use these unsatisfying food situations to get curious and discover more about your body. What is going on that day (or that week)? Why might you not feel super satisfied? Do certain foods or food components satisfy you more than others? Are there other circumstances that play into making you feeling satisfied? If you are not allowing yourself to have foods that you really want, it's unlikely that you will feel satisfied. Sometimes this may a conscious decision that can be the result of diet mentality, like not keeping ice cream in your house because you're afraid you'll eat it all. Other times, you might be subconsciously restricting by thinking things like, "I'll do better tomorrow," or, "I can't believe I ate all of that."

This is where a common fear often arises: "But if I eat all the foods I enjoy, I won't ever make healthy food choices!" Truthfully, when you loosen the reins on your rules and restrictions and allow yourself to eat pleasurable foods, your body will naturally find a balance because, ultimately, pleasure and enjoyment come from eating foods that both taste good *and* make our bodies feel good. But first, you need to give yourself unconditional permission to unapologetically eat.

CHAPTER 9

Moving from Scarcity to Abundance

Diet culture has taught us that our appetites are too much—that we can't trust our bodies around food and, unless there are guardrails in place around what, when, and how much we eat, we'll go off the tracks. These beliefs cause us to shrink ourselves—and our appetites. They keep us distracted, which means we are more apt to "stay in line" and not challenge the status quo (which is exactly how those in power want it).

Recall in Chapter 1 when I shared how early Protestantism, combined with the rise of the slave trade, associated "overeating" with ungodliness and greediness, gluttony with sin, and fatness with immorality? I bring up the racist, classist, sexist roots of diet culture again to remind you that there is not a problem with *your body*—there is a problem with *our culture.* Your body is not wrong, and your appetite is not too much or out of control—it just feels that way because that's what our culture has taught you. To build back your inherent body trust and honor your hunger, you also need to give yourself *unconditional permission* to eat unapologetically.

Restriction because of external rules and guidelines about what you can and can't eat causes you to feel out of control around food. Restriction and deprivation breed guilt, and your body perceives that starvation is on the horizon. Your drive to eat increases, which eventually leads to more cravings and greater likelihood of binge-type eating behavior. Whenever you limit the amount or type of food you eat, you're setting yourself up to crave more of those foods in the future. Restriction and rules around food may feel like a way to take control in the moment, but those constraints are what end up keeping you feeling so out of control and entangled with food.

The remedy: Try to allow yourself unconditional permission to eat—and enjoy—food. By doing so, you can (eventually) end your body's feelings of deprivation, pull yourself out of the dieting cycle, and rebuild trust with your body. Here's what I mean when I say "unconditional permission":

- Releasing any physical and mental food restriction that you may still be holding onto
- Noticing any diet mentality that you may still be partaking in and letting that go
- Allowing yourself to eat what you want when you want it
- Creating abundance with food, both physically and mentally
- Adjusting your language to make all foods neutral

Once you stop depriving yourself and put all foods on an even playing field, you can tune in to your body's inner wisdom to figure out what it is you *really* want to eat. Although it doesn't happen overnight, and it's usually not easy, it is possible to get to a place where your decision of what to eat—or not to eat—is based on self-care and comes from a mindset of abundance, rather than self-control, deprivation, or restriction.

The Honeymoon Phase

A few months ago, I was out to dinner with a group of people, some of whom were strangers. In typical first-meeting fashion, I was asked about the work that I do. As I explained my food and body philosophy, I got head-nods from the women around the table. "That makes so much sense," one of them said, "I've struggled with food and my body image for so many years." The others murmured agreement. Then came the line that I've grown used to by this point, "What you're saying sounds great, but the problem is, if I allowed myself to eat whatever I wanted, I'd just eat pizza for dinner every night!"

Ah, yes—the old "my intuition tells me to eat a pint of ice cream every night" retort. This is a common misconception of intuitive eating, and it describes what is often referred to as the *honeymoon phase*. When first reintroducing or allowing foods that were previously considered off-limits, most people go through a phase where they *do* eat pizza every night for dinner or polish off a pint of ice cream most evenings. This honeymoon phase is not only completely normal, but it is actually a necessary and important step in the intuitive eating journey.

Whenever you avoid certain foods, whether it's to follow a formal diet plan or because you're trying to "eat healthier," you're restricting yourself in some way. When you release that restriction and allow yourself to have "off-limits" foods again, you'll most likely eat a quantity of them that feels "not normal" or uncomfortable. During this initial honeymoon period, these foods feel new and exciting to your brain and your body. Depending on how long you've been preventing yourself from eating these foods, they may really *be* new and exciting. Take Alicia, a client of mine who had been following the Paleo diet on and off for several years. When she stopped restricting and began asking herself, "What do I want to eat?" her answer was almost always a carbohydrate of some kind: bagels, pasta, sandwiches, you name it. She allowed herself to eat these carbs but also had moments of panic—she felt like she was eating "way too much." But this desire for all the carbs was a totally *normal* response. Alicia had been depriving her body of carbohydrates for so long, no wonder it was all she wanted!

This novelty factor drives a lot of the eating that occurs during the honeymoon phase. Other elements that come into play include deep-rooted diet mentality and mental or emotional food restriction. You may feel like you are physically allowing yourself to eat whatever you want, but the diet mentality is so ingrained that you may still have some subconscious rules or restrictions that you are trying to follow. Or you may be allowing yourself to eat whatever you want, whenever you want it, giving yourself *physical* permission to eat—but not fully giving yourself *mental* permission.

Remember, having an increased appetite and desire to eat is a *normal* response to any type of restriction. Imagine being underwater for several minutes: When you finally come up for air, you gulp for air and take panicky breaths. Coming up for air from diet culture feels similar, and your initial eating experiences are going to have this panicky, out-of-control feeling as well. But this stage is an essential part of the intuitive eating process, and you have to move through it to get to the other side and be able to trust your body (and have it trust you).

The length of the honeymoon phase varies. Some people find that this period is rather brief, and they move through it over several weeks. For people who have been chronically dieting, who may have experienced significant body trauma, or who may be in more of a deprived state, this period can last a while—for several months to a year or longer. The phase will also be longer if you are giving yourself only physical permission without working on releasing your mental and emotional restriction. (I'll talk about how to do this shortly.) It is also common to go in and out of the honeymoon period, sometimes repeating this phase as you reintroduce different previously restricted or off-limits foods. None of these situations are good or bad, right or wrong, so try not to compare yourself to others on this journey. Just know that you are going through a normal and crucial part of the process.

You may feel somewhat out of control during the honeymoon period, especially at the beginning. You may feel tempted to restrict to get back in control. "What if I just don't keep sugar in my house, but still let myself eat it when I'm out?" one client asked me recently. Okay, so that may help you to feel more in control in the moment, but what is that going to do long term?

Recall the science of food habituation that I mentioned back in Chapter 2. The more you are exposed to a food, the less your brain cares about it, and your desire to eat it diminishes. While *restriction* leads to an increased desire, *permission* yields a decreased desire. Say you were told you could eat a burger and fries for dinner every night. Although that might sound great on night one, by the fifth or sixth night of eating the same meal, it will likely have lost its allure. You will adjust and get habituated to different foods the more you eat them.

Needless to say, the opposite is also true. When you don't have access to certain foods, your brain focuses on them more. For instance, if you've ever been on a trip without access to your favorite foods, what's the first thing you feel like eating when you get home? For me, it's all the foods that I missed while I was traveling. This happens to me no matter where I am visiting. At first, all the new foods are exciting, and I can't wait to check out all the restaurants, but after a week or two of eating out for all my meals, I'd give anything for some peanut butter toast. So although keeping sugar out of your house short term may feel like it will help you be more "in control," it will only lengthen the habituation period.

The same thing happens when you label food off-limits. As soon as you tell yourself that you can't have something—say, dessert, candy, or chocolate—your brain will focus on those foods. It's totally counterproductive because you eventually end up thinking of nothing but this food (or foods) that you can't have until you finally "give in" and eat it. At that point, the restriction has been so strong, and your body doesn't know when you'll let it have the food again that you have a hard time stopping. I can't tell you how many people have told me that after a month (or less) of following the Whole30 diet, all they wanted was a burger and fries. (Seriously, I've heard this *exact* food craving from dozens of people.) Labeling foods off-limits or limiting when you can have them keeps you swinging back and forth in the deprivation-binge pendulum as you go through periods of deprivation and restriction followed by rebound overeating. Back and forth, back and forth.

One of the clearest personal examples of this came with chocolate. I always considered myself to be "obsessed" with chocolate, and my obsession was a constant joke among my family and friends. I even put that description in my AOL instant messenger profile (ha, who remembers those?) during college and, later on, my online dating profile. I'd limit myself to a certain amount of chocolate each week, and every day I'd obsessively think about when I could eat it next and how much I should "let" myself have. Whenever I did allow myself to eat chocolate, I'd often end up bingeing; then I'd feel incredibly guilty, beat myself up, and vow never to do *that* again.

As a chocolate lover, I always felt like I "had" to have it every day. My cravings were so real. Yet, I never allowed myself to have most forms of chocolate in my house. I would never buy ice cream, chocolate bars, candy, or cookies. "I won't be able to control myself," I thought. "I'll eat it all!" The only form of chocolate I'd keep in my house was a certain brand of small dark chocolates (never milk chocolate) that I'd "allow" myself to have each evening.

Then came the summer when my roommate's boyfriend began stocking our freezer with ice cream every time he'd visit. At first, I felt out of control and ate a ton of ice cream almost every day. But he kept bringing more and more, and eventually, I made my way through the honeymoon period and habituated to the ice cream. I got so used to it being there that I eventually completely forgot about it. One afternoon, I opened the freezer to take out some meat to thaw and was shocked to realize that there was still a pint of ice cream inside. I had finally gotten to the point where I knew—and trusted—that it wasn't going anywhere, and the urgency to eat it dissipated. And those tiny dark chocolates that I thought I loved so much? Turns out, I don't enjoy them much at all; they had just tasted so good in the moment because I had been keeping chocolate off-limits. I still love chocolate, but I crave it much less frequently, and I know the types that I really enjoy the taste of, which makes it all the more satisfying.

As Alicia continued allowing herself carbohydrates, she did find that almost every morning, her answer to "What sounds good to me?" was a bagel. This trend continued for several months, but she kept allowing herself to have a bagel if she wanted it. At the same time, she worked on eating whenever she felt hungry, finding satisfying foods, and reframing her mental restrictions. Slowly, as she continued to build back trust with her body, she habituated to bagels. She still eats them, or some other form of carbohydrate, at breakfast, but the urgent need dissipated, and many mornings, Alicia craves other foods instead.

To move through the honeymoon phase and get to the other side, you need to work on rebuilding body trust. This takes time, but you've got to trust the process and know that it *will* pass, and you *will* get to the place where the thought of eating pizza feels as neutral as the idea of eating a salad. Once you learn to give yourself *full permission* both physically and mentally, view all foods neutrally, and find ways to show abundance, it will come.

Write Yourself a Permission Slip

What are some of the food rules or restrictions that you are struggling to let go of? Write yourself a permission slip and put it somewhere to remind you that you have permission to eat and enjoy *all* foods.

Some examples:

- I have permission to eat carbs at every meal.
- I have permission to eat after X o'clock at night.
- I have permission to eat whenever I feel hungry.
- I have permission to snack between meals.
- I have permission to eat what I want and not compare myself to others.

How to Make Peace with Food

When you allow yourself to eat all kinds of foods *consistently*, your body begins to know and trust that it can have these foods when it wants it. Then something magical happens: Food loses its power over you. In intuitive eating, this concept is referred to as *making peace with food*. Part of the peace process involves allowing yourself to have access to the foods that you have been physically restricting. Permitting yourself to eat these foods releases the physical restriction and creates an environment of abundance.

One of the first things people do when they start trying to practice intuitive eating is they give up all their rules related to food. "I'm done dieting!" they say, and then proceed to eat whatever they want. For some people who have the support of a therapist or dietitian, haven't been restricting very long or intensely, and who don't have complex body trauma, this may work really well. However, I find that many people at this stage end up feeling overwhelmed and out of control. If this is you, know that it is normal (remember—it's the honeymoon period!) and that going from restriction to a free-for-all may not be the best or safest way for you to reintroduce certain foods.

For people who have been restricting for a while or have a long list of "forbidden" foods, it can be overwhelming to allow unconditional access to all of them at once. It may be helpful to go slowly and introduce a fewer number of those off-limits foods at one time.

Challenge: Reintroduce Your Off-Limits Foods ___

1. Make a list of all the foods that are most appealing to you. What are your favorite foods? Which foods do you just love eating? This can be any type of food; don't limit yourself here.

2. Go through and put a check mark by any of the foods you currently allow yourself to eat regularly.

3. Circle the foods you have been restricting—whether consciously (like on a diet) or subconsciously (through food rules, keeping the food out of your house, feeling guilty for eating it, and so on).

4. Pick one or two of the off-limits foods that you circled in Step 3 to start with. Go to the store and buy those foods and keep them stocked in your pantry. If possible, buy enough of the items so that you have them in abundance, like three bags of chips or four bags of peanut butter cups (an actual example from a client of mine).

5. Once you have those foods at home, allow yourself to eat them whenever you want. When you eat them, check in with yourself: How do they taste? How does it feel in your body? If you really like it, buy it again.

If this process feels daunting, start by picking one food that feels the least anxiety-provoking to you and see how it feels to have that food available in abundance. Continue repeating with each of the foods from your off-limits list until you feel habituated to each of them. Remember, this process can take many weeks or even months. If you are financially unable to afford purchasing larger quantities of these foods, do the best you can to allow yourself to eat enough and eat satisfying foods.

Mental and Emotional Food Restriction

Now, if at this point you're thinking, "I don't know what I'm doing wrong! I'm trying to eat intuitively and allowing myself physical access to all sorts of foods, but I just keep binge-eating!" then you probably are still holding on to some mental and emotional restriction. A common sticking point in intuitive eating involves releasing *physical* restriction of foods while still *mentally* or *emotionally* restricting. Here's what that can look like: You decide to give yourself unconditional permission to eat, begin to allow yourself to eat whatever you want, and keep all the foods around, but after several weeks (or months), you still feel out of control around food, binge, and have a hard time feeling that you're "done" eating.

To truly let go of dieting and the diet mentality, it's not enough to make the physical change of letting yourself eat what you want; you need to make mental and emotional shifts, too. Even if you allow yourself to eat all the things, if you're still mentally restricting, then you'll still feel out of control around food. For those of us who are privileged enough to be food secure, food is probably never truly *scarce*. Often food is all around you yet, psychologically, you may operate from a place of scarcity. Even if there is plenty of food available, this mental scarcity causes your body to feel restricted and sets off a starvation response in your body—just as if you were physically restricting.

Examples of mental restriction include thoughts like

- ◆ "I'm not going to snack this afternoon; I always eat so much."
- ◆ "I'm only going to eat when I'm hungry today."
- ◆ "It's okay that you ate the cupcake, but you can't do this every day."
- ◆ "This food is so unhealthy; I need to try to do better tomorrow."
- ◆ "I've been eating so terribly; I've got to get a handle on this."

All of these thoughts send your body the message that *restriction is coming*. Your body senses an impending scarcity, *even if* food is physically available to you. This type of mental or emotional restriction has the same effect as physically restricting food: It causes your appetite and cravings to increase, and you'll continue to feel out of control around food.

Monica had made huge strides in recovering from disordered eating by the time I met her. Yet she still was going through periods of restricting followed by bingeing and felt "stuck" when it came to giving herself unconditional permission to eat. We started working together on bringing awareness to all of the thoughts and feelings Monica was having about food. A light bulb went off: "I was so surprised at how much diet mentality was still buried in my brain. I know that physical restriction doesn't work, but I also still have some underlying fantasy of being thin," she shared. This sneaky diet mentality, including some hope of using intuitive eating to lose weight, was keeping Monica in the dieting cycle. "I feel so guilty whenever I feel like I'm eating 'terribly.' So eventually, I gather up my discipline and try to be super good about everything," she told me. "I'll feel in control for a bit, until I feel out of control—and then I go back to whatever food behavior I told myself I shouldn't do. Like snacking at work—it's this war of, 'I want to go get a snack,' and then, 'but I shouldn't.'" Monica realized that her guilt and the subconscious rules she was still hanging onto only served to make her feel *more* urgency to eat.

Monica also realized that, although she was telling herself she could eat whatever she wanted, at the end of the day, she was running through her day's worth of food and judging herself for being "good" or "bad." Then would come the tomorrow-I-won't-do-this thought. Monica's body was still getting the restriction message, so it's no wonder she was still bingeing and felt so out of control around food.

Find Neutral Language to Describe Food

Another form of mental restriction comes in the language that we use to describe food. Labeling a food as *bad, junk, garbage,* an *indulgence,* a *cheat meal,* or a *treat* places a judgment upon it. It demonizes certain foods and elevates other "good" ones. (Remember: This is binary thinking.) The subtext of all of these negative labels is *this is a food that you shouldn't have that often,* which your body interprets as—guess what—*restriction.* And what happens when there is any type of restriction? You are more driven to eat those foods and you may feel out of control around them.

Plus, if you label a food as *bad* or *junk* or *garbage* or *crap,* then eating them is probably going to come with a heaping side of guilt and self-judgment. This guilt counteracts any pleasure you would have otherwise felt from eating the food, which makes it tough to enjoy the food and often means you won't feel satisfied. The judgment of the food may transfer to a judgment of the person who's eating the food; in other words, eating a bad food translates into "I'm a bad person" followed closely by "I shouldn't have done that." Your body senses this mental restriction and fears starvation is on the horizon, even if it clearly is not. It gets the message that you may not allow yourself these foods again because they're so "bad," which makes it that much easier to devour an entire bag of chips (because what the hell—the day is already "shot," right?). This guilt, shame, and judgment disconnect you from what your body truly wants, and it undermines your ability to listen to—and trust—yourself.

Food descriptors like *guilt-free* and *sinfully delicious* can also serve to disconnect you from your body's wisdom. These words are external judgments of food, albeit ones that pose these foods as "healthier," which can lead us to think, "It's better for me, so I can eat as much as I want." This mindset may cause you to eat based on external factors, rather than responding to your feelings of hunger, fullness, and satiety. I used to love a local New York City frozen yogurt shop and would visit it regularly, serving myself a big cup piled with toppings. I almost always ate to the point of feeling very uncomfortable, and then I would feel so guilty. However, once I started tuning in to my body, I eventually realized that *I didn't actually like frozen yogurt.* What I thought I "loved" was really just a response to my diet mentality, where I believed frozen yogurt to be better for me than ice cream. Now, I always opt for ice cream instead of frozen yogurt because that is what I know I like and enjoy. Sure, I still sometimes eat ice cream to the point of feeling uncomfortably full, but it happens less frequently (and without a side of guilt) because I've removed the "bad" judgment from it, and I trust that I'll allow myself to eat it whenever I want.

Even words like *healthy* and *unhealthy* can have a similar effect. This isn't necessarily because of an issue with the words themselves but because the moral connotation our culture has given them. *Healthy* now equals *good* (and often is equated with boring and tasteless), whereas *unhealthy* equals *bad*, which means labeling foods as *healthy* or *unhealthy* can also prompt some mental restriction. The same goes for the common phrase, "everything in moderation." I used to say this often, and it took me a while to realize that in reality *moderation* is still putting a restriction on food. "People would often tell me to eat in 'moderation,' and it was such a trigger word for me," a woman shared with me. "As soon as you say I can have three cookies at night, which seems like moderation, all of a sudden I want ten. And as soon as I eat more than three, I feel like I've failed, so I end up saying 'screw it' and binge." Moderation is subjective, and for someone who is trying to move away from external diet rules, it can feel limiting and restrictive. Not to mention that "eat in moderation" has been completely co-opted by diet culture. So by trying to eat a "moderate amount," you continue to be under a restriction on how much you can or can't eat, which keeps you in the diet cycle.

Although some type of moderation does end up defining what many people naturally land on, that only happens by not putting restrictions on yourself and figuring out—sans rules—what feels good for you. Moderation looks different for everybody, and getting to that place still requires unconditional permission to eat all foods (which at times doesn't look like what you may think "moderate" is). When it comes to the language you use with food, shifting your mindset to view foods as neutral will allow you to make choices that are based on self-care and satisfaction and come from a place of abundance rather than scarcity.

Shift from Scarcity to Abundance

To remove the mental (and physical) restriction from food, it can help to think of shifting your mindset from one of *scarcity* to one of *abundance*. Keeping foods off-limits, labeling foods as good or bad, and having thoughts of "I'll do better tomorrow" all are types of scarcity mindset. Although you may have access to plenty of food, any form of scarcity can spark a feeling of restriction in your body, which is interpreted by your brain as *starvation is coming*. Instead, if you can consider all types of foods as allowable and abundant, the sense of scarcity will be alleviated, and you can make decisions on what to eat based on your body's intuition and wisdom.

To create an environment of abundance, consider both physical and mental forms of scarcity. Physical scarcity can be in the form of keeping certain foods out of your house or office for fear of eating them all. It can also include times in which you feel hungry, yet don't have any food around you that you can eat—like when you're out running errands or stuck in a work meeting. As much as you can, you want to try to create a physical environment of food abundance. Here are a few suggestions for how you can do this:

- Eat enough food consistently throughout the day.
- Keep your house stocked with a variety of food that you enjoy.
- If you are frequently in the car or at an office, keep some shelf-stable foods there.
- Give yourself permission to have more food later if you want it.

222

By eating consistently throughout the day, you help build back trust with your body (and avoid getting to the place of ravenous hunger). Stocking up on a variety of enjoyable foods at home, at the office, and in the car (or a bag or purse if you're on the go) will help waylay feelings of scarcity. Having food readily available naturally creates a sense of abundance; often, just knowing food is available in case you get hungry can decrease anxiety or feelings of urgency. When you eat a meal—or snack—and you feel full, you can show abundance by telling yourself, "You can eat some more later if you still want it." This can help you be able to stop when you feel "done" rather than falling into a scarcity-driven I-don't-know-when-I-can-have-this-again binge. You can use this whether you're home (by keeping more food available or saving leftovers) or out to eat (by boxing up the food and taking it home with you).

I often do this even if I'm not certain I want the food. For example, I recently went into a coffee shop to order a latte. I wasn't feeling hungry, but some of the baked goods looked really tasty. I couldn't decide if I actually wanted them, so I bought a couple in case. As soon as I purchased them, the slight feeling of scarcity I had over potentially not having them went away. The key here is to make sure you do allow yourself to eat the food later—even if it's within thirty minutes or an hour after you stopped eating it. If you are thinking about eating it, give yourself permission, and *let your body have it*. This will help to show more abundance and build back trust with your body.

It is also important to notice any mental scarcity and make a mindset shift toward one of abundance. Here are a few ways in which you can do this:

- Notice any food labels, call them out as unhelpful, and shift your language to make all foods neutral.
- Catch any mental restriction (like thinking, "I'll do better tomorrow") and reframe that thought to show abundance.
- Become aware of any sneaky, deeply rooted diet mentality and challenge it by doing the opposite of what it says.

You can release mental restriction by reframing any critical or judgmental thoughts you have about food into more helpful, positive statements that reflect abundance. Here are a few examples:

Instead of "I can't believe I ate so much today; I totally screwed up."

Reframe to "I'm learning how to listen to my body and trust myself with food. There is no screwing up."

Instead of "I didn't pay attention to what I was eating at all this week. Why can't I do better?"

Reframe to "This was a rough week with a lot of stressful things going on at work. It makes sense that food was a bit chaotic this week."

Instead of "I really shouldn't eat that. It has so much sugar."

Reframe to "I'm allowed to have it whenever I want."

Instead of "This is such a binge-food for me. I should just eat it all now to get it out of the house."

Reframe to "If I want some later, I can have it again. It will still be there."

Shifting from a mindset of scarcity to one of abundance requires releasing *both* physical and mental restriction. For example, I worked with one woman who never kept chocolate in her house because she would end up eating the whole bag in one or two sittings. (Just as I had once thought about myself.) She committed to creating an environment of abundance and bought two big bags of her favorite chocolate. In addition to showing physical abundance, she also practiced reframing her thoughts to demonstrate mental abundance. She told herself, "I can eat the chocolates whenever I want to. If I eat some and then want more later, I can eat them again." And if she wanted more, she ate more. By establishing physical *and* mental abundance, she was able to eat the chocolates when she wanted them, without any guilt, and she didn't require any willpower or self-control.

Shifting your mindset is an active process; it does not happen overnight. It can take many weeks to months, but the more you practice *noticing* your thoughts and *shifting* to a framework of abundance, the easier it will become.

Reframe to Create an Abundant Mindset_____

Notice any conscious or subconscious mentally or emotionally restrictive thoughts that you have during the day. Get curious: How are these thoughts or beliefs affecting your eating behaviors? How might they be getting in your way of connecting to your body? The next time you notice these thoughts, call them out as unhelpful diet mentality; then reframe them, like so:

- I'm allowed to have ____ whenever I want.
- When I'm hungry, I can eat again.
- The food will be there later if I want to have it then.
- I had more sweets than felt good, but I had lots of other foods, too.
- This is a process; every eating experience is a learning experience.

Employing Mindfulness

You'll notice that I've said several times already that you can try to *notice* and *observe*. Mindfulness skills are really useful when you're working on giving yourself unconditional physical and mental permission to eat. The more you can be *aware* of the thoughts that you have related to food and *notice* how those thoughts affect your behaviors, the more you can work on actively shifting your attention and responding with abundance instead of scarcity.

A big part of this process involves experimentation. Try things one way, and then try them another and observe (nonjudgmentally) what happens each time. Each eating experience is a learning experience in which you can get curious and notice things like the following:

- What happens when you allow yourself to eat a food that was previously off-limits?
- How does it taste? How is the eating experience?
- What thoughts or feelings come up for you?
- What happens afterward?

Sometimes you may not be sure whether you truly don't want the food or some sneaky diet mentality is telling you not to eat it. Remember the tip I shared in Chapter 4: *Do the opposite* of what your mind is telling you—in this case, eat the food in question. Challenge that inner diet mentality by doing what it's telling you not to do. Then get curious and notice what happens and how you feel. The next time this situation arises, and you can't decide whether you should eat the food, try a different approach, and don't eat it. Again get curious and notice what happens. By challenging these inner diet mentality voices, you get to test whether diet mentality is talking or your inner wisdom is talking. It's only by experimenting—and showing abundance—that you can tease the two apart.

How to Make Food Decisions with an Abundance Mindset

When you are deciding what to eat, ask yourself the following questions:

- What sounds good to me right now?
- What does my body feel like eating?

Allow yourself to have what sounds good. Check in with your body as you eat and once you finish the food. Notice what happens: Are you satisfied? What thoughts are you having? How does your body feel?

What Happens If You Really Can't Eat Whatever You Want?

One question is inevitable: What if you aren't able to eat what sounds good to you in the moment? Realistically, you're not going to be able to eat the exact thing you want every time you eat, just like it's not always possible for every meal to be satisfying. But this doesn't mean that you can't listen to your body and practice intuitive eating. Intuitive eating does not mean "you always have to eat exactly what you want," just like it does not mean "eat only when hungry, and you have to stop when you are full."

There will be times when you don't have access to the food that sounds good because it's out of season, not sold at your local supermarket, or not available at that time (like my craving for French pastries when I was living in the middle of rural Vermont: not happening). It could also be that you don't have the financial security to eat whatever feels satisfying. Intuitive eating is a privilege, so there may very well be times when eating exactly what sounds good doesn't fit into your food budget. Or you may have food allergies or food intolerances, or you may be required to follow a medically necessary diet, in which case you *can't* eat certain foods safely. And what about times when you meal plan or have to pack a lunch at 7:00 a.m. to bring to work when you have no idea what you'll be in the mood for later?

The difference between these scenarios and diet mentality is that you are not *purposely* depriving yourself; you may just have to eat what is available. That doesn't mean you still can't find ways to show abundance. The key is to approach the eating situation with flexibility. Start by checking in with your body to ask, "What sounds good right now?" If the answer is something that is not an option in that moment, can you find a similar food that will still be satisfying? Or is there something else you can add to your meal to make it more enjoyable, even if it's not the exact food you had in mind? Experimentation comes in handy here. Approach food with curiosity and flexibility, and you can start to figure out some go-to foods that will generally keep you full and satisfied. That way, if you can't have exactly what you want in the moment, you have a toolbox of other food options that you know will be satisfying.

Meal Planning

When it comes to meal planning, shopping and preparing food ahead of time can seem counterintuitive to the concept of unconditional permission and abundance. The reason has less to do with what meal planning is and more to do with what diet culture has turned meal planning into: something rigid, structured, and stemming from a place of restriction or dieting or staying "in control." I always picture those awful "inspirational" images of a week's worth of containers, each filled with grilled chicken, vegetables, and a minuscule amount of brown rice. Meal planning does *not* have to be like that.

Meal planning can be flexible and take into consideration your satisfaction and food preferences, and you can do it loosely without rules. When figuring out what you're going to make for the week or pack for lunch, think about what foods are usually satisfying and enjoyable. If you're able to, keep a variety of foods in your house or bring several additional snacks with you to work. Then remove the pressure: If you aren't craving that meal in the moment, and there is other food available, permit yourself to eat something else instead (and save the other meal for later in the week).

You can also be flexible if what you prepared ahead of time doesn't sound good, *and* there are no other options. It's normal to have experiences when you eat what is available, even if it's not the most exciting, enjoyable meal. You're not intentionally depriving yourself of satisfying foods because you're dieting or trying to become smaller; you're just dealing with real life. Sometimes self-care means fueling your body and moving on with your day, knowing that you can aim to maximize satisfaction at the next meal (which is a great way to show abundance).

Abundance and Food Allergies

Food allergies can be traumatic and have a lasting impact on your relationship to food and your body. You may have had a scary allergic reaction or visited many doctors and done multiple tests, feeling sick and confused as you tried to figure out what foods were causing your symptoms. All of these experiences can create a disconnect and distrust in your body.

Although some of the language used for discussing intuitive eating may make it seem like it's not something you can do if you have food allergies, intolerances, or sensitivities, this is not the case. The principles of intuitive eating can be really supportive in helping you safely reconnect to your body and create a more peaceful relationship to food while catering to any allergies or intolerances that you may have.

Creating a flexible eating environment and giving yourself unconditional permission doesn't mean making yourself feel unsafe or ignoring food allergies. Instead, it's about liberalizing other areas of your diet to minimize stress and reestablish eating as an enjoyable experience. Use the idea of abundance and flexibility to find foods that you enjoy, outside of diet mentality, that are food-allergy-friendly. Try different substitutes, experiment with new recipes, or taste-test new products that don't contain your food allergen. Allowing yourself the flexibility to experiment and try new things can help prevent you from feeling too restricted or stressed about what you can eat or not eat.

It can also help to shift your intention from "I'm not allowed to have that food" to "I get to choose foods that I like and that make me feel good." Rather than creating a hard rule reminiscent of dieting or restriction, think of it as a choice that is informed by your experience with this food or knowledge of how this food feels in your body. Remember, you are working *with* your body, not against it.

Abundance and Medical Conditions

Intuitive eating is for *everyone*, even if you have a medical condition that is exacerbated by certain foods. The problem with diets, even if for specific health issues, is that unless you've healed your relationship to food, any restriction will still cause you to feel deprived and send your body into starvation mode. I can't tell you how many people I've seen who were told by their doctor to follow a specific diet, say for diabetes or high blood pressure, who fell into the same diet-binge cycle. Unless there is truly an immediate life-threatening situation, working through the honeymoon phase of unconditional permission will get you to a place where you can see foods as neutral and make decisions about what to eat—or not eat—for your health from a place of self-care instead of restriction. When you get to that place, it is a much more sustainable way to eat, support your health, and take care of your body (compared to diet advice of just "eat fewer carbohydrates" or "lose weight").

For example, I recently worked with a client with prediabetes who was trying to "watch" her carbohydrate intake. She was limiting the foods she allowed herself, measuring specific portions, and trying to keep her blood sugar stable. This plan would work for a little while, but she'd "fall off the wagon" eventually. This cycle continued for years. When we started working together, she began working on permitting herself to eat whatever she wanted as she also tuned in to her feelings of hunger, fullness, and satisfaction. In the short term, she ended up eating lots of carbohydrates, but eventually, she got to the other side of the honeymoon phase, and many of her cravings went away because she habituated to them and let go of the scarcity mindset. She then was able to implement some gentle nutrition to help support her health and balance her blood sugar. Her decision to eat foods that supported her health came from a place of self-care and abundance rather than self-control and restriction. Because she had worked through connecting with her body's inner wisdom and gave herself unconditional permission, eating fewer carbs didn't set off the same starvation response.

So for someone with diabetes, working through the unconditional permission phase could mean craving a donut, eating it, and then noticing—without judgment—how it makes you feel. Do you have an energy crash after? Does the donut taste good, or did you not really enjoy it? Also, notice what happens to your blood sugar. Then, as you start to habituate and build back trust with your body, you can figure out what foods give you maximum enjoyment *and* help you feel your best. This approach can work with any medical condition; however, if you do require a medically necessary diet, I recommend seeking out a weight-inclusive dietitian who can help you eat to support your health in a nonrestrictive way. I'll also share more about using gentle nutrition in Chapter 12.

Moving from Allowing to Feeling

Diet mentality can be deeply ingrained in your subconscious mind, and it takes time to rewire your brain's programming. Your brain gets used to doing and thinking one thing so that those old thoughts can feel safe, even if your conscious mind knows you'd be better off letting go of them. Just as your diet mentality thoughts and behaviors took root through repetition, you also need to repeat new thoughts and behaviors over and over (and over) before they will begin to take hold.

Be patient with yourself; the process of giving yourself unconditional permission to eat may feel really scary. Your mind may try to send you back toward what it is comfortable with (aka dieting), with thoughts like, "See, I knew this wasn't going to work," or, "You should be further along by now; what's wrong with you?" Use your mindfulness skills to notice when your mind is going down that road and take a step back to say, "Okay, there it goes again; it's just my mind doing what it does," and try to let it go.

Continue to work on challenging the diet mentality by shifting your behaviors. Guilty thoughts or feelings of shame may still be present, but the more you can practice making behavior changes anyway, over time, your thoughts and feelings will begin to shift as well. For example, you may have the thought, "This is too many carbs," or, "What will people think if I eat all this?" But you can change your behavior by eating the food anyway, *despite* feeling guilty or judged.

Slowly, positive eating experiences will go from few and far between to regular and consistent as you build back more trust with your body. As one of my clients said to me, "I really never thought I would get here. I know you said to trust the process, but I didn't think it was possible for me. But wow—I finally made it to the other side, and it's like a switch flipped: Now I can just eat and move on—no more anxiety or obsessing." (Note: It took many months before the "switch flipped" for this client, which is very normal.) Unconditional permission is like a mountain: It feels incredibly challenging on the way up, and you will frequently want to turn back. The only way to the top is with time and patience.

In the next part, we will move from *allowing* uncomfortable sensations to arise without trying to "fix" them to *feeling* and sitting in this discomfort.

PART 3

Feeling

CHAPTER 10

Self-Care and Sitting with It

Erica spent years trying to eat "perfectly" and keep up appearances. If she could appear perfect, then she would prove that she was worthy and get the external validation and approval that she craved. "I realize now that I started controlling food and my body at a very young age in an effort to distract from the trauma I was experiencing at home," she explained to me. "Now, it's become such an ingrained habit, and I've never done the work to unpack the feelings underneath this guise of perfectionism."

Dieting is a great distraction, as is perfectionism. Many people use these tools, and others, to avoid facing painful situations, feelings, and emotions. When you stop trying to "fix" yourself through dieting and let go of that distraction, a lot of thoughts, feelings, and memories can rise to the surface. Also, as you strengthen your interoceptive skills to connect more with feelings of hunger and fullness, you will likely start to feel more feelings. The reason is that your ability to feel your body sensations correlates with your ability to feel other feelings. Having all sorts of feelings arise during this process is normal, but it can be wildly uncomfortable. The goal at this point is not to make the discomfort go away but instead to *sit with* the discomfort. The emotions that have been hidden beneath years of dieting and restricting need to be uprooted, felt, and processed.

It would be great if we could just stop using dieting as a "fix," allow ourselves to heal our relationship to food, and then go straight to body acceptance, but, alas, this isn't how it works. To move from dieting and body fixing to body acceptance, you have to make space for grief, which involves bringing any deep-rooted shame and fears to the surface and allowing yourself to feel the emotions that you've been suppressing. It means grieving the loss of your old body or a body that society deems "acceptable" (i.e., thin) and giving up a feeling of control. It may also mean grieving the reality that you may very well be treated differently by society if you're in a fat body. This long, often painful process involves what Brianna Campos, LPC, calls "sitting in the suck." As she says, "You can't bypass body grief and go straight to body acceptance. You have to sit in the suck."[1]

I recently asked a handful of clients what sorts of things they'd been "sitting with," and they said

- Giving up a feeling of control
- The fear of finding a partner
- People judging me based on my body size
- Missing the validation I got when I was in a smaller body
- Not being respected because I'm in a fat body
- Knowing I'll be treated differently
- Being ashamed of the way I look
- Giving up the idea that I'll one day achieve the thin "ideal"
- Missing the idea that losing weight will solve all my problems and make everything better
- Logically knowing I don't need to be in a smaller body to feel free, but still struggling to unlearn the body ideal that I've been conditioned to believe is "better"
- Never being able to fit into my old clothes
- Being worried about how others will see me if I gain weight or don't lose weight
- Feeling like I need to justify my body size by achieving "perfect" health
- Never being accepted by certain people
- Knowing I'll always have a body that society deems to be "wrong"

It is human nature to want to push uncomfortable feelings away, but it's also not helpful (especially long term)—or realistic. When we are unable to sit with discomfort, we then end up bypassing the feelings. Some people try to bypass by numbing—whether through binge-eating, substance use, or overworking. Others try to get through the feelings by attempting to "fix" them through behaviors like dieting, compulsively exercising, people-pleasing, or perfectionism. All of these things can relieve discomfort temporarily, but they don't help in the long run. Avoiding your feelings can make the emotions you don't want to deal with seem even scarier. All the while, the feelings are still there, just pushed further down.

How Do You Bypass Feelings? _____

When you start to notice an uncomfortable feeling arise, what do you do? Do you ever try to avoid the feeling by numbing or fixing (or perhaps a combination of both)? What effect does bypassing the feelings have in the short term? What about the long-term effect of bypassing?

The ability to be present in your body, feel your feelings, and tolerate discomfort without turning to harmful coping mechanisms requires time, support, and safety. All of these things, especially safety, are privileges, and I recognize that not everyone is at the point where they're able to do this. In this chapter, I explain how to develop self-care and positive coping strategies, which are essential before you dive into bringing your feelings to light and processing any body grief.

Self-Care Is Self-Preservation

Self-care has become a ubiquitous term, and its meaning has been watered down from the original intent. Today, self-care is often thought of as "me time," and it has been commodified and packaged as a way for women to "beautify themselves" (think face masks, waxing, massages, mani-pedis), but it actually originated as a radical political concept. In her 1989 book *A Burst of Light and Other Essays*, Black poet and activist Audre Lorde wrote, "Caring for myself is not self-indulgence. It is self-preservation, and that is an act of political warfare."[2] Lorde's ideas about self-care included race, gender, and class dynamics, and BIPOC people and queer communities embraced the concept as an action of defiance in a world that oppressed anyone with those identities. To try to preserve and care for yourself in a world that tries to tell you you're not valued and don't have the right to care is to assert yourself and your needs.

In this way, self-care is a practice of nurturing your physical, mental, and emotional health to prioritize and protect your well-being. Self-care is sometimes hard and can be painful, but in the long run it helps to keep you physically, mentally, and emotionally healthy. It includes a wide range of activities that you use to meet your needs, and, contrary to what you may see on social media, it's not all about bubble baths or massages or mani-pedis (although those things can be forms of self-care, too!). Self-care goes beyond superficial, feel-good activities and includes things like going to the doctor, eating consistently, setting boundaries, drinking water, budgeting money, or taking time to do nothing. Those may be more "boring" than the self-care we read about online, but in reality, these small, daily practices help us to improve and protect our physical, mental, and emotional well-being. As Rachel Helfferich, a non-diet dietitian and yoga teacher, said to me, "Self-care includes choosing what makes me feel good on a *soul level*."[3] Here are some other examples of self-care:

- **Physical:** Physical activity, resting when tired, eating nourishing foods, taking a shower, wearing clothes that fit comfortably
- **Mental:** Going to therapy, learning a new skill, meditating, spending time in nature
- **Emotional:** Spending time with friends or family, standing up for yourself, journaling, going to support group meetings

When thinking about self-care, it can be helpful to think about connecting to an inner caregiving part of yourself. Rebecca Scritchfield developed the Body Kindness® philosophy as a way to practice mindful self-care by cultivating your inner caregiver voice. She uses the term *spiraling up* to describe the process of making self-care choices that come from a place of love (rather than shame) and connection to your body, so you notice what you need and can make decisions that care for your well-being. "Choice by self-care choice, your mood and energy spiral up," Scritchfield writes.[4] "Choices that energize you and open you up, like an expanding spiral, and build positive emotions and a strong mindset one decision at a time."[5]

When you find yourself going downward into a "doom spiral," as one of my clients calls it, think about one self-care practice that you can do to help yourself begin to spiral up. Take getting enough sleep as an example. A part of you may want to continue watching TV or working late into the night while your inner caregiver recognizes the importance of rest, even when it's hard to stop what you're doing. Easing yourself into bed is a self-care choice that may help you feel more energized, clear-minded, and creative for the next day, hence "spiraling up." Although going to bed may seem simple enough, it can often be hard to care for yourself in the present moment when you also feel drawn to extend other activities for any reason.

"The practice of body kindness is a practice of being good to yourself. When you make feel-good choices, your energy spirals up," says Scritchfield. "You're happier and more emotionally resilient to the normal ups and downs of your day-to-day. This resilience strengthens you even more, preparing you to handle hard things that inevitably come up."[6] As Lorde said, self-care is self-preservation.

Build a Self-Care Toolbox

What is one physical, mental, and emotional self-care practice you can start regularly doing?

Schedule these self-care practices on your calendar to remind yourself to dedicate time each week to care for yourself.

Cultivating Coping Skills

Aside from taking part in regular self-care practices, it's important to cultivate multiple coping skills that you can use when you struggle in a more acute way. What are the signs that difficult things are coming up for you? What thoughts, feelings, behaviors, or sensations do you pick up on when things are not going so well? How do you cope with the stress, anxiety, or other emotions that arise? How do you take care of yourself when things feel difficult?

I ask these questions the first time I meet with my clients, and the vast majority of the time, I get a blank stare or a short laugh and a response along the lines of, "I don't really have any good coping strategies." Sometimes, people tell me they exercise to cope with stress but that it's the only tool in their arsenal. Others will tell me they emotionally eat, but that often it doesn't actually help them to feel better.

As you move through the process of healing your relationship to food and your body, difficult thoughts, feelings, and emotions are going to arise. Sitting with these can be uncomfortable and sometimes deeply painful. As one of my clients said to me, "Feeling my feelings sucks." She's not wrong; it can be really challenging to feel all the things, especially if you've been avoiding or distracting yourself from them. This is where you use coping skills: the strategies for responding to an emotion, stress, or trauma to help you tolerate, deal with, and process your emotions.

Positive Versus Maladaptive Coping Mechanisms

Not all coping skills are created equal. Coping mechanisms should help to relieve some of your suffering and can even be a temporary distraction, but you ideally are not using them as a way to completely avoid dealing with reality. When coping strategies become a crutch used to deny the problem, they can be maladaptive.

Maladaptive coping mechanisms are counterproductive. They may make you feel better in the short run but can cause bigger problems down the road and be harmful to your well-being. These strategies are also usually ineffective, meaning they don't actually make you feel better, or they don't help you to face the uncomfortable situation or emotion. Examples can include using alcohol or drugs to escape, withdrawing from people, exercising excessively, and restricting food or dieting. Dieting is commonly used as a way to cope because controlling food can provide a false sense of security and make someone feel better temporarily. However, we know that dieting and restricting do the opposite in the long term. Those things strip the pleasure away from food, disconnect us from our bodies, and cause us to feel worse over time.

Positive coping mechanisms, on the other hand, are those that help you to tolerate and deal with difficult feelings and situations. They can help you to get some space and feel better psychologically so that you can work through a tough situation or process difficult emotions. They allow you to "sit with" your discomfort so that you can move through it and come out the other side. Sometimes positive coping mechanisms are those familiar and safe routines that enable you to temporarily distract from difficult emotions, like binge-watching a favorite TV show or playing video games.

TV often gets a bad rap as a coping strategy, but it can be a really helpful way to relieve stress and anxiety. (True story: I once encouraged a client to play *more* video games when she was going through a difficult period.) Other examples of positive coping strategies include reading, writing, drawing, spending time outdoors, seeking support from friends or family, meditating, engaging in physical activity, deep breathing, listening to music, or eating.

When we are in the midst of a stressful situation or emotion, we tend to turn unconsciously to our unhelpful, maladaptive coping behaviors—even if we know that they don't work. My maladaptive coping behavior is what my partner calls "doom scrolling." When I'm feeling shitty, my go-to behavior is to whip out my phone and spend hours going down internet (usually Instagram) rabbit holes. While this feels good in the moment, after a few hours I feel even worse. However, when I'm already down and I have no bandwidth to come up with better options, my brain falls back to this already-wired connection of "feeling crappy $\longrightarrow$ scroll Instagram." Consequently, developing a coping plan before you run into a situation in which you need to use one is helpful, and often necessary.

Create a Coping Plan

A single coping strategy will not work for every emotion you feel or uncomfortable situation you go through. By cultivating multiple coping strategies, you can have different tools in your arsenal depending on what part of you needs attending to—body (physical or biological needs), mind (emotional needs), or heart (spiritual or community needs). Coping strategies can fall into several different buckets, including *connection, relaxation or calming, pleasure, movement or energizing,* and *release.* Depending on what you are feeling—and whether your body, mind, or heart needs attending to—you may find certain strategies more helpful than others.

Here are a few examples of each:[7]

- **Connection** (mind, heart): Call a family member; go out to dinner with a friend; play a game with your kids; play with a pet; visit a local coffee shop or bookstore to be around other people; explore a new area of town; pray; visit a local spiritual organization; look at pictures of people, places, or things that bring you joy; find a support group

- **Relaxation/calming** (body, mind): Meditate, do some deep breathing, use progressive muscle relaxation, give yourself a massage, light a nice-smelling candle, listen to music, read a book, color or draw, take a bath, put on a lotion that smells good, sit under a weighted blanket
- **Pleasure** (body, mind): Eat a favorite yummy food, put on a comfy sweater or cozy pajamas, sit outside in the sunshine, watch a funny television show, listen to an enjoyable podcast, watch adorable baby or animal videos online
- **Movement/energizing** (body): Take a walk, go for a run, put on music and dance, do some yoga or other stretches, clean the house, do the laundry (yes, chores count!), cook a nourishing meal, garden
- **Release** (body, mind, heart): Have a good cry, punch or scream into a pillow, journal or free write, dance it out to your favorite angsty music

Coping can also look like saying "no" and setting boundaries with work, family, and friends to prioritize your mental and emotional well-being. I'll be talking more about setting boundaries in Chapter 16.

Create a Coping Plan _____

Make a list of all of the coping strategies that you can try—including connection tools, relaxation tools, pleasure tools, movement tools, and release tools. Put the list somewhere where you can easily access or see it. The next time you are feeling down or upset, pull out the list and pick one of the tools. It will take some practice and experimenting, but over time you will get better at both identifying the emotion you're feeling and picking a strategy that you know will help you feel better.

Food as a Coping Mechanism

Emotional eating constantly gets a bad rap, but food *can* serve as a positive coping mechanism. The key is to try to use food in a way that helps you to feel better rather than just using it as a distraction or a way to numb your emotions. For food to be a helpful coping tool it generally needs to be

- Something you really enjoy eating
- Something you eat in a (somewhat) mindful way
- Free from guilt or shame

If you are using food to cope but don't pay attention to how it tastes, are mindlessly eating until you feel sick and uncomfortable, and/or are feeling guilty or ashamed after eating, then it is probably more of a maladaptive and ineffective coping strategy. Start by making a list of all of the foods that taste good and that you enjoy eating (never mind whether they are "healthy" or "allowed"; write down any food that comes to mind). For example, my list includes peanut butter cups; soft chocolate chip cookies; thick, chewy brownies; and Talenti gelato. The next time you choose to eat in response to an emotion, pick one food that you really love. Sit down with the food and pay attention to how it smells, how it feels in your mouth, and how it tastes. At the same time, use the tools I discussed in Chapter 6 to notice and reframe any negative, guilty voices so that you can feel more neutral about the food that you're eating. Remember, shame causes a stress response and can mitigate any positive feelings that the food would have given you. When you can eat a delicious food without a side of guilt and allow yourself to experience pleasure fully, it can help you cope with feelings in a positive way.

Do a Support System Inventory

Asking for help is not a sign of weakness but a strength. During difficult or stressful periods, having people that you can ask for help and who can provide emotional support is crucial. I touched on this earlier under *connection* coping tools, but it's important to specifically build out a support system of people you can talk to. This may include your partner, a family member, a friend, a therapist or counselor, a weight-inclusive dietitian, or another trusted health professional. Ideally, you'll have at least a handful of people you trust to be open and vulnerable with. Do an inventory:

- What support systems do you have in place?
- Which people in your life could offer you support if difficult things start to come up?
- In the event you need more support, what is your plan?

For example, my first line of support is to talk with my partner or my mother. If I can't reach either of them, I have a friend whom I trust and who is a really great listener. If I talk with these people and use some of my other coping strategies but still find that I'm struggling, my plan is to make an appointment with my therapist. If you do not have any close friends or family members who you can talk with, I recommend trying to find a counselor, therapist, or support group. Check out Psychologytoday.com for listings of therapists, teletherapy options, support groups, and treatment centers.

Bring Your Feelings to Light

Once you have a coping plan and support system in place, you can begin to allow those deep, dark feelings and shame stories to come to light. When you bring these thoughts, feelings, and beliefs to the surface, you can face them, feel them, grieve, and begin to let go of the feelings and heal. Now, if you're used to avoiding or distracting from your feelings, initially, you may find it hard to identify what emotions you are experiencing. That is okay; it takes patience, practice, and a willingness to sit in the suck.

Our bodies tell us a lot of information about our emotional world and our deeper experiences. When we can connect to our bodies, they can be a conduit through which we feel our emotions and explore our fears. When you notice emotions arising, reflect upon the following:

- What sensations do you feel in your body when you experience that emotion?
- Where do you feel those sensations?

If you're unsure, try doing a head-to-toe body scan, checking in with each body part to see how it feels. For example, one of my clients noticed that anxiety and stress provoked the sensation of something feeling lodged in her chest. Another client felt a thickness in her throat, and a third felt an uncomfortable sensation in her belly. One woman found that anxiety and excitement felt similar in her body, like a jumpy sensation. Yet when she explored more, she noticed that happy emotions, like excitement, meant she used her hands, whereas unhappy emotions, like anxiety, meant her limbs felt more weighed down.

This practice can be done for both happy, pleasant emotions as well as sad, painful ones. If you are struggling to stay with your body while experiencing uncomfortable emotions, try it first when you experience happy feelings. As you begin to understand how your body communicates, you can figure out what emotion or feeling you're experiencing.

Unpack, Explore, and Dialogue

I received a message on Instagram from a woman who said, "I've realized that the reason I want to be thin is because I want to be admired for being beautiful. I'm guessing this is a completely normal desire, but it's holding me back from being accepting of my body as it is right now. What can I do to stop feeling this way?"

As I shared in Chapter 5, start by unpacking and exploring where this desire came from. Yes, it's understandable that someone would want to be beautiful and admired for it because our society places a premium on thinness and youthfulness and equates that with beauty (especially in women). But try to go deeper. Think back to childhood: Why might those beliefs have started to form? What did you see? What did you experience? What were you taught (explicitly or implicitly)?

Engaging in an inner dialogue can also help to get at the root of why you feel that way. A great way to practice this is by using the *if/then exercise*, something I learned from Fiona Sutherland and Marci Evans in their Body Image Training for Clinicians course.[8] In the case of the woman who messaged me, she would say, "If I was beautiful and admired, then _____." Continue the pattern with at least four more "if _____" statements and "then _____" answers; move each "then" response you landed on into the next "if" spot.

Here's an example from Adriana, a client I've worked with. Initial thought/feeling: I'm afraid of staying at this size.

If I stay at this size, **then** I won't be able to fit into my clothes.

If I'm not able to fit into my clothes, **then** I'll feel insecure about myself.

If I feel insecure about myself, **then** I'll be unhappy.

If I'm unhappy, **then** I'll go back to comparing myself to other people.

If I compare myself to other people, **then** I won't feel worthy.

If I don't feel worthy, **then** I won't put myself out there.

If I don't put myself out there, **then** I will end up alone and will never have a partner.

On the surface, Adriana believed her fear of not losing weight was about her ability to fit into her clothes, but when we dug deeper, she discovered that it was really about her desire for a life partner. As we continued our discussion, she realized that deep down, she was feeling biological and social pressure to meet someone and have children—even though she wasn't sure she wanted kids. Talking about this was very emotional for Adriana, and she'd never actually said any of it out loud before. But by bringing her fear to the surface and sitting with it instead of trying to "fix" her body, she was able to connect more deeply with herself. About a year after this initial conversation, Adriana said, "It was scary to reveal all of those things that I had held inside of me for so long. But by doing so, I began to question all of the things I thought I 'should' want and have now been able to explore what it is that I *actually* want. It has been terrifying, and I have shed many tears, but I have also never felt so much joy."

Exploring Your Feelings

What are some uncomfortable feelings that you are having about your body? Use the if/then exercise to come up with at least five if-then statements. What is really at the root of this feeling?

Processing Body Grief

When I met Elena she had discovered intuitive eating the previous year after dieting for several decades. She had begun to find a more peaceful relationship to food but was still struggling with her body image. Elena had grown up an extremely good athlete in a fit, conventionally attractive body. "For so long, beauty and athleticism were the tools with which I navigated the world," she shared with me. "Now, both of those things are going away; at fifty-six years old, I'm no longer considered a beautiful woman, and my body is not athletic." Elena realized that beauty and athletic ability were crutches that she had relied on for many years, and now that they were gone, she wanted to develop a new skill set for navigating the world in her current body. Before she could do that, she needed to mourn the loss of her younger body and sit with what it means to be middle-aged in a changing body that no longer felt like her own.

Grief is defined as deep, sharp sorrow and mental suffering or distress over loss.[9] It can encompass a range of feelings, everything from deep sadness to anger, denial, and even regret. In her 2008 paper, "Size Acceptance as a Grief Process: Observations from Psychotherapy with Lesbian Feminists," Jeanne Courtney, wrote

> *As women let go of the idea of control, we experience loss. We lose any hope of making ourselves exempt from social and internalized contempt for imperfect bodies. We lose hope for the social and economic rewards promised to thin women. We lose the belief that we can eliminate health or mobility problems with weight loss, especially troubling when medical practitioners have offered it as a single, simplistic strategy. On a primitive level, we lose an exhilarating, grandiose fantasy that somehow, someday, through willpower and self-deprivation, we can gain absolute control over how our bodies look, how they feel, and what they can do.*[10]

As we process the reality that we can't control our bodies and face the fact that we may never achieve an "ideal" body, the feeling of loss can bring about grief. This sense of grief is magnified for those who live in bodies that are routinely marginalized. When you live in a society that deems fat (and Black or Brown, disabled, gender nonconforming, and aging) bodies "wrong" and oppresses people who hold those identities, giving up on attempting to force yourself into fitting into an arbitrary, Eurocentric beauty and body standard is not an easy thing to do. For some people, changing their body may be a matter of survival. As one of my clients living in a very fat body shared, she was grieving the fact that she would never be respected as much or treated as well by others as she had been when she was in a smaller body. For people navigating chronic illness or gender nonconformity, accepting a body that brings constant pain or doesn't look like who you know yourself to be can feel impossible.

Processing body grief acknowledges all of these realities. Finding your way back to body acceptance does not mean that any fatphobia, ableism, ageism, homo- and transphobia, racism, or sexism you've experienced is okay. But by processing your feelings, you can honor them and move past them, finding new belief systems and taking actions that best serve you and the life you want to live. Doing so entails noticing your feelings of loss and hopelessness, connecting to those emotions, and holding space to feel those feelings while finding ways to cope as you move through the process.

Notice: Using mindfulness skills, notice what thoughts arise when you think about not dieting and no longer striving for the thin ideal. What comes up when you think of sitting with not trying to change your current body? Knowing that permanent weight loss is not possible for most people, how does that make you feel?

Connect: What emotions do you feel when these thoughts arise? Where do you feel it in your body? What does it feel like?

Feel: Try to sit with these uncomfortable emotions without trying to distract or numb. Where do these feelings originate from? How have you felt them in the past? Do you remember the first time you felt this way? What beliefs have you internalized that contribute to these feelings? Journaling or talking aloud to a trusted person or therapist may help you process and work through some of these feelings.

Cope: What can you do to mitigate some of the discomfort you're feeling?

Exploring Body Grief

When I asked Elena to notice what came up for her when she thought about never getting back to her previous body, the first thing she mentioned was that she felt "gross" and uncomfortable in her current body. It was hard for her to connect with her emotions about this, and she said that she often just pushed these feelings aside without dealing with them. With my encouragement, she practiced sitting with her feelings of discomfort in her body and unpacking exactly what that meant and felt like to her.

Elena's discomfort of "my body feels so gross" was a concrete example of what it felt like to be in her body, yet it was so much more complex than that. As we explored it some more, Elena realized that beneath the "gross" feeling was a fear of aging, of losing her identity as a young, beautiful, athletic woman. Along with this, she was in the midst of a big life transition because many of her friends had moved away, her job had shifted to be a work-from-home situation, and her kids no longer lived close by. She wanted to meet new people but felt self-conscious and was worried about others judging her for her body size and age.

Elena's feelings about her changing body did not magically improve overnight. However, as she opened up and allowed herself to feel vulnerable and expose her deeper fears, she began the process of moving through body grief.

Let's walk through another example of this using my client Nari, a thirty-eight-year-old who had let go of her disordered eating behaviors and had been honoring her inner body wisdom by eating enough and eating what she wanted. Several months into our work together, she was in the midst of "sitting in the suck" and grieving the loss of the body that she always thought she would someday "achieve." Here was what Nari shared with me as she worked through letting go of trying to fit herself into society's arbitrary thin body ideal:

Notice: My fantasy body has always been something a little curvier, with big boobs and a butt, full hair, smoky eye makeup, and red lipstick. But always with a flat stomach. I really fantasized about looking sexy. Or, I suppose, what the media and society have deemed as "sexy." I want to exude sex, energy, liveliness, and passion. In my head, those things go together—and only can happen if I'm in a thin body. When I look in the mirror, I instead see someone who is dumpy, pudgy, and tired.

Connect: While I'm starting to feel more neutral about my body, I'm sad that I'll never be that "glamorous" ideal that I've always wanted. When I think about that, I feel a tightness in my chest and in my throat—it feels a little scary. But also, I'm pissed at the people (aka society and the media) who've told me I need to be in a smaller body in order to be happy or accepted. Fuck them. When I get angry, I notice my breath quickens, and my hands reflexively ball into fists. But I'm still sad, too. It feels like a weighed-down, heavier kind of sensation. Like I'm holding a lot in.

Feel: I've had this internal fantasy ideal for as long as I can remember—probably elementary school or middle school. While part of me wants to not feel so shackled by what I think I must do or must look like, in my head that also involves being thin. I guess that makes sense, though—all the advertisements I saw where beautiful, glamorous young women in thin bodies were riding off into the sunset without a care in the world. Everything I internalized, from my family to the media I consumed, linked together a small body and an ideal, happy, successful person. Logically, I know I don't need a thin body to feel free, but it's really hard to separate the two.

Cope: I talked about this in therapy and cried a lot, which helped me let go of a lot of the tightness and heaviness I was holding in. Walking my dog in the park also helped me feel better. He was so happy and excited to run around that I couldn't help but smile. It felt nice to connect and spend time with him. Plus, moving my body helped me to get some of my emotions out as well.

Exploring Body Grief _____

How would life change for you if you were in a smaller body?

What do you need to grieve about your current body, your old body, and/or perhaps never having a body that society deems "acceptable"? Make a list.

Stages of Grief

Moving through grief is not a linear process; it's not something you "do" and then never deal with again. While the discomfort body grief brings can certainly lessen over time, there will still be waves of grief brought on by certain experiences. As one client said to me, "I wish I could just grieve and move on! Instead I grieve, feel neutral about my body for a while, then have something happen that causes me to feel intense self-loathing. Then I get pissed off at the patriarchy, grieve, and feel neutral again."

The Five Stages of Grief model was developed in 1969 by Elisabeth Kubler-Ross as a way to explain the experience of bereavement. The model has since been adapted to describe other forms of grief. The five stages, as described by Kubler-Ross, include denial, anger, bargaining, depression, and acceptance. In the paper I mentioned earlier, Jeanne Courtney applied the five stages of grief to the process a woman goes through when she discovers the concept of body size acceptance and lets go of society's fatphobic thin beauty ideal. I was first introduced to Jeanne's work in a blog post entitled "Body Acceptance Begins with Grieving the Thin Ideal" by Meredith Noble, a food and body peace coach.[11]

I find the stages of grief model to be a helpful illustration of how *knowing* our anti-fat beliefs and *recognition* of our biases about race, gender, weight, and health is not enough to find peace with our bodies. Intellectually knowing and understanding these concepts only gets you so far. You can learn about how our culture's racist beliefs were what led to widespread fatphobia and understand how the thin beauty ideal serves to keep anyone with a marginalized identity oppressed and in line, but you may still desire weight loss. Let's take a closer look at how each of the stages of grief can apply to the process of letting go of dieting and finding body acceptance.

Stage 1: Denial

When first learning about the insidious roots of diet culture and the lies we've been told about weight loss and health, it's common to reject these ideas. Kubler-Ross describes this denial as the "No, not me" and the "It cannot be true" stage. It's hard to believe that these truths about diet culture and body size might be accurate because it's so counter to mainstream beliefs about health and well-being. In some ways, denial functions as a form of coping. If you deny that any of this is true, then you don't have to deal with the inevitable pain and sorrow that will arise from processing the reality of what you've been taught about your body. In this stage, you may continue to diet despite understanding that long-term weight loss is not possible for the vast majority of people. You may still be focusing on external cues to dictate what you should and should not eat and are disconnected from your body and your feelings. Although part of you may be beginning to process all of the harm that diet culture has inflicted, it's often easy to turn back toward dieting and attempting to "control" your body because it's all you know.

Stage 2: Anger

As you start to process the fact that dieting doesn't work long term for weight loss and that it is the probable cause of your disconnected relationship to food and your body, you may feel angry at yourself. "No, not me" gives way to "Why me?" During this stage, I often hear women beating themselves up for ever starting to diet, blaming themselves for their food and body issues and thinking "Why did I ever diet and do this to myself?"

At this point, when you notice anger turning inward, it's important to remind yourself that you are not to blame for falling into the diet cycle. The blame can be placed squarely on our patriarchal, white-supremacist society that breeds diet culture and taught you that to be worthy and accepted, you needed to be in a small body. It is not your fault that you spent so much time, energy, and money trying to change yourself; it's diet culture's fault. This is where you can turn that anger toward the incredibly messed up culture that got you here. The anger stage is a really important part of the grief process when you learn to show yourself compassion and then get mad as hell at the society that taught you that your body was wrong. Get angry at the white men that long ago set standards by which all women are judged. Get angry at the $70 billion diet culture that has profited from your body hatred. Get angry at the lies that fatphobic media tells about weight loss and health. Feel that anger, express that anger, and process that anger. And remind yourself that this is not your fault.

Stage 3: Bargaining

As the anger wears off, you are left with the pain of grief. At this stage, you may have seen how hard it will be to move away from diet culture. You may have started to let go of dieting but are now feeling out of control and scared. This is where some people may decide to try *just one more diet* and think "Once I lose weight, I'll try intuitive eating." You may begin to negotiate—to try to come up with something that isn't as "bad" as dieting but isn't as hard as completely giving up on weight loss. Some people tell themselves they are dieting for health reasons or that they'll just try to "eat healthier" to "feel better" when the real underlying motivation is weight loss—and a sense of control. Even if you've done some processing of your body grief, there may still be a part of you that really wants to be thin. In the bargaining phase, part of you may believe that losing weight will help you feel better, happier, and less ashamed. You may be remembering times when you had success losing weight while forgetting (or refusing to think about) how awful you felt during that time.

Stage 4: Depression

This stage is when reality sinks in. It's becoming clear that bargaining is not an option. Feelings of hopelessness can arise when you realize that you may never have the body you've always hoped for or the one that society has taught you that you "should" have. You may feel a lot of sadness when you reflect on the time, effort, energy, and money you've spent trying to be thin and all that you've missed out on because of diet culture. Depression can arise when you face the reality that, even if you can accept your body, you still will be living in a racist, sexist, fatphobic world, which is not an easy place to exist. Some people find themselves retreating inward during this stage as they process their feelings of grief related to having to accept their current body and having to do so in a society that judges and oppresses fat bodies.

Stage 5: Acceptance

In this fifth stage, you stop resisting your body and instead begin to accept it. It's not that you no longer feel pain or sadness; it's that you are no longer trying to change things. You come to terms with the idea that attempting to force yourself to fit into society's standards of what is "acceptable" won't be freeing or liberating and won't help you embrace or connect to your body. You accept that dieting doesn't work and start to work with your body instead of against it. Part of this acceptance phase also includes acknowledging the rampant anti-fat, anti-Black, ableist, sexist attitudes in our society. Body acceptance doesn't exist in a vacuum. We can do the internal work but also need to understand the systems in place to police and oppress our bodies. This is why so many folks who are working on their own body acceptance also get involved in social justice activism. Because until *all bodies* are liberated, no one is free.

Most people do not move linearly through the stages of grief. While the process is different for everybody, the lines between each of the stages are often blurred, and going back to earlier stages is common. You may have days where you feel accepting of your body, and then other days where you fall back into depression or bargaining. This is a completely normal part of the body acceptance process.

How to "Sit With" Your Feelings

Processing our body grief involves learning to sit with—rather than push away—difficult emotions. You can use the four mindfulness steps that I shared in Chapter 6 to help you sit with, explore, and move through whatever emotions are coming up for you.

1. Notice that you're feeling an emotion. Don't try to change the way you feel or judge yourself for it. Judgment distracts from feeling the actual emotion and prevents you from processing it. If you notice any judgment arise, acknowledge it and set it aside.

2. Create a "pause" and shift your attention: identify the emotion and acknowledge that you are feeling that way. Notice where you feel the emotion in your body. What does it feel like? Does that sensation change over time?

3. Get curious: What might be causing you to feel this way? What happened now, or in the past, that made you feel this way? What beliefs or assumptions do you have that led you to feel this way? Where did those beliefs come from?

4. Notice any negative self-talk, self-shaming, or judgment and respond with self-compassion. Validate and accept your emotions. Remind yourself that it is okay to feel this way and that emotions aren't permanent; it will pass. Ask, "What do I need right now?" and consider using one of your coping mechanisms.

As you bring your feelings to light, practice letting them flow through you. Don't try to hold on to the emotion or attach to it. Instead, ride the emotion like a wave, feeling all the feelings and then releasing them. If you feel anxious about getting carried away with uncomfortable emotions, practice dropping anchor using the technique that I described in Chapter 6. When a storm of emotions is swirling, dropping anchor allows you to feel grounded and not get overwhelmed by your feelings. This technique can help you remain in the present moment and sit with your feelings rather than avoiding them or pushing them away.

Try practicing with less intense emotions first. The more you practice, the more capacity you will have to sit with the tougher, more uncomfortable feelings. In addition to dropping anchor, it may also be helpful to move while you are processing your emotions. Some people find it helpful to go for a walk or fidget and shake their bodies a bit. Emotions are stored in your body, so movement can help to discharge them. It can also be helpful to do some journaling and write down what it is that you are feeling. Often, we get caught up in our heads, so getting the feelings out on paper can help to release and process them.

Feeling your feelings can be really tough. But the more you can allow yourself to feel them, sit with them, and explore them—without pushing them away—the quicker they will dissipate. All feelings are impermanent; none will last forever. As you work through your feelings over time, you'll gain confidence that you can ride out the storm and make it to the other side. The next time a painful emotion arises, you'll remember that—although it feels awful in the moment—you *can* get through it. The more you go with your feelings, rather than against them, the more practice and trust you will build. You *can* do hard things. In the next chapter, you'll learn a skill that will help as you practice sitting with your feelings.

CHAPTER 11

The Power of Self-Compassion

During moments of pain and discomfort, it often can feel easier to run away rather than sit and deal with what is going on. Self-compassion is a tool you can use to *be with* yourself and your uncomfortable feelings rather than distracting from or avoiding them. In the simplest terms, self-compassion involves treating oneself with kindness rather than criticism or judgment.

For many of us, that is easier said than done. Any misstep, mistake, or perceived "failing" is met with internal commentary from a loud, angry, judgmental inner critic. This is the critical internal voice that says things like

- You're such a terrible person.
- You're so stupid.
- You look awful.
- There's something wrong with you.
- You'll never be successful.

This inner voice often criticizes who you are and how you behave, including commenting on your emotions, appearance, food choices, intelligence, and work ability. Even when you try to push it away, the voice can persist as nagging thoughts that you are not "good enough." The inner critic voice often leads to feelings of shame, low self-esteem, and self-doubt, which can undermine your ability to connect fully with yourself and others.

Why do we find it so hard to stop beating ourselves up?

Development of the Inner Critic Voice

Earlier in the book, I shared how some of our most basic survival instincts exist to ensure our social group accepts us. Thousands of years ago, to be rejected and abandoned by others was literally a matter of life or death. Although that's not so anymore, the development of a self-critical voice can be seen as a type of safety behavior designed to ensure acceptance within one's social group.

This process begins during childhood as children receive feedback from their caregivers. A child's inner critic voice is shaped based on the ways they are spoken to and the feedback they receive, whether loving and encouraging or angry and critical. These words are imprinted in their minds. For people raised with critical caregivers, those criticisms can quickly become internalized. Children learn that to protect themselves from criticism, they need to ensure there is nothing to attack. The self-critical voice begins to develop to keep them "in line," preventing them from making mistakes and thereby being criticized. Given that children are dependent on their caregivers for survival, this inner critic voice likely did serve them at one point in time. One of my clients grew up in an abusive household and realized that her inner critic kept her under the radar and out of trouble so she could remain safe as a kid. Another client shared that, by criticizing herself first, her parent's inevitable criticism didn't hurt quite as badly.

This latter example is evident when many of us, as full-grown adults, continue to apologize for ourselves. The classic preface of, "I have a stupid question," or, "I know this is silly," can serve to blunt our sense of inevitable criticism. When it comes to appearance, many women feel the need to apologize for how they look by saying, "I didn't have any time to get ready or do my hair; I'm such a mess today." I can't count the number of times I've heard, "I'm sorry I didn't have time to put on makeup before our call," during the many video calls I've had as a clinician over the years. If we beat others to the punch and put ourselves down before they get a chance to criticize us, we may not feel as embarrassed.

Western society also plays a role in both the development and maintenance of our inner critics. In a society that stresses individualism, perfectionism, and binary thinking (all characteristics of white supremacy culture),[1] it is common to point out how someone is wrong, bad, or inadequate. Making a mistake becomes a shameful personal failure, rather than something to learn and grow from. Capitalism demands productivity and output, so perfectionism is rewarded. When we see the "best" get rewarded and appreciated, the focus becomes competition rather than collaboration, and perfectionistic tendencies are further honed. Yet this perfectionist mindset is what continues to breed our inner critics; when things are not "good enough," we feel we have no one to blame but ourselves. In this way, the adult inner critic becomes a tool of capitalism and white supremacy, functioning to keep everyone "in line" by perfecting, producing more and more, and ensuring continued progress and wealth accumulation for those at the top.

Self-criticism can also arise out of a person's desire for control. In a society that grooms us to feel personally responsible for all of our failures, we learn that falling short of perfection is something that *can* and *should* be avoided. The inner critic voice can then serve as a mechanism of control—if we can just keep ourselves from screwing up, others won't think we are failures, and we'll be accepted.

Although your inner critic may have served to keep you protected and safe at certain points in your life, chances are it's become vastly unhelpful in other areas. Perhaps your inner critic stops you from being vulnerable with others, taking chances at work, or speaking up to set boundaries. Consider how that inner critic has been harmful to you—both in life in general, but also specifically related to your relationship to food and your body. "My critical voice is always telling me that in order to be good, successful, loved, and happy, I have to be in a thinner body," one client told me. "It helped me in certain ways when I was a child, but as an adult, all it's done is disconnect me from my body, isolate me from friends and family, and held me back from doing what I really want in life."

Understanding how your inner critic voice developed and how it may have helped or protected you in the past can allow you to have compassion for it—and for yourself.

Explore Your Inner Critic _____

What contributed to the development of your inner critic voice?

What are some of the common words or phrases that your inner critic says?

Does your inner critic voice sound like anyone you know?

How might your inner critic have helped you in the past?

How has your inner critic held you back or harmed you?

Evolution of the Food Police Voice

A specific type of inner critic voice is referred to in the book *Intuitive Eating* as the *food police*.[2] The food police voice comes from all of the externally driven rules and beliefs about food that have become internalized deep within your brain. This voice judges what you eat, when you eat, and how you eat. The food police voice sets the rules by which anything you eat (or don't eat) is judged. These rules pop up daily as the food police voice monitors your food decisions, like declaring you "good" for eating a salad and "bad" for choosing the burger. Other common food police thoughts may include

- No eating after a certain time at night.
- You already had a cookie last night; you can't have another today.
- I know your stomach is growling, but it's not time to eat yet; you have to wait for dinner.
- You can't have that bagel; it has way too many carbs.
- That meal was too big—better make sure you go to the gym to burn it off.
- You ate a sandwich for lunch, so no bread at dinner.
- You've eaten so well this week—you deserve that dessert.

Although some of these rules might not *seem* bad, they can be harmful because they use external factors rather than internal ones to dictate food choices. Even if you're not dieting, your inner food police voice is still around and usually causes mental restriction. These daily reminders make it tough to view eating as a normal, pleasurable activity. Instead, any time you eat becomes a situation in which you've either succeeded or failed. Choose a salad for lunch, and you've been "good." Have fries with your burger, and you're "bad." This food police voice sets impossible standards and, when you "break a rule," sets you up for overeating (as in the "what the hell—the day is already shot; I might as well just keep eating" thought).

Just as you didn't come into the world with the inner critic voice, you are not born with this judgy food police voice. This inner monologue develops through exposure to years of diet culture messages, whether through family, friends, healthcare professionals, or the media. The more diets you try, the more rules you internalize. Many people come to me exasperated and at their wit's end. They've tried many diets with food rules that completely contradict one another, and they now have no idea what to eat. Learning to notice and then reframe the food police voice allows you to make food choices based on *your body's* health and satisfaction rather than on external diet rules or deprivation. I'll share more about how to reframe your food police voice later on in this chapter.

Bring Awareness to Your Food Police _____

Spend one day keeping track of any food police thoughts that pop into your head. Write down any words or phrases that the food police voice says that try to dictate what, when, or how you eat. Do you notice any patterns?

Are You "Shoulding" All Over Yourself?

Another common way the inner critic shows up is through "shoulds":

- I should exercise more.
- I should lose X pounds.
- I should be better at this.
- I should do my hair.
- I should be productive today.
- I should put on makeup.
- I should settle down.
- I should meditate more.
- I should drink less.

- I should spend more time with my kids.
- I should be happier.

These "shoulds" often stem from societal beliefs that you have internalized. The main message behind them is that you're not good enough, and you need to be better. It's a type of binary thinking—I should or I shouldn't—that then becomes "rules" that must be followed. The outcome of binary thinking tends to be one of two things: It goes well, and we feel righteous; it doesn't work out, and we feel like a failure. There is no space to exist in the gray area in between.

"Shoulds" can lead to disconnection from yourself, your body, and your values. When you spend so much time listening to the "shoulds," it becomes difficult to distinguish what you really *want*. Often, what you think you *should want* is very different than what you *actually want*. This is true with food decisions, but it can also be the case with so much more in your life. As one woman said to me, "At first, this journey was all about rewriting my relationship to food and my body. Then it became about how I was spending my time and what I enjoyed doing. I realized that I'm more of an introvert and allowed myself to stay home rather than listen to the voice that said I 'should' go out. Now, I'm at the point where I'm questioning all of the things I thought I 'should' want: Do I even want a long-term partnership? Do I want kids? All these things I thought I had no choice in, and that I thought were necessary for a 'happy ending,' I'm now realizing that is not the case."

By determining the difference between *should* and *want,* you can figure out who you *really are* underneath all of the societal expectations of who you *should be*. You then get to decide how you *want* to live.

Bring Awareness to Your "Shoulds" _____

Spend one day keeping track of your "should" thoughts. Any time you have a "should" (or "shouldn't") thought, write it down. At the end of the day review the list. What themes or patterns do you notice?

The Lie of Laziness

It used to be really hard for me to do nothing. For years, if I wasn't working, reading, going to the gym, spending time with friends, or doing anything I deemed "productive," I felt lazy. And *lazy* was synonymous with *bad*. Much of my self-worth was tied up in my ability to multitask and how much I was producing. If I was lazy, then I wasn't doing enough. If I wasn't *doing enough*, then I *wasn't enough*.

Grind culture perpetuates this idea that if we are not hustling and busy every minute of the day, then something is wrong with us. At the root of these beliefs: capitalism and white supremacy. Productivity is at the heart of capitalism: If you aren't producing, you're not of value. This is one of the reasons why ageism is so rampant in Western culture; young folks are more valued in a capitalistic society because they can produce more. People who work sixty-, seventy-, eighty-hour weeks are not just normalized; they are often celebrated. Being able to function on just a few hours of sleep is seen as something brag-worthy. Multitasking is a superpower. "If I'm not doing two things at once, it feels like a waste of time," a woman said to me recently.

Tricia Hersey founded The Nap Ministry in 2016 and embraces napping as a political act. Hersey, a Black speaker, performance artist, preacher, and activist writes, "The everyday pace of our culture is not healthy, sustainable, nor liberative. We are living and participating in violence via a machine-level pace of functioning. This toxic space has been accepted as the norm. Anyone who goes against this pace is living as an outlier and a risk-taker."[3] Any form of rest is therefore seen as lazy. "Rest is a form of resistance because it disrupts and pushes back against capitalism and white supremacy," says Hersey.[4]

When you feel lazy, what is it that you are really worried about? Recently, I dug into this with a client who realized that her desire not to be "lazy" came from her constant need to please others and not wanting to look like a failure. "In order to be successful, I have to do everything: do my job well, keep the house clean, cook the best dinner, keep my body looking good. I have to be a wonder woman." Another woman I worked with told me that she was afraid if she let herself take a break, she'd go to the extreme and never get off the couch. These are the lies that our society tells us to keep us productive. In a society that rewards productivity and constantly sends the message that we are not enough, it's no wonder so many of us struggle with "shoulds."

In reality, allowing yourself to listen to your body and to rest when you need to is an act of self-care and kindness. Resting can be a way of honoring your body. You don't need to earn rest or justify why you are resting. And you don't need to feel guilty when you skip the gym, sleep in, or have a day when you do absolutely nothing "productive." Sleep and rest *is* productive. As Hersey says, "This is not just about naps. It's about trying to disrupt and dismantle a toxic system that says you're not enough."[5]

Practice Resting

I realize it may sound funny to think about "practicing" rest, but if you're like most people, you're probably not really resting. If you're watching TV while checking email or listening to music and doing the dishes, you're not resting. Schedule small amounts of time to rest each day and larger chunks of time to rest over a week. For example, try to schedule ten- to fifteen-minute breaks several times throughout the day. Then, a few times per week, allow yourself to rest several hours at a time. When I say "rest," I don't necessarily mean that you have to lie down and nap, although you can certainly do that. Resting is doing anything that you enjoy but that is not you being "productive" in the classic sense—e.g., reading, lying outside and watching the clouds, listening to music, playing video games, or watching a favorite TV show.

How Self-Compassion Can Help

Although your self-critical voice may have developed during a time of need, in the long run, it breeds shame. Shame is what creeps in and makes you feel like *something is wrong with me*, or *I'll never be good enough*. Criticism and shame lead to pain, disconnection, and isolation, getting in the way of any meaningful growth or change.

When your inner critic voice pipes up, it can generate cortisol, one of the stress hormones, and launch you into a fight-or-flight stress situation. When a stress response occurs, it is really difficult to move forward in a helpful, positive way. This is where self-compassion comes in. Kindness, not hate, breeds connection, happiness, and self-growth. Research has found that people with strong self-compassion skills have more of some qualities and less of others, as shown in the following chart:

More	Less
Coping skills	Perfectionism
Resilience to stress	Anxiety
Intrinsic motivation	Depression
Positive health behaviors	Self-criticism
Body appreciation	Fear of failure
Personal accountability	Rumination
Likelihood to try again after a mistake	Neuroticism
Empathy and compassion	Feelings of shame

In terms of body image, research has found that being kind, compassionate, and understanding toward oneself can decrease dieting and disordered eating behaviors, lower body shame, decrease body comparisons, and improve body appreciation.[6] People with strong self-compassion skills inherently believe that their self-worth is *not* contingent upon their appearance, and they are less likely to internalize the thin body ideal. In other words, self-compassion is essential to improving your relationship to food, your body, *and* yourself.

The Three Components of Self-Compassion

In the book *Self-Compassion: The Proven Power of Being Kind to Yourself,* Dr. Kristin Neff explains how self-compassion has three core elements: mindfulness, self-kindness, and common humanity.[7] There was a reason I put the chapter on mindfulness before this chapter about self-compassion. If you aren't aware of how you speak to yourself, then it is much more difficult to shift your inner voice from a critical one to a more compassionate one. The *mindfulness* piece of self-compassion involves noticing and bringing awareness to your inner thoughts and feelings. It requires you to notice any painful feelings that arise as you observe them nonjudgmentally rather than getting caught up in the thoughts. It's only after you notice and acknowledge your inner thoughts and the pain and shame they bring that you can then practice responding kindly.

The second element of self-compassion is *self-kindness*. Once you are aware of your inner negative, critical, unhelpful thoughts, you can speak or act toward yourself in a warm, kind, gentle way. You may find this difficult because, in all likelihood, your self-critical voice has gotten a lot of work over the years, whereas your self-compassionate voice has not. One helpful technique is to think of speaking or responding to yourself and your thoughts as you would to a friend who was going through a similar experience. What would you say to a friend who messed up or made a mistake? My guess is that it would *not* be, "Wow, you are such a failure; no wonder you can't [get a job, lose weight, find a partner]." Most of us say cruel, hurtful words and phrases to ourselves all of the time, yet we would never dream of saying them to another person we care about. As you practice speaking more kindly to yourself, it can often help to conjure up the voice of a loving family member or friend. One of my clients, when she was first working on strengthening her own self-compassionate voice, found it helpful to think about what I would say to her or what her grandmother would say to her. For a while, the woman would have our voices pop into her head to say kind things until she began to develop her own self-compassionate voice. Later in this chapter, I'll share some ways you can practice responding to critical thoughts with kind ones.

The last component of self-compassion is *common humanity*. Shame thrives in secrecy, and if we isolate or hide when we experience pain, then it can feel like we alone are suffering. When you can remind yourself that *all* humans make mistakes, that *all* humans fail (or are made to feel as though they are failing), and that *all* humans experience pain, it can help quiet your inner judgy voice. No one is perfect, and no one should expect to be perfect. The experiences you go through are not happening to you alone; others are feeling and experiencing similar things. Instead of keeping your pain inside, opening up and sharing your vulnerabilities to a safe, trusted person can help you experience this feeling of common humanity. I see this occur daily in an online community that I moderate. Members are often nervous about speaking up, and they feel like they are the "only ones" experiencing what they are going through. Yet immediately after posting, a chorus of people comment and chime in with some version of, "I feel this way all of the time, too!" As one of the members posted recently, "I've felt so alone this past year as I've tried to work on body acceptance. Everywhere I turn, diet culture is there. I'm so grateful to have found this group for support." I'll share more about cultivating community in Chapter 13, but for now, continue to tell yourself, "I am not alone in this experience; we all suffer."

Common Misconceptions of Self-Compassion

At this point you may be thinking, "But if I'm easy on myself, I'll just let myself off the hook." Most people think that they need to be hard on themselves, or else they'll never accomplish anything. Self-compassion can feel like giving up or making excuses. One client of mine was adamant that if she weren't tough on herself, she would never exercise. "I need that critical voice in order to stay on track and stay motivated," she told me. When we did more exploration, she realized that the harsh inner voice caused her to feel so stressed and anxious that she would shut down, turn on the TV, and just zone out. Being hard on herself wasn't actually helping her to be more active; it had the opposite effect.

Criticism and shame are not good motivators for changes. I once heard someone say, "You can't take good care of something you hate." Although shame and judgment may motivate you in the short run, over the long haul, they create stress and disconnection in your body and can keep you feeling stuck. In contrast, self-compassion is linked with more intrinsic, or internal, motivation. Self-compassion isn't being "easy" on yourself, and it doesn't mean you are being "weak." In fact, it's just the opposite: People with strong self-compassion skills can put things into greater perspective and are grounded in a strong sense of who they are. In other words, self-compassion can help you to feel better about yourself *without* having to compare yourself to anyone else and *without* needing external validation (or fearing external judgment).

This is why self-compassion is different than self-esteem. As Neff explains in her widely viewed TED Talk, "Self-esteem is a global evaluation of self-worth."[8] It becomes a binary judgment of "am I a good person or a bad person?" You can make this evaluation only if you compare yourself to another person, which means to have high self-esteem, you need to feel as though you are *better than others* in some way. As Neff shares, this is not a helpful thing because we only feel good about ourselves if we meet some "ideal" standard; otherwise, we've failed and have low self-esteem. When it comes to body image, in a culture that has created an unrealistic beauty ideal, we're basically screwed if we try to measure up against it. Our self-esteem is contingent upon how we measure up to others, so it ends up always fluctuating depending on whether we are doing "well" compared to some arbitrary standard set by society.

In contrast, self-compassion requires no external comparison to others. It holds that all humans are worthy—"flaws" and all. By embracing this fact, we can seek personal growth without fear of failure and without holding others back. Also, you are much more likely to take good care of something that you love, understand, and feel connected to versus something you hate.

Building Your Compassionate Voice and Silencing Your Inner Critic

Most people's inner critic has been honed over decades, which means counteracting it with a compassionate voice isn't going to happen easily and won't occur overnight. Cultivating self-compassion is an active process that consists of four parts: noticing, acknowledging, responding (with kindness), and remembering common humanity.

Step 1: Notice Your Inner Critic Voice

Before you can shift to self-compassion, you need to be aware of how you talk to yourself. Using the mindfulness techniques from Chapter 6 bring your attention to your inner critical voice. What does your mind say when it is judging or criticizing you? What key words or phrases commonly appear? Many times, the inner critic voice uses similar judgmental statements, and it can help to notice patterns. Whose voice does it sound like—your own or someone else's? For some people, the voice reminds them of someone from their past who was critical of them. When is the inner critic voice more or less likely to appear? Are there certain experiences that cause it to get louder? It is only once you are aware of how you are speaking to yourself that you can begin to respond to that inner critic and build a more helpful, self-compassionate inner voice.

Step 2: Acknowledge the Outcome of Being Self-Critical

Once you are aware of your inner critic voice, including when and how it speaks to you, then you can evaluate its effect. Is this voice helpful or unhelpful? In other words, what happens when you are self-critical? Does that inner voice motivate you to make changes? Or does it send you down a negative shame and judgment spiral? Don't worry so much about testing the voice—i.e., analyzing whether what it says is true or untrue. Instead, be more interested in whether the voice is *helpful* or *unhelpful*. Is self-criticism helping you to live a rich, meaningful life in alignment with your values? Or is it doing the opposite, perhaps by causing you to disconnect, withdraw, or spend time and energy on things that are not important to you? How might your life be different if your inner critic didn't affect you in the same way?

Step 3: Respond with Kindness

When you recognize that the inner critic is trying to pull you down into a shame spiral, remind yourself that your mind is trying to keep you safe but that you don't need it to do that anymore. It can be really difficult to be nice to ourselves when we're in pain. However, with mindfulness, you can actively practice creating a "pause" between recognizing the inner critic voice and reacting to it. This allows for space to respond with kindness. Make an active effort to soften the voice in your head. As I mentioned earlier, try to consider how you would speak to a friend who was going through a similar tough experience or who may have messed up or made a mistake. What would you say to that person? Can you speak to yourself similarly? Until you build up your own self-compassionate voice, it may help to imagine the voice of someone who loves you or cares about you. What would that person say to you?

Self-compassion includes both kind thoughts and kind actions. Kind thoughts can be statements that you say to yourself when you notice your inner critic voice speaking and shame starting to creep in. The inner critic might say, "What is wrong with you? You're such an idiot. You need to do better." Compassion steps in to respond, "I know you're trying to keep me safe, but the harsh judgment isn't helping." Some other examples of self-compassionate statements include

- I'm doing the best that I can in this moment.
- It's okay for me to feel upset, but I don't have to go into a shame spiral. I can use some coping tools.
- I'm learning how to recognize what my body needs.
- I'm listening to my own internal authority, not some arbitrary external authority.
- Feeling pain and discomfort is difficult, but I can get through it.

Self-compassion also can take the form of kind actions that you do for yourself when you are struggling. As with the kind statements, it can help to think of what you do for a loved one when that person struggles. Perhaps you hold their hand, hug them, or put a hand on their shoulder. Physical touch activates the parasympathetic nervous system, which is responsible for helping us calm down and relax. Research has found that hand-holding and hugging decrease the levels of the stress hormone cortisol, lowers blood pressure, lowers heart rate, and promotes the release of oxytocin, which helps you feel more trust and connection.

You can do what Neff calls "supportive touch" to give yourself some physical reassurance.[9] While it may feel silly or awkward, your body and your brain can't tell the difference between a supportive touch that comes from another person or yourself. That means you can do simple self-compassionate actions to soothe and calm your nervous system:

- Hold the sides of your face
- Place your hands over your heart
- Firmly press your fingertips one at a time
- Self-massage your neck and shoulders
- Cross your arms across your chest and give yourself a hug
- Cup your hands in your lap
- Stroke your arms gently
- Use a heating pad for warmth
- Hug a pillow
- Cuddle with a pet

As you do these things, take a few deep breaths in through your nose and out of your mouth. Using a combination of kind actions with kind words and statements can help to silence the inner critic and strengthen your inner self-compassion voice.

Step 4: Remember Common Humanity

When your inner critic voice is talking loudly, remind yourself that you are not alone in this experience. Everyone has painful experiences where they feel less-than; everyone makes mistakes; everyone feels embarrassed and ashamed. Reflecting on the ways your experience is connected to other people's experiences can help diffuse shame. It's also important to remember that your inner critic voice developed in response to a fatphobic, racist, sexist, ableist, queerphobic society. If we didn't live in such a society, we wouldn't beat ourselves up so much. Remind yourself how your inner critic voice developed and have compassion for yourself. It is not your fault.

Create a Self-Compassion Toolbox

It is often hard to be nice to ourselves in the midst of a painful moment. Do some brainstorming so that the next time you struggle, you have a list of self-compassionate language and actions that you can use.

- Make a list of self-compassionate words or phrases you can use when you are going through a rough time. If you have a hard time coming up with language, think about what you would say to a friend.
- Make a list of self-compassionate actions you can try the next time you are struggling.

Utilizing Affirmations and Mantras

I know the words *affirmation* and *mantra* sound a little woo-woo, but try to stick with me for a moment. Although the idea of doing these things may feel silly (that was certainly my first thought), they can have tremendous benefits on your overall well-being. Participants in a group program I run are encouraged to record themselves saying a variety of affirmations aloud to listen to when they are having a tough time. Several of the women were resistant at first, and they were more than a little skeptical that it would have any benefit. The next day, though, one of them shared that listening to her voice recording had an instant effect on her, both physically and mentally.

Research supports what the woman experienced. Using affirmations or mantras consistently can help rewire and reprogram your brain, meaning your inner critic voice quiets down while your self-compassionate voice strengthens. Saying positive affirmations aloud to yourself breaks the pattern of negative, inner critic thoughts. In moments of pain, when your brain is filled with negative, unhelpful thoughts, affirmations provide some go-to self-compassionate or helpful words for you to use instead. For example:

- I am strong and confident.
- I am not more valuable if I take up less space.
- I am getting better at recognizing what my body needs.
- I am not measuring my success by my weight.
- I am okay just as I am.
- I am doing enough.
- I am making decisions based on self-care and self-compassion.
- My feelings are real and valid.
- My worth and value is not dependent upon my weight.
- I am funny and kind.
- My body is fine the way it is.
- I am allowed to rest.
- It is okay to be right where I am; I don't always need to be striving or improving.
- I am unlearning what society has taught me to hate about my body.
- I am not going to be intimidated by someone else's vision of what I "should" look like.

Create Your Own Affirmations

Write five to ten positive affirmations that resonate with you and challenge your inner critic thoughts. Use present tense and self-compassionate language. Once you have written these statements, try recording yourself saying the affirmations aloud (using your phone's voice memo feature or any other recording device). Save the recording and listen to it once a day, or whenever you notice your inner critic voice getting loud. You can also write affirmations on sticky notes and put them around your house or office as daily reminders.

Reframing the Food Police Voice

Since the food police voice is a specific type of inner critic voice, you can use the same steps I described earlier to reframe this unhelpful voice into a more helpful, supportive one: notice, acknowledge the outcome, respond with kindness, and remember common humanity.

Step 1: Notice the Food Police Voice

What judgments is your inner food police voice making about what you are (or are not) eating? Notice any absolutes that you use to describe food (or yourself), like good/bad, should/shouldn't, or clean/junk. When do these thoughts appear? Are there certain times of the day, week, or month when they are louder? Where did you learn these rules?

Step 2: Acknowledge the Outcome of the Food Police Voice

What happens when the food police voice pipes in to judge your food decisions? Is the voice helpful or unhelpful? For many people, the food police voice causes disconnection—when you're trying to listen to an external food rule, it's hard to pay attention to what your body really wants and needs. The food police voice can also result in all-or-nothing thinking and can keep you in the deprivation-binge pendulum. Either you're following the food police voice rules, or you're saying "eff it" and eating whatever you want. What happens when you hear the food police voice but don't "do" what it says? Does it cause guilt and food obsession? How might your relationship to food be different if the food police voice didn't have as much of a say?

Step 3: Respond with Kindness

Once you've identified the food police voice's unhelpful rules and beliefs, you can challenge those thoughts by reframing them to something more helpful. Replace any absolutes with words like *may, can,* or *is okay,* as in, "I can eat whenever I'm hungry," or, "It's okay to have dessert tonight." You might also notice judgmental "should" statements and replace them with "could": "I should go to the gym today" becomes "I could go to the gym." This allows you some space to check in with yourself rather than following the lead of the inner critic voice. Likewise, you can replace "shouldn't" statements with "can." "I shouldn't have another piece of pizza" is reframed as "I can have another piece of pizza if I want to."

Think of several self-compassionate statements that you can say to yourself when the food police voice pops in, such as

- I had many times this week when I honored my hunger.
- I am learning to trust myself with food.
- I am learning to include foods I find satisfying and enjoyable.
- I am learning to overcome past food rules.
- This is a process, and I am learning a lot about myself.

It also helps to use curiosity and be able to make *observations* rather than *judgments.* For example, "I can't believe how much I ate at lunch today," can instead become, "I notice that when I don't have enough carbs at breakfast, I become ravenous by 11:00 a.m. and have a hard time stopping when I'm full at lunch."

Step 4: Remember Common Humanity

Given the rampant diet culture we live in, it's next to impossible to go through life without developing an internal food police voice. You are not alone in this struggle, and beating yourself up only makes it worse. Remind yourself that it is not your fault, and show yourself some compassion to diffuse any shame that arises.

Challenge the Food Police _____

The next time you notice the food police voice telling you to eat or not to eat something, challenge it by doing the opposite. Then observe, nonjudgmentally, what happens. You can practice challenging "should" statements in the same way: Do the opposite of what you think you *should* do, then see what happens and how you feel.

It takes a lot of time, practice, and patience to quiet your self-critical voice and strengthen your self-compassionate voice. Some of these critical thoughts may never dissipate completely; they may always be around in some capacity. But over time, as you practice actively noticing, shifting your attention, and responding with kindness, the amount of brain space these thoughts take up can decrease dramatically. Continue to practice using self-compassion, and try not to let guilt or shame get in the way of your growth or allowing yourself to honor and respect your body.

CHAPTER 12

Honor and Respect Your Body

When Robyn was a child, she often felt rejected by her family. "They provided food and shelter, but emotionally they abandoned me from a very young age," said Robyn, who's now forty-six. When Robyn and I started working together, she had given up dieting years prior but still struggled to listen to her body cues. "I can understand what my body wants, but I feel stuck in this place of rebellion where a voice inside me prompts me to do the opposite of what my body says. I know I'm not treating my body well, but I keep doing it anyway." Several weeks later, Robyn had an aha moment: She was not respecting her body.

"For a long time, I used dieting as a way to abandon, shame, and punish myself," Robyn explained. "When I discovered intuitive eating, I was thrilled that I could eat all the foods that I had kept off-limits. Yet I still had a part of me that felt like rebelling. For example, if I wanted an apple, I would actively choose to eat chocolate instead because I felt the 'rules' of intuitive eating said I should. But now I can see that this is just another way in which I am abandoning myself. Instead of abandoning myself in the name of dieting, I have substituted abandoning myself in the name of intuitive eating." Robyn realized that it was never about the food. She was still punishing her body with food, though this time under the guise of eating whatever she wanted. She was continuing to abandon her inner wisdom to outside forces, just as she had been taught as a child.

Respect is defined as "due regard for feelings, wishes, rights, or traditions of others."[1] Mutual respect is an essential part of any meaningful, healthy relationship. If one of your relationships lacked respect, most people would consider it to be an unhealthy or harmful dynamic. When we withhold respect from others, we tend to treat them poorly. When you disrespect someone, the implication is that the person is not worthy or valuable to you. And when someone believes that they are unworthy, they are less likely to take care of themselves or treat themselves well.

The same thing happens with your body. You are in a relationship with your body; it is a two-way street where information and experiences are communicated back and forth. A healthy relationship with your body cannot exist without mutual respect. When you speak badly about yourself, ignore your body signals, or put others' needs in front of your own, you send your body the message that you don't respect or value it. Most people try to avoid disrespecting someone they care about. Yet how many of us stop to consider how we might be disrespecting ourselves? Some examples of body disrespect include

- Ignoring your body's inner signals—e.g., not eating when you are hungry
- Following others' cues on what to eat or how to exercise, rather than your own
- Doing a form of exercise that you don't enjoy or that doesn't feel good
- Body-bashing or body-checking
- Wearing uncomfortable or ill-fitting clothing unnecessarily
- Beating yourself up for any perceived mistake or "failure"
- Comparing yourself to others
- Not following your intuition or gut feelings
- Suppressing your feelings and not allowing yourself to feel things deeply
- Putting other people's needs ahead of your own
- Not setting boundaries and letting people walk over you
- Silencing yourself and your feelings to please others or avoid conflict
- Altering yourself to please others

When you disrespect your body, the disconnect between yourself and your body grows wider. It is really hard to listen to and take care of something that you don't respect. Loving your body is not a prerequisite for respecting it. You can respect your body no matter how you feel about it because respect begins when you recognize that you are valuable and worthy of care *just as you are today*—regardless of how your body looks, how it works, or how you feel about it. Respecting your body doesn't start when you feel good about your body; it starts when you realize your worth as a person is inherent and everlasting.

We can show respect to others through listening to them, serving them, showing kindness, and expressing appreciation for them. Body respect means that you do all of those things for your body. You can *listen* to your body, *serve* your body by caring for it physically and mentally, *be kind* and compassionate to your body, and *appreciate* your body as it is right now.

Relationship Review

Think of a person with whom you have a healthy, positive relationship, and do the following:

1. Make a list of the core traits present in that relationship. What do you value about that person?
2. Look at those traits and list which ones you currently feel like you have in your relationship with your body. Which ones do you not have?
3. Ask yourself how you can start to cultivate those traits with yourself and your body.

Body Respect: Listening

Dieting and making food decisions based on external cues often means ignoring what your body cues tell you. In contrast, when you listen to what your body is communicating to you and honor your internal cues, you show body respect. As mentioned in Chapters 7 and 8, listening to your body means responding to your hunger cues by eating consistently, eating enough, and eating satisfying foods. It also means giving yourself unconditional permission to eat, thus allowing you to experiment and discover what foods sound good and feel good in your body. When you allow your body to have what it wants to eat rather than being influenced by diet culture and diet mentality, you are respecting your body.

Behaviors That Impede Listening

Certain experiences can pull you outside of your own body and make it difficult to listen to your body cues. Two common behaviors that do this are *body-checking* and *body comparisons*. Body-checking involves compulsively scrutinizing or monitoring your body, weight, or shape for any changes. There are many ways that people body check: weighing themselves on a scale, trying on a certain pair of pants, pinching their skin, looking at specific body parts in the mirror, or taking "progress" photos. People often body check in an attempt to feel more in control, yet in reality, it has the opposite effect. When we don't receive the feedback we want, anxiety, fear, and worry come rushing in because that information reinforces the belief that our bodies are the problem or that something is wrong with us. Our desire to get rid of those feelings and "fix" our bodies causes us to push our internal signals away and fall right back into the dieting cycle.

Take my former client Krysten, who struggled with body-checking her stomach. She would study herself in the mirror, measure her waist, and physically pinch and manipulate the fat on her abdomen. Whenever she would walk by a window or other reflective surface, her eyes would immediately go to her midsection. All these body-checking behaviors triggered her inner critic voice, which would say, "You are so disgusting," or, "Look at all your gross rolls; you need to get it together." When Krysten and I began working together, she was able to make huge strides in reconnecting with her body cues and listening to her body, yet one glance in the mirror would send her spiraling. She'd disconnect from her inner wisdom and feel pulled back toward external rules and restrictions to "get it together."

Body comparisons have a similar effect. Comparison is an innate human characteristic. Although some comparisons can be healthy and helpful, people who frequently compare themselves to others have lower self-esteem, are more self-conscious, and have higher rates of anxiety and depression. Another client, Sam, frequently compared herself to her brother and sister-in-law. "He is super fit, and his wife is so tiny; I just feel so huge next to the two of them," she told me. Whenever Sam was around them, one of two things would happen. Either she would feel the diet mentality coming on strong and have the urge to restrict, or she would think, "Screw it," and binge-eat until she felt sick. In both scenarios, the body comparisons pulled Sam out of her experience and caused her to ignore or override her body cues.

The current media landscape and immediate access to thousands of images at any given time make body comparisons all the more widespread and damaging. The vast majority of people in the mainstream (Western) media and with large followings on social media are young, thin, white, and "traditionally" beautiful. Yet in the real world, fewer than 5 percent of people actually look like this, and even among those who are considered "beautiful," Photoshop is pervasive and commonplace. Almost all of the images we see on social media, as well as on television or in magazines and advertisements, are edited to make the person's body fit into the "perfect" aesthetic that we are used to. There's also widespread use of minimally invasive plastic surgery, like Botox and fillers, among the people in those photos. What we are exposed to on social media can make this beauty and body ideal seem real, normal, and attainable; however, the standards that these images uphold are anything but.

Reduce Body-Checking

You can begin to reduce body-checking by raising awareness of your body-checking behaviors. Make a list of all the methods you use for body-checking, whether that's weighing, measuring, trying on clothes, looking in mirrors, or physically manipulating your body. Even if you've gotten rid of your scale, you may still be keeping tabs on your body's shape in subtle, sneaky ways. Notice all of the different ways that you take part in body-checking. Reflect on the following questions:

- Why do you feel the need to body check?
- Are there certain situations, thoughts, or feelings that cause you to do more body-checking?
- How do you feel after body-checking?
- How does body-checking affect your ability to respect your body?
- When you have the urge to body check, what is it that you really need?

Once you've raised awareness of your body-checking behaviors, work on resisting the urge to body check. In the short term, it may help to hide the scale, cover mirrors, and wear looser clothing so you are less inclined to body check. When you feel the urge, ask, "What do I need right now?" Pull out your list of coping tools and use one of those instead. Over time, as you challenge your body-checking behavior more, the urges will become less and less frequent. By body-checking less often, you will create more space to be able to connect with and listen to your body cues without as much anxiety over how your body looks.

Reduce Body Comparisons

To curtail your tendency to make body comparisons, begin by identifying what situations, experiences, or people cause you to compare yourself to others in a negative, judgmental way. Common culprits include magazines, television or movies, social media, family members, friends, or coworkers. Then, when you are in those situations or around those people, be aware and notice when body comparisons creep in. Pause and check in with yourself: What is going on right now? For example, although Sam had decreased her body comparisons overall, her brother and sister-in-law still provoked strong comparisons. When we discussed this, she reflected on the fact that her brother had a lot of things that she didn't have—a house, a family, a dog, a stable career—all things she associated with success and happiness. Sam realized that she was conflating her brother and sister-in-law's small, fit bodies with these outward symbols of success and happiness.

For people who live in bodies that are marginalized by society, body comparisons are often tougher to navigate. When you have to navigate a world that is built to exclude you, you are reminded of how your body compares to others no matter where you turn. For example, a fat client of mine constantly worries that she won't be able to find a chair to hold her body in every restaurant or office she walks into. Or a woman with a disability who has to maneuver her body through an inaccessible physical environment like steps, curbs, or narrow hallways every time she leaves her house.

Although it's almost impossible to completely stop comparing yourself to other people, once you notice that you're doing it, you can practice inserting a "pause" and choose how you want to respond rather than react. Use self-compassion and remind yourself that body diversity is inherent. Bodies come in all shapes, sizes, colors, and abilities, and all bodies are worthy and valuable. Shift your language from comparison or judgmental phrases to observational words. For example, if your initial thought is, "She is so much skinnier than me," change that thought to, "She is thin." If it feels safe, bring your focus back to you and your body sensations. Try to stay true to yourself instead of being swayed by external factors. What do *you* need in this moment?

Diversify the Media You Consume

It takes just two minutes of looking at images for someone to start to have a negative perception of their body, and most people these days spend way more than two minutes per day looking at photos of other people. When the majority of the images feature people that look a certain way, you may start to believe those images portray what real life is. The photos set an unrealistic bar against which you may end up measuring (and then feeling terrible about) yourself. Western culture has normalized one specific standard of beauty (i.e., young, thin, light-skinned, flawless complexion). When it comes to bodies, though, there is no such thing as one "normal." Remember, two-thirds of women in the United States are sized 14 and up, and less than 5 percent of the world looks like the thin, "perfect" body that we see so much of in the media.

Start to be a conscious consumer of media you watch, read, and look at. Pay attention to who is featured: Does everyone look similar, or is there diversity? If there are fat people, people with disabilities, or people of color, how are those characters portrayed? I was standing in line at the grocery store recently when I picked up a women's magazine that I used to read voraciously throughout high school and college. As I flipped through it, I was immediately struck at how every image—whether a photo accompanying a story or an advertisement—featured almost-identical-looking thin, white, traditionally beautiful women. The only photo of a person in a fat body was included as part of a before and after weight-loss article (ugh). Representation matters, and magazines, television shows, movies, and social media accounts that feature only certain types of bodies send a message about what types of bodies are valued in our society.

Although I'm not saying you need to give up your favorite television shows, I am suggesting that you start to notice how the types of media you consume affect you. If you notice that a certain magazine, TV show, or social media account causes you to fall into the comparison trap, can you stop reading, watching, or following it? For example, a few years ago, I realized that looking at the Instagram account of a fitness professional whom I know socially always made me feel bad about my physical fitness. This wasn't something I was conscious of right away, but over time I noticed how I'd watch his Instagram stories and then feel guilty for not working out that day. I'd feel ashamed that I, as a health professional, wasn't in better shape. Once I made this connection, I decided to "mute" his Instagram stories so that they wouldn't pop up on my feed. Immediately I noticed a difference in how I felt during the day: my guilty feelings and comparison-itis completely went away.

Make a point to diversify the media that you consume—read books that feature fat, Black, or queer main characters. Follow social media accounts that feature a diverse range of body shapes and sizes. (See Appendix B for suggestions.) By following people of all different shapes, sizes, genders, abilities, and colors, you widen the definition of what a "normal" body is. The more you see images of people that feature fat bodies, hairy bodies, saggy bodies, bodies with stretch marks and acne, belly rolls and cellulite, the more you begin to realize that all this is *normal*. We are all normal. Make a conscious effort to add these images of reality by including better representation in any media you are consuming. By doing so, you'll be less inclined to make negative comparisons. And less comparison means you will be better able to stay with your body experience and listen to what your body is telling you it needs.

Social Media Cleanout _____

Be a conscious consumer on social media, especially on image-centric apps like Instagram. Start by unfollowing accounts that do any of the following:

* Make you feel bad about yourself or your body
* Feature extreme exercise or dieting behaviors
* Promote cutting out certain foods or food groups
* Feature lots of images of thin, young, and/or white bodies (even an account that is technically "anti-diet" can still be harmful and can cause comparisons)
* Talk about "clean eating" or "good" foods and "bad" foods
* Give unsolicited diet advice
* Share before and after photos
* Propel the myth that weight loss = health (because remember, it does not)
* Cause you to compare yourself to them

Then diversify your feed by following accounts that feature a more diverse range of body shapes, sizes, genders, races, and abilities. For a list of accounts, check out Appendix B on page 378. The more you normalize looking at a range of bodies, the more comfortable you can begin to feel with your own body.

Body Respect: Serving

In this case, *serving* means showing your body you care about it by doing what you can to take care of yourself physically, mentally, and emotionally. Instead of making decisions based on self-control, restrictions, or judgments, body-respect choices come from a place of self-care, curiosity, and self-compassion.

As I discussed in Chapter 10, self-care encompasses physical, mental, and emotional practices that show your body respect. In this section, I'm going to focus on two methods of self-care that have historically been co-opted by diet culture: nutrition and exercise. Many of us have learned the vast majority of what we "know" about nutrition and exercise through the lens of diet culture—that 70 billion–dollar-per-year industry that capitalizes on our society's racist, sexist, classist beliefs and our desire to feel accepted and in control. We are taught how to use nutrition and exercise to manipulate and control our bodies but never learn how to eat or move in a way that truly nourishes us physically and mentally. This is where the intuitive eating concepts of gentle nutrition and joyful or intuitive movement can be helpful.

One important note before I jump into these concepts: Not everyone will be in a place where they are ready or able to incorporate gentle nutrition or joyful movement. If that is the case for you, it *does not mean* you are disrespecting your body. As I'll discuss shortly, diving too quickly into gentle nutrition before you've had a chance to connect to your body's interoceptive cues and release feelings of restriction or scarcity can pull you outside of your body and can then be the opposite of body respect. You can work to show body respect in multiple ways, so if you decide not to use gentle nutrition or movement (right now, or ever), that is okay. You know yourself and your body best, and you can do what is most supportive for you.

Gentle Nutrition

As I shared earlier in this book, when you decide to stop dieting and let go of external rules around food, it is very common to do a total 180 and start eating everything in sight. Especially if readily available foods are ones that you have been restricting. In her book *Landwhale*, Jes Baker describes running straight from Diet Land to Donut Land where she lived her "best and most delicious, rebellious life."[2] (Therapist and fat activist Deb Burgard developed the concept of the Diet Land to Donut Land pendulum.) Yet she eventually realized that, although she was eating whatever she wanted, she was still making food decisions based upon external influences. "Was I making decisions based on what *I* wanted every day? Sometimes, yes, and it was amazing. But more often than not, my choices were simply reactions to Diet Land, a place I hated and thought I had left behind...but that shit lingers."[3]

Going from Diet Land to Donut Land is like the swinging pendulum. On one end of the pendulum, you have diets, with all sorts of rules about what you can and can't eat. On the other end is donuts—and any other food the Diet Land actively demonizes. This opposite end of the pendulum is where we go when we are actively rebelling against diet culture. Body respect is not in Diet Land or Donut Land; it's the place that falls in the middle. This is where gentle nutrition, the term used by the authors of *Intuitive Eating*, comes into play.[4] There is a lot of nuance required here because diet culture has co-opted nutrition and turned it into an externally driven set of

282

rules and restrictions. Even the whole "It's not a diet; it's a lifestyle change" philosophy is a wolf in sheep's clothing (where the main message is still that you need to follow external rules and lose weight). In contrast, *gentle nutrition* involves using nutrition knowledge alongside your body wisdom as a form of self-care. The use of the word *gentle* reflects the flexibility and permission that is inherent and integral to respecting your body.

Gentle nutrition uses both your body knowledge *and* your brain knowledge to make food choices that honor your body cues *and* your health. Your body knowledge includes your inner wisdom, such as your ability to feel hunger cues, know what foods satisfy you, and understand how different foods make you feel. Your brain knowledge is built from your eating experiences and incorporates some external wisdom. For example, you may feel like eating a donut and know that it will satisfy you. But you also remember that the last time you had a donut for breakfast, you were hungry soon after and experienced an energy crash in the late morning. Brain knowledge might also pipe in to remind you that it's been several days since you had a piece of fruit and suggest that maybe you can add it to your meal today.

Gentle nutrition is the tenth and last principle of the intuitive eating framework for a reason. When you are disconnected from your body's inner wisdom and hold a lot of internalized diet mentality, trying to make decisions based upon a food's nutrition composition can pull you outside of your body's needs. When we try to incorporate brain knowledge about nutrition before doing the work to reconnect to our bodies and rid ourselves of diet mentality, we usually end up disregarding or overlooking our body knowledge. Once you've worked through the process of reconnecting with your body cues, made peace with food, and reframed the food police inner voice, then you are more able to consider both your brain and body knowledge. Then a decision about nutrition can come from a place of self-care rather than self-control.

That said, there is often a very fine line between making a decision based upon self-control and diet mentality or upon self-care and gentle nutrition. Sometimes the outcome—what you choose to eat or not to eat—will be the same, which can make it even more confusing. To differentiate between the two, consider the question, "What is my *intention* behind this food choice I am making?" For example, the choice to eat a salad could come from a place of lingering diet mentality ("I shouldn't eat more carbs today"), or it could come from a place of self-care ("Vegetables make me feel good").

Part 3: Feeling

One way to tell the difference is to ask yourself how you feel after the meal. Are you able to eat, feel satisfied, and move on? Or do you continue to think about what you did or did not choose to eat? In the case of choosing a salad, if you eat it and then proceed to think about the burger or pasta that you did not have, then chances are the decision to eat the salad was rooted in diet mentality. On the other hand, if you eat it, enjoy it, and can move on, the decision was likely made by listening to your body.

Very often, it is not one or the other—*just* diet mentality or *just* self-care—that informs your food choices; it's a bit of both. This is normal, and it is okay—your diet mentality may have been ingrained for years, so it doesn't just disappear overnight. Think about approaching your food decisions with curiosity instead of judgment so that you can begin to tease out the different factors going into your meal or snack choice. Ask yourself questions such as these:

- What thoughts went into my decision to eat (or not eat) that food?
- Could any lingering diet mentality thoughts have played a role?
- Was there a part of me that tried to restrict what I was eating under the guise of listening to my body?
- Did my brain knowledge override my body knowledge?
- Is this choice coming from a place of self-care or a place of self-control? Or a bit of both?
- Was there any black-and-white or all-or-nothing thinking involved in this decision?
- Would I have made the same food choice if I knew there was zero chance it would change my body?

Gentle nutrition sits in the middle of the pendulum where you are no longer eating for outside reasons—whether that be *following* diet rules or *rebelling* against diet rules. Diet Land doesn't get to have a monopoly on salads and hummus, just as Donut Land doesn't have an exclusive license to donuts and sweets. Instead of *either/or*, gentle nutrition is *both/and*. It is the place where you can find a natural balance of eating what you want *and* nourishing your body. If you feel ready to start practicing gentle nutrition, the following sections offer a few tips for beginning.

Focus on *Adding* Rather Than Removing

Instead of trying to restrict what you eat, think of ways that you can *add* more nourishing foods or ingredients to your meals. Take a look at what you currently eat. Are there any areas where you could add more nutrition? For example, can you have the pasta and *add* a side of vegetables? Or a bowl of cereal and *add* a handful of berries? Maybe you've never craved vegetables or always associated them with boring, bland diet food. This could be a fun time to start exploring new recipes and cooking techniques. (See Appendix B for a list of cookbooks and recipe websites.) Spoiler alert: Veggies taste freaking amazing when cooked with butter (and YES, this still "counts" as nutrition!).

Focus on the Bigger Picture

Your body is not a clock that resets every twenty-four hours. You don't need to eat vegetables every day or have X grams of protein at every meal to be healthy. (And remember that you do not need to be healthy to be deserving of body respect.) Take a look at your overall eating patterns. Are there places where you would like to add more nourishing foods? Or are there times when you want to try to eat a wider variety of foods? For example, during a stressful period where all that sounded good was quick-digesting carbs and comfort foods, I didn't touch a vegetable, fruit, or whole grain for over a week. When I noticed this, I decided to work on incorporating more vegetables. My intention came from a place of gentle nutrition—"vegetables provide me with fiber and nutrients that my body needs"—rather than a diet mentality place of, "Oh, crap. I have to eat more vegetables or else I'm not going to be healthy/skinny/lose weight/etc."

Try a Loose Structure with Meals and Snacks

Meal planning is often a technique used in dieting for crafting a rigid structure for our days and our foods. But moving away from dieting doesn't mean that you can't have any structure for meals and eating. Instead, it's about doing it in a way that promotes flexibility while you still listen to your body. Meal planning can ensure you have enough food on hand, that you can save time on busy weekdays, and that you can make meals that both taste good and feel good in your body. You might find it helpful to have a loose structure for meals, like carbohydrate + protein + fat + fiber. Or you might realize that making a few meals ahead of time cuts down on week-night stress. Try to think about your intention behind meal planning and approach it from a gentle, flexible, self-care place.

Be Flexible

Watch out for rigid, all-or-nothing thinking. Maybe eating a combination of carbs, protein, fat, and fiber feels best in your body, but that doesn't mean that every single meal needs to include all of those things. Or maybe you brought a homemade lunch to work, but when your lunch break rolls around, someone brings in pizza, and you'd rather have that instead. A key part of gentle nutrition is flexibility, and knowing that one (or several) food decision doesn't make or break your health (there's that gray area again!).

Stock Up on the Essentials

When you have a wide variety of foods available to you, it's easier to make decisions using both your body and brain knowledge. When you go grocery shopping, try to get a combination of staple food items along with quick grab-and-go foods and foods that you both enjoy and find satisfying. If you've been shopping on autopilot or approaching it with some leftover diet mentality, it can take some experimenting to find new foods that you enjoy. One of my clients realized that her typical path through the grocery store was one that she developed years prior when she was dieting. Although she had been taking active steps to move away from diet culture, her weekly grocery trip still looked very similar to her dieting days. Once she realized this, she actively tried to adjust by taking a new path through the grocery store, walking down every single aisle, and picking out at least two new foods each time she shopped.

Exploring Gentle Nutrition _____

Pick one meal that you've eaten recently, and then answer the following questions:

- What was your intent behind this food choice? Why did you choose to eat this?
- Do you like this food?
- Did you enjoy eating it?
- Did you have any feelings of guilt when eating it?
- After eating, what happened? Were you able to move on? Or did you continue to think about food and eating after you were done with the meal?
- Do you think this food choice came from a place of self-care or self-control?

After working on the other pieces of the intuitive eating framework, most people find that their urgent, obsessive cravings eventually begin to dissipate. When you feel more neutral about all foods, you can better know (and trust) what, when, and how much you want to eat. This doesn't mean that diet culture or diet mentality completely goes away or that getting the pendulum to swing gently in the middle between Diet Land and Donut Land is an easy task. If you struggle with this, remember that feeling challenged is normal and, most importantly, it is *not your fault.* It takes a lot of time to unwind all the baggage that's been put on you from society, and there is no shame in that. Some people find that they naturally get to a place where (assuming they have adequate food access) they are eating a large variety of foods, including high-nutrient foods that support their physical health and fun foods that support them emotionally. Other people have to spend a little more energy incorporating gentle nutrition. Neither is right or wrong, and both can support body respect.

Gentle Nutrition Practice ─────────

Pick one of the following to try:

- What is one food you can try to add to your diet?
- If you always eat the same types of foods, choose a different variety of grains, protein, vegetables, and/or fruit the next time you're at the store.
- Spend ten minutes on your favorite (non-diet) cookbook or recipe website, and pick out one new recipe that you'll try this week. In Appendix B, I offer some suggestions of cooking and recipe resources.

───────────────────────

Intuitive Movement

Much like nutrition, exercise and fitness have been co-opted by diet culture. They're often sold as a way to lose weight, get lean, or change your body shape. Even when the premise is "getting in shape" or "being healthier," the subtext is still *exercise to get smaller.* From the fitness instructor who encourages you to "burn off those weekend calories" to a personal trainer who gives you a strict workout plan, it's hard to avoid. We are often taught that only certain activities "count" as exercise or that you have to exercise for a certain amount of time; otherwise, it's not worthwhile.

No wonder most of us approach exercise as something we "should" do or a task to check off our list. We can know it's good for our health, yet it still becomes something we dread, force ourselves to do, or struggle to do at all. Under the veil of diet culture, exercise can become an unpleasant requirement instead of something we *want* to do. This is part of the reason why it is so hard for many people to start or maintain a consistent exercise practice.

Moving your body has a long list of beneficial effects, all of which have nothing to do with weight or body size. Physical activity can help increase energy, sleep quality, strength, balance, and stamina while decreasing stress, anxiety, and the risk of several chronic diseases, including type 2 diabetes and high blood pressure. Exercise has both physical and mental benefits, which means it can be a wonderful way to practice body respect. But how do you do it without falling down the diet culture rabbit hole?

This is where intuitive movement comes in. Intuitive movement is the practice of connecting with and listening to your body to figure out how it feels and what type of movement it needs that day. Instead of picking what type of exercise you think you "should" do, you use your body's internal cues to figure out the best type, length, and intensity of the workout. Instead of exercising to burn calories or lose weight, intuitive movement is about exercising because of the self-care, health, and mood benefits you see. Instead of forcing yourself to do X days of cardio and X days of weight-training, you get to explore movement that feels good in your body. This shift in mindset allows exercise to become more enjoyable and less stressful, so it can be something to look forward to rather than dread. Just like with nutrition, exercise must be decoupled from weight loss for you to find a sustainable movement practice. Practicing intuitive movement can help you nurture a healthier relationship to exercise and with your body.

For a wonderful example of joyful, intuitive movement, watch young children. They will run around for hours, chasing leaves or bubbles, playing games, or rolling around in the grass. Call them in for dinner, and you often hear a chorus of, "But I want to keep playing!" Children's perception of physical activity isn't as a chore or something they *have* to do because they are moving their bodies in ways that feel natural and enjoyable. Somewhere along the way, we've lost that sense of moving our bodies because it feels good or is fun. Intuitive movement requires you to look *inward* for inspiration and to determine what types of movement would be best at the moment rather than relying on extrinsic motivation. This means asking yourself questions like

- What does my body need today?
- What type of movement do I feel like doing?
- What type of exercise would be most beneficial or supportive to my body today?

Some days, you may do an intense spin class, whereas other days, you might prefer restorative yoga or a short walk. Intuitive movement is flexible, not rigid, and gives you the space to explore what feels good in your body. It involves shifting the focus from a form of punishment or self-control to a form of kindness and self-care. In the following sections, I suggest a few ways to incorporate intuitive movement.

Find a Form of Movement That You Enjoy

If you find yourself dreading your workout, it's a sign that you may not be engaging in forms of movement that make you or your body happy. If you're not sure, ask yourself what form of movement you'd want to do if exercise didn't have any effect on what your body looked like. If you can't think of any type of movement that you like doing, then do some experimenting. Look into different classes, whether it's in-person classes (think yoga, Pilates, kickboxing, ballroom dancing, spin class, water aerobics, belly dancing, and so on) or online streaming workouts or videos. Or get outside and try hiking, biking, walking, jogging, tennis, or—in the winter—cross-country skiing or snowshoeing. Don't discount smaller daily movements like walking the dog, cleaning the house, gardening, or jobs that require frequent movement or prolonged periods of standing. These "count" as movement, too.

Pay Attention to How Movement Makes You Feel

Check in with yourself after you finish exercising. How does your body feel? Did your workout or movement that day leave you feeling energized? Do you feel stronger or have less pain? Focus on the internal, intrinsic benefits that you notice. Note: Feeling extremely fatigued and drained after your workout is usually a sign that you've overworked and pushed your body too far and that you may need a rest day. If your workout routine is causing you any stress or anxiety, then it's going to be counterproductive to any possible benefits.

Think About Your "Why"

What is your *intention* behind exercising? Are you exercising because you want to lose weight or change your body or because you think you "should" do it? Do you feel guilty when you miss a workout? Notice when those "shoulds" or guilty voices pop-up and get curious about them. Then focus on finding a reason to move your body that has nothing to do with weight loss or calories, such as because of how it makes you feel, for the physical health or mental benefits, or because you know it will help you get a good night's sleep. Reframe exercise as something that you are doing to take care of your body rather than punish it. If having goals helps you, strive for non-body-based goals like lifting more weight, being able to run further, or improved flexibility.

Watch for All-or-Nothing Thinking

Intuitive exercise is flexible, not rigid. Challenge the idea that you have to exercise for a certain amount of time for it to "count." One of my clients realized she would only exercise if she could commit to a certain amount of time, so she challenged this thinking by doing shorter workouts. If you skip a workout or have a few weeks where you move less than normal, show yourself some compassion (then move on). Remember, it's the bigger picture that matters more than the day to day.

Don't Be Afraid of Rest Days

Rest days are just as important as active days because they allow your body to recover and heal. When you begin to strengthen your interoceptive awareness skills and build back trust with your body, you can learn to accept whatever it is your body needs that day. Trust that when your body needs a rest day, it *needs* a rest day.

Don't Force Yourself

Often, people have a fear of "If I don't force myself to exercise, I'll just sit on the couch and never move!" This is similar to the "I'll just keep eating and eating and eating" fear that can come with letting go of dieting and giving yourself unconditional permission to eat. Both fears imply a lack of trust in your body (and perhaps also a narrow definition of "exercise").

In reality, *not moving* all the time probably isn't going to feel very good for most people. Several years ago, chronic hip and shoulder pain sidelined my usual workout routine. After a few months of thrice-weekly physical therapy, I was "discharged" to continue the therapeutic exercises on my own. While I find those exercises incredibly boring, I quickly realized that whenever I went more than a couple of days without moving, my hip and shoulder pain immediately came back. Of course, I still have days (and weeks) where I don't do much activity, but I know that moving more helps my joints feel better. This is what now motivates me to get up and move during the day. Sure, my exercise routine looks very different than it did several years ago, but it's overall much healthier (both physically and mentally) and sustainable, and it no longer causes me any stress or anxiety.

Explore Your Relationship to Exercise _____

Consider journaling on the following questions:

What has your relationship been to exercise in the past? What is it like now? What thoughts and feelings come up when you think about exercise? Do you have any rules or rigid ideas of what "counts" as exercise? Which types of movement or exercise do you enjoy, and which types do you not enjoy? How do you feel after you move your body? Write down all the "whys" for moving your body that have nothing to do with body size or appearance.

Based on what you came up with here, write down one action step you could take to begin incorporating intuitive movement into your life.

Body Respect: Being Kind

Respecting your body means treating it with kindness and compassion. As I shared in Chapter 11, self-compassion can take the form of both *words* and *actions*. Body respect involves noticing any negative inner self-talk, including body bashing or self-criticism, and stopping it in its tracks. Respect your body by replacing those negative thoughts with more positive, kind affirmations.

Another way you can treat your body with kindness is by dressing it in comfortable clothes that fit your here-and-now body. Wearing clothing that is uncomfortable or that doesn't fit properly can be an unmistakable physical reminder of your body size. If you're in the earlier stages of this journey and are gaining weight, the constant reminder of your changing body size can make it hard to move forward in this process.

Dressing the body that you have right now is a way that you can show your body respect. As one of my clients told me recently, "Not having the extreme anxiety or body bashing because of tight clothes has made me feel 1,000 times better. I had to get past the fear of going up a few sizes, but now that I have the clothes, it was SO worth it."

I understand that for many people, buying new clothes may be easier said than done. Although the average American woman is a size 14 to 16 and more than half wear larger than a size 16, most clothing manufactures don't carry more than a size 12 or 14 in stores. This is a form of discrimination as clothing manufacturers only cater to the "ideal" thin, straight up and down body type. The larger your body, the more difficult it is to find clothing that fits, let alone get cute, comfortable clothing that you like. Things are starting to improve as more retailers begin to offer expanded sizing options, but only about 16 percent of retailers offer "plus-size" clothing (and the vast majority of these options are only online). Also, purchasing new clothes can still be difficult if you struggle with finances. Clothing items like leggings, flowy tops or dresses, and pieces with some stretch in them can help to make the pieces last longer if your body size is still fluctuating.

Try to view buying new clothes not as a failure of your body but as a way to be kind, compassionate, and respectful of your body. It is *not* your job to fit into certain clothes; it is the clothes' job to fit you. You are not better or worse for wearing arbitrarily sized jeans. Clothing sizes are not standardized, and, even if they were, there are no "standard-size" people, which is why you can wear one size in a certain brand of clothing and have to go four sizes up to fit into a different brand. Fashion industry expert Lynn Boorday analyzed data from a 2002 study of almost 11,000 people and found that in women with a size 28-inch waist, which is most often associated with clothing size 6, the average hip girth varied by more than 12 inches.[5] But stores only carry one size 6, so they have to pick the proportions that they want to make the clothes for. Clothing companies decide for themselves what a specific size "looks like," and most target specific (aka thin and white) demographics. All this to say that if a piece of clothing doesn't fit you, that says more about the clothing company than it does about your body. And if the size on the tag bothers you, you can always try cutting it out so you don't have the constant reminder.

If seeing your old clothes in your closet causes you to feel sad, anxious, or go down a shame spiral, consider doing a closet cleanup. Now, I know this is often easier said than done as many people are resistant to change, and getting rid of clothes you love can be a hard pill to swallow. But ask yourself whether seeing a whole bunch of clothes in your closet every day that no longer fit is *helping* or *hurting*? In a recent conversation with a client, she realized that as sad as she was to give up her old clothes, opening her closet was giving her a lot of anxiety, and it often ruined her whole day. If you aren't ready to completely give up your old clothes, a good intermediate step is to box them up and put them out of sight, so you don't have that daily reminder. Use self-compassion and remind yourself that your body is worthy of kindness and comfort no matter what size it is.

How to Deal with Photos of Yourself

If you struggle with feelings of sadness or shame whenever you see a photo of yourself, you're not alone. For most people, seeing a less-than-flattering photo of themselves can send them down an awful shame spiral. The next time this happens to you, pull out your trusty mindfulness and self-compassion skills, and try the following:

1. Notice what thoughts arise when you see a photo of yourself. Take a step back, pause, and detach yourself from your thoughts. "I'm having the thought that I look awful in this photo." What is the story that you are telling yourself about your body? Where did you learn these thoughts or beliefs?

2. Employ self-compassion. Would you say the things you are thinking about yourself to a friend? What kindness can you show yourself instead?

3. Recall what was happening and how you felt at the moment the photo was taken. What memories from this moment do you want to remember when you look at this photo? For example, instead of focusing on how you look, can you think about the fun that you had that day?

4. Remind yourself that it is just a photo, and it says nothing about your worth. Think about all the other aspects of you that the camera does not capture.

If you see old photos of yourself in a smaller/different body and begin to feel sadness, shame, or regret, ask yourself the following questions:

- What did you have to sacrifice to maintain that body or size? Was it sustainable?
- How was your mental health at that time?
- Were you truly happy with your body at that time, or were you still trying to change it?

Remind yourself that your body is not meant to stay the same size, shape, or appearance all of your life.

Body Respect: Appreciating

I recently took an online fitness class with Lauren Leavell, a National Academy of Sports Medicine certified personal trainer. At one point, she said, "Can you think about what your body *is doing* rather than what it is *not doing*?" In that moment, I realized that I had been much more focused on what my body wasn't able to do in class, and I hadn't been paying any attention to what it actually was doing. I turned my focus away from how tight my hips and shoulders were and turned it toward appreciating what was happening. My lungs were breathing in and out; my back was stretching; my hips were able to get easily into child's pose; my body was able to relax.

Often, we are so focused on what our bodies are *not* that we forget to stop and appreciate them for what they *are*. We can show respect for our bodies by appreciating the ways they show up for us every day. When you notice a negative or critical body-related thought pop into your head, pause and redirect: remind yourself that your body is more than something to be looked at. Replace that critical body thought with a statement about yourself that has nothing to do with your appearance—for instance, *My legs carry me wherever I need to go, I'm curious and love to try new things*, or *I'm compassionate and have wonderful, deep friendships*.

You Are More Than an Object

Make a list of at least fifteen things that you like and appreciate about yourself and your body. The catch: None of them can be specifically appearance related. If this is difficult, think about the things that you appreciate in your friends. Do you hold any of those traits, too? You can also think about what your friends would say that they appreciate about you. Write those things down.

As I discussed in Chapter 6, a regular gratitude practice can also help to redirect your brain's negativity bias. Instead of focusing on the things about you that you wish were different, actively work to express gratitude for the things about yourself and your body that you are thankful for. Write those things down daily, and you may be surprised at some of what you unknowingly take for granted. Actively practicing gratitude can help you gain perspective of what is truly important in your life.

Body respect begins with the small ways in which you show up for your body every day. Instead of trying to change or shrink your body into something that society deems "acceptable," can you start to listen to it, serve it, be kind to it, and appreciate it, just as it is today? In the next chapter, I'll share more about how you can begin to redefine the relationship that you have with your body.

CHAPTER 13

Redefining Your Relationship with Your Body

I spent so long trying to control and change myself.

When I was twelve, I got a perm.

At fourteen, I started straightening my hair (and continued to do so for well over a decade).

My boobs were nonexistent, so I wore padded bras.

My skin was pale, so I went to tanning beds.

I didn't have abs, so I compulsively exercised.

My butt was flat, so I did hundreds of squats.

I wanted to fit in, so I spent hours stressing about what to wear.

I thought my brown hair was "boring," so I dyed it blond.

When I hit puberty and gained weight, I went on a diet.

I began to get wrinkles, so I spent a ton of money on skincare products (and *almost* got Botox).

I spent years contorting myself and my body to try to fit into the type of body and beauty ideals that society deemed "attractive," "good," and "worthy." Years trying to control myself and my body. Years spending so much time and energy attempting to change my body so that I would be perceived a certain way. Yet all I was really doing was burying my true identity underneath all the things I *thought* I needed to be so that I'd be accepted.

We do not arrive in this world with a negative view of our bodies (or anyone else's). At birth, our relationship with our bodies typically starts out simple and easy. Babies love touching, exploring, and looking at their bodies. They don't bemoan the size of their bellies or the rolls in their legs. Toddlers are not ashamed of what they look like, and they don't feel the need to change their appearance. At one point, you also had this type of unencumbered relationship with your body. It may be impossible to recall, but there was most likely a time in your life when you enjoyed your body. Hence, any animosity, shame, or loathing that you may feel about your body today was not of your creation. It was handed down to you from society and people around you. Body shame is something that is learned, which means it can also be unlearned.

What Is Body Image?

Body image is often (incorrectly) thought of as *thinking you look good*. In reality, how "good"—or "not good"—you think you look has very little to do with your body image. Body image is a person's *perception* of their body, as well as the *beliefs* they hold that inform that perception, and the *thoughts* and *feelings* that they have about that perception.

Perception is defined as "to see, hear, or become aware of something through the senses."[1] When it comes to thinking about our bodies, we often let our minds dictate our perception. Yet our minds don't become aware of our bodies in a void; we take in the influences of the society we are a part of and the people and systems that surround us. Most people take the thoughts and beliefs that they have about their bodies as fact without stopping to question where these thoughts or beliefs came from or critically think about the social constructs and systems that informed them. We are so quick to project our thoughts and beliefs (which are really society's thoughts and beliefs) onto our bodies. When we think we are seeing our bodies, what we are really seeing is society's perceptions that we have internalized as our own.

Your body experience doesn't exist in a vacuum. You weren't born with the desire to shrink certain body parts (and perhaps grow others)—this inclination came from somewhere. What would your body image be like if you hadn't been receiving messages from society all of your life? Without social constructs and external world comparisons, there'd be no such thing as a "positive" or "negative" body image.

Body image—that is, how we perceive our bodies—often determines how we live our lives. The way we view our bodies can govern how we feel about ourselves and how we show up in the world. The vast majority of women—at least 90 percent—report some level of body dissatisfaction, which means that women, as a group, are often not fully experiencing or taking part in their lives.[2] The effect occurs not just on an individual level but in the collective sense as well.

When someone has poor body image, they are less likely to be able to completely participate in the world. Women with higher levels of body dissatisfaction have lower self-esteem and self-worth, have higher rates of depression and anxiety, and are more likely to suffer from eating disorders. Many people put their lives on hold because of how they feel about their bodies. They put off dating, socializing, applying for a promotion, going back to school, having a family, or traveling. Body dissatisfaction is also associated with worse health outcomes because people with poor body image are less likely to take care of their bodies. Dealing with poor body image is a time and energy suck. Just imagine how much more women would do—and how much better our world would be—if we weren't taught to be so preoccupied with our bodies.

Body Image Baseline

How would your life be different if you felt better about your body (without having to change what you look like)? How would you know if you had a positive body image? How would you treat yourself differently if you felt better about your body? How important is it to you to improve your body image?

The Body Image Healing Process

You were born into a loving relationship with your body. At one time, you enjoyed your body, loved your body, and were one with your body. At some point, your attitude shifted, and a disconnection occurred. Healing your body image involves rebuilding your relationship with your body. As Sonya Renee Taylor writes in *The Body Is Not an Apology*, "Radical self-love is not a destination you are trying to get to; it is who you already are."[3]

The process of healing your body image isn't a quick snap of the fingers or forcing yourself to "love" your body. Instead, it is about shifting from rejecting, avoiding, or trying to "fix" your body to allowing your body to *just be*. In the first two parts of this book, I spoke about how to stop fixing and start allowing. This shift is the foundation that can begin the body image healing process. After which, you can begin to build more awareness about what your body is communicating to you and what it needs. This is *body image healing*, which involves developing more insight into the ways you relate to your body and how your body gives you a sense of who you are. How do you talk to your body? How does it talk to you? Can you understand what it is communicating to you? Do you listen to what it has to say? Rather than forcing your body to feel one way or another or ignoring it completely, you can instead begin to feel and explore.

Body image is fluid. It isn't the same from day to day or even moment to moment. The way we feel about our bodies, and in our bodies, fluctuates during our lives—sometimes changing with each passing hour. Body image responds to changes in age, body size, emotions, experiences, environment, and more. As we move through life, our bodies naturally shift and change, and we have different experiences that can affect our body image. I've noticed my body image change as I went through a breakup, tried on a new pair of jeans, adjusted to a new work schedule, and every month when I get my period.

Body image is a moving target, which means it isn't something we can just fix or heal and then never think about it again (as much I wish this were the case!). Rather, healing body image is an active process. It is about learning to be present in your body and be able to tolerate discomfort when it arises rather than pushing the feelings away or trying to "fix" your body. Body image healing also involves questioning and unlearning all of the thoughts and beliefs that society has taught you about bodies. In many ways, body image healing is an ongoing process of navigating life's changes and challenges.

Goals of Body Image Work

Healing your body image and reclaiming your body doesn't necessarily mean weight loss, body love, or an end to all body discomfort. The goal of body image work is not to feel 100 percent positive about your body all the time; for most people, that wouldn't be realistic or necessary. Instead, the goal can be not to let how your body looks, what size it is, or even how you feel about it hold you back from living out your values. Can you learn to be present in your body, take care of it, and show up for yourself every day—no matter how you feel about your body?

One of my clients compared body image to a bad hair day. "When I have a bad hair day, it sucks for a bit, but I don't let it stop me from going about my life. It doesn't change what I do, or don't do, that day," she told me. "I know that I'll wash it again in a few days, and I'll feel better about it. What if I could do that with 'bad body image days,' too?" If a bad body image day were like a bad hair day, you could acknowledge it in the morning—"Okay, this sucks; I'm feeling crappy about my body"—and then move on with your day. This is the goal: Being able to feel crappy about your body *and still live your full life.* Bad body image days—just like bad hair days—are part of the human experience. They're going to happen, and you can't stop that, but you can stop how much it matters in terms of your self-worth.

Body Image Development

Do you remember when you first started to become aware of your body? Most children recognize themselves in mirrors and begin to develop a sense of self-awareness around age two to three.[4] This is the age that many kids start to voice strong preferences for what they want (or, more often, do not want) to do, wear, or eat. My nephew Riley's favorite word at age three was some variant of "mine." TV remote: "Mine!" Cup of coffee: "My coffee!" Glass of wine: "Riley juice!" (My response: "No, my love, this is Auntie's juice.") Around this time, kids also begin to demonstrate body awareness. They start to understand their bodies as distinct objects, separate and different from other people's bodies. At this age, my niece Isla loved to show people all her different body parts. "My belly, my nose, my hair"—she'd point and repeat over and over again.

But when does this intuitive recognition of the body as "mine" transform into something with value attached to it? When does "mine" become *better* or *worse* than another person's? When is "mine" taken from us? When does "mine" become something for another person to look at, value, measure, judge as palatable, approve or disapprove, accept or not accept, love or not love? When does "mine" become a judgment for *just being*?

Around age three, children begin to notice similarities and differences between themselves and others. "That person has different color skin than me," or, "We both have brown hair," they may say. Questions may pop-up: "Why is that person not walking?" they ask about someone in a wheelchair. Although their observations may initially be neutral, they don't stay that way for long. Children assign meaning about these similarities and differences in the context of a culture that is full of bias.

Through media messages, family, and peers, kids learn to compare themselves to others. They are taught to assign a value of "better" or "worse" based upon a socially constructed body hierarchy. By age five, children already show a preference for thin, light-skinned, conventionally attractive people. It is around this age that girls begin to profess a desire to be thin, whereas boys often want to be muscular.[5] At this point, children have internalized the messages they've been hearing since birth and begin to express body dissatisfaction.

Increased weight concern around age five often shows up as dieting by age nine (which is also when we start to see the onset of clinical eating disorders). By nine years old, 50 percent of girls have dieted or restricted their food intake in some way. According to research cited by the National Eating Disorders Association, 42 percent of first through third graders want to be thinner, whereas 81 percent of ten-year-olds are afraid of being fat.[6] The majority of kids are more afraid of being fat than they are of cancer, war, or losing both their parents. These statistics are both heartbreaking and horrifying, and they also show how deep our society's anti-fat bias runs. Children see how people who don't fit into a thin, light-skinned mold are treated in society. As I discussed in earlier chapters, fat people are routinely stigmatized and discriminated against in a variety of ways. It's no wonder children are afraid of being on the receiving end of oppression and hate.

In my practice, I see much of the same: The majority of my clients started their first diet around age nine or ten, usually in response to comments from family members, doctors, and/or bullying from their peers. My client Kaja, now forty-two, remembers bingeing and eating so much that she couldn't breathe as early as age eight. "My parents always told me I was too chubby and warned me that I shouldn't get 'too fat,'" she said. "I went on my first diet at age ten. For months, I wasn't allowed to eat anything without telling my parents, and they made me walk laps around the house. I lost a bunch of weight, but the second I got praise—and freedom—I started bingeing again."

Humans develop knowledge of their bodies in a social context. From a very young age, you were taught to evaluate yourself (and others) based upon certain societal and cultural appearance standards. This means that perceptions we have about our bodies are learned, not innate. So are the thoughts that arise in response to that perception. Most of our judgments about bodies—both our own and other people's—are not objectively true; they are molded by socially constructed ideas and beliefs. You didn't pop out of your mother's womb with a preference for, say, flat stomachs, cellulite-free thighs, smooth skin, and toned arms. You learned all of these body ideals. We don't *inherently* believe our bodies are bad; society *conditions us* to feel this body shame and hatred.

Factors That Impact Body Image

Struggling with your body image is not a personal flaw or an individual issue. You don't feel like crap about your body because you are broken; you feel like crap because you have been swimming in a culture that tells you that you're only worthy if you look a certain way. Healing your body image involves critical examination of both social constructs and your body experiences over time. Rather than focusing on what is *wrong* with you, can you look at what has *happened* to you and what you were *taught*?

A variety of factors affect body image development, including

- Body size
- Weight stigma or discrimination
- Physical ability or disability
- Gender identity
- Culture and race
- Parents/caregivers who emphasize or desire thinness
- Peers who diet or express body image concerns
- Social supports and acceptance (or lack thereof)
- Degree of societal privilege or power
- Bullying or teasing, especially related to appearance or weight (regardless of actual body type)
- Interruptions in a person's body experience, including trauma
- Media messages
- Lack of representation of certain identities and bodies
- Documentation status

In Chapter 5, I suggested you explore some of the ways your upbringing, your family or caregivers, and your experiences as a child affected how you feel about your body. Now let's take a look at some of the ways systems of oppression can play a role in the development of body image.

Body Image and Systemic Oppression

A body hierarchy exists in Western societies. White, cisgender, heterosexual, able-bodied, young, thin people are at the top and set the standard against which all other bodies are measured. This inherently means that Black, transgender, queer, disabled, chronically ill, older, fat bodies are at the bottom of the hierarchy. The more one deviates from the social standard, the further down the hierarchy they are, and the more systemic oppression they face. The closer someone is to the top, the more privilege and power they have access to. In 1989, Kimberle Crenshaw, a Columbia law professor and scholar, coined the term *intersectionality* to describe this dynamic.[7] Although it was originally used to highlight the specific discrimination that Black women face, this framework is now used to help explain how all the different aspects of a person's identity intersect with one another. This includes race, class, gender, physical ability, sexuality, age, nationality, religion, body size, socioeconomic status, and more.

Intersectionality helps to describe the ways that people with varying identities and backgrounds encounter the world. As Crenshaw explained in her seminal paper, when you treat someone as purely a woman or purely Black, this ignores the specific challenges that Black women as a group face. The combination of several different identities affects a person more than if they were living with just one at a time. For example, a person is not only Black, fat, a woman, or a person with a disability. She is a Black fat woman living with a disability. Somebody who is Black is going to experience the world differently than someone who is white. Somebody who is fat is going to experience the world differently than someone who is thin. Somebody who is cisgender is going to experience the world differently than somebody who is transgender. People with different individual characteristics face discrimination; when you combine two or more characteristics, it explains how certain people are pushed even more toward the margins of society. The more marginalized identities one has, the more oppression one faces. Intersectionality also describes how various systems are set up to keep those at the top of the body hierarchy in power and continue to discriminate against and oppress those at the bottom.

Everyone in our society is affected by our culture's fatphobia, which means that people of all sizes struggle with their body image, although not in the same way. Virgie Tovar, an activist and the author of *You Have the*

Right to Remain Fat, developed the concept of the three dimensions of fatphobia to explain the differing types of body injustice that people face.[8] "[The three dimensions] are intrapersonal, how you feel about your body; interpersonal, how others feel about and treat your body, [and] institutional—how well you're allowed to maneuver society and systems, such as clothing, employment, medical care, buildings, etc. based on your body."[9]

The more intersecting identities that you have, the more systemic oppression you face, and the more body injustice you experience. For people in straight-sized, socially accepted bodies, body image healing involves mainly the internal work of unlearning social constructs and shifting their mindset. But for those in bodies with marginalized identities who have to navigate life in a fatphobic, sexist, racist, ableist, homophobic, transphobic society, doing the internal work can only go so far. As Shira Rosenbluth, LCSW, an eating disorder therapist, shares, "When your body is oppressed and it's a barrier to receiving healthcare, employment, travel, safety, clothes, etc.— it's not a matter of just learning to love yourself. You can't love yourself out of societal oppression."[10] And as anonymous essayist Your Fat Friend writes, "Fat people who are sad, who eat well, who eat poorly, who exercise, who don't—we all live our lives in the pressure cooker of fatphobia. Our bodies are epidemics, our disease communicable, our lives quarantined. Of course we defend ourselves, give up, give in, deny, push back. We are products of a system that is dead-set on isolating us, shaming us, dividing us, shunning us."[11]

In my twenties, I—as a thin, white, cisgender, able-bodied woman—experienced body image issues. I had many negative thoughts about my body, and I spent so much time and energy trying to change it. But when I stepped out into the world, I was not treated any differently because of my body compared to how I would have been if I were in a fat body or a Black body or a queer body. As I worked to heal my body image, I didn't have to contend with the world continuing to tell me that my body was "wrong." I could go to the doctor and not be told that I needed to lose weight "for my health." I could walk into any store and buy cute, stylish clothes right off the rack. I could post photos of myself as I ate pizza or burgers or ice cream and be congratulated for "normalizing" eating. Yet when someone in a fat body or Black or Brown body or gender nonconforming body does those same things, they get a very different response from society. Many colleagues of mine who share the same messages that I do are publicly attacked because they are fat. They are accused of "glorifying obesity" or "spreading dangerous lies" while thin practitioners like myself are applauded for "helping people love their bodies." My colleagues get trolled online and receive dozens of malicious, hateful comments whenever they post a photo of themselves. That has never happened to me, and, if it ever were to, I know it would not be related to my body or identity.

If it's not clear yet, a person's body image is not just about the size of their body or how they perceive themselves to look. Things like race, gender, and sexuality are all body image issues. A person's body image is shaped not just by how they view their body but by how *others* view (and treat) their bodies, including their skin color, gender, and sexuality. As Christyna Johnson, MS, RDN, LD, shared recently in a social media post, "It's exhausting living in a body that [is] viewed as a threat. It's exhausting living in a body that is objectified, commodified, bought, and sold. It's exhausting living in a Black body."[12]

Body Image and Representation

In earlier chapters, I wrote about how the vast majority of images that we see in the media seldom portray realistic bodies. Yet these images still shape our views of reality. Exposure to these images can lower self-esteem and increase feelings of inadequacy. Often people feel like they need to "fix" themselves and attempt to "conform" to this body ideal through dieting and weight loss. Although the people we see in the media represent a body type that less than 5 percent of the population holds, we still compare ourselves to them. Bodies of marginalized identities are rarely seen in the media, and this lack of representation affects a person's body image, too. When fat people or trans people or BIPOC people are not seen, the underlying message is that these bodies are not worthy or that they don't belong. On television, in movies, in books and advertisements, white, conventionally attractive people get to live rich, full lives. If and when people of other identities exist, they tend to reinforce negative stereotypes and biases. The erasure and negative portrayal of fat people, people of color, people with disabilities, and queer and trans folks adversely affect how people with those identities see themselves.

Critically Examine the Systems

Despite constant negative messages, lack of representation, or threats to your safety, you can still pursue a better relationship with your body. Your worth is inherent, no matter how society treats you. As Christyna shared with me, "Despite being traumatic at times, there is plenty of joy to the experience of living in a Black body."[13]

To help you truly heal, begin to question the systems in place that have caused you to feel the way you do about your body. Remember, so much of how you feel about your body (and others' bodies) is the result of social constructs. Your beliefs about what bodies are "good" are not objective realities but the result of human interaction. Much of what you may take as "truth"—like thin bodies, flat stomachs, and big butts being most attractive—is actually socially constructed. When you take these socially constructed ideas as fact without examining them, they can begin to seem fixed and unchangeable. Yet this is not the case. When you start to critically examine these socially constructed body ideals, you can unlearn some of your perceptions of what types of bodies are "good." And the more people who do this, the more we can start to shift what society and the culture deems as acceptable and "good," too.

Healing your body image requires you to dismantle your internalized anti-fat beliefs and unlearn biases about race, gender, weight, and health. Through this process of unlearning and working through any body grief that you experience, you can move toward reclaiming your body. Approaching this process with a sense of openness, self-compassion, and curiosity will be important. Pay attention to what thoughts, feelings, and emotions arise in your body and your mind. Try not to judge yourself so that you may take a step back and think critically about the connection between the societal factors and your body image. Remember, rather than focusing on what is *wrong* with you, examine what has *happened* to you, how you've been *treated*, and what you were *taught*.

Understanding Your Body Image ─────────────

Explore all of the different factors that have affected your experience in your body over time. Make a list of the different experiences, events, feelings, or people that have affected how you came to feel the way you do about your body. Consider the following questions:

- When do you first remember having negative feelings about your body?
- Where do your beliefs about bodies or body size come from?
- What attitudes or beliefs did your family have about body shape or size while you were growing up?
- How have your identity and lived experiences affected your body image?
- What sort of discrimination or oppression have you faced that may have played a role in your body image?

After reflecting on these questions, consider creating a body image timeline. Beginning from your earliest memory, draw a timeline of the factors that affected your body image over the years. Don't worry about interpreting or analyzing; instead, try to explore all the things that have caused you to come to feel the way you do in your body. Note: This is not about your weight but about how it has felt to be in your body.

Body Image Versus Body Positivity

Everyone has a relationship with their body. No matter their size, age, gender, ethnicity, or sexuality—everyone can struggle with body image. But working on your body image, or attempting to have a more positive outlook about your body, is *not* the same thing as body positivity.

Body positivity grew out of the fat liberation movement (also referred to as the fat acceptance movement), which was grounded in the civil rights movement of the 1960s.[14] The fat liberation movement began in response to the discrimination and systemic prejudice that people in fat bodies faced. It advocated for the rights of fat people, raised awareness about how dieting and intentional weight loss was harmful, and sought to reclaim the word "fat" as a neutral descriptor. The movement got widespread attention in 1967 when a man by the name of Lew Louderback published a piece in *The Saturday Evening Post* entitled "More People Should Be FAT."[15] This article attracted the attention of William Fabrey, who then went on to found the

National Association to Advance Fat Acceptance (NAAFA) in 1969. One of NAAFA's goals was to undo the systemic fatphobia and size oppression that existed across all facets of society, including in the workplace, schools, and advertising. The movement cemented fat acceptance as a political concept because it argued for human rights for fat people. Another fat liberation group, The Fat Underground, which spun off of NAAFA in the early 1970s, was led by fat, queer, Jewish women. They held a feminist worldview and focused on confronting the medical establishment about the lack of efficacy of dieting and raising awareness of the "double oppression of fat women in society" (i.e., intersectionality).[16]

Body positivity was one facet of the fat liberation movement. It began a way to center and celebrate the bodies that were historically relegated to the margins of society. This differs greatly from the body positivity we see today, which has become watered down to the point of being almost unrecognizable. What started as a radical underground movement led by fat, Black, and queer women is now full of straight-sized, young, conventionally attractive white women posing in bikinis or hunched over to show off their belly "rolls." As Tovar writes, "Fat activism is really interested in all three of these dimensions [of fatphobia and body injustice: intrapersonal, interpersonal, and institutional], but perhaps primarily it's interested in the institutional dimension. With body positivity, the schema is inverted, with interest primarily residing in the first dimension: how you feel about yourself."[17]

While it's encouraging to see the idea of body positivity become more mainstream, the current iteration of it doesn't look anything like what its founders originally intended, and current-day body positivity now excludes the people who first started the movement. It has become a buzzword that centers the stories of young, straight-sized (i.e., thin), white, cisgender, heterosexual women. Body positivity has also become commoditized by capitalism and the media to sell clothing and make certain brands seem "woke" and inclusive. Thin influencers in socially acceptable bodies profit from showing their "imperfections." What began as a human rights issue is now centering the stories and experiences of women who can tuck their fat "rolls" right back into their yoga pants. Body positivity is no longer synonymous with fat liberation and fat acceptance (let alone fatness itself). For this reason, many people may find the term *body liberation* to be a more useful descriptor, which I'll talk about more shortly.

Reclaiming Your Body

Reclaiming your body is a process of deindoctrination. Through the unlearning of society's messages, you get to reclaim for yourself that which is true and real. When you reclaim your body, you can take back power from society and return it to where it belongs: with you.

There are many different expressions used to describe the ways you can approach this reclamation. Some options may feel more helpful or authentic to you than others. For example, for some people, the idea of "love your body" makes it seem like this is yet another thing that is impossible to achieve, whereas other people find this concept of body love helpful. Either way, remember that a positive body image isn't a specific destination or end goal. It doesn't mean achieving a certain body. Having a better body image does not mean loving your body or even liking how you look. You can feel better about your body without loving it (and without changing the way you look). When you have a positive body image, how you feel about your body doesn't hold you back from living your life. A positive body image means being free and embracing yourself and your body, no matter what you look like (and no matter how you feel about what you look like).

At this point, I often hear from people that they are afraid of "letting themselves go." Or, more accurately, they are worried that *other people* will think that they have let themselves go. To which I say yes, you have let yourself go. You've let yourself go do other things rather than worrying about your body or food all of the time. You've let yourself go do more creative, meaningful, joyful things. You've let yourself go be powerful, content, and unapologetic.

In the end, you have the autonomy to decide what relationship you want to have with your body as a result of this process—whether that be body love, body peace, body acceptance, body liberation, or something completely different. In the next sections, I've described several of the different phrases or expressions most often used. Feel free to take what is helpful to you and leave what is not. Ultimately, it's all about feeling okay with yourself (at least more of the time) exactly as you are.

Body Love/Body Positivity

I lumped these two terms together because body positivity began as a social justice movement, but it has since become somewhat synonymous with body love. Some people find the idea of body love or body positivity to be helpful. One of my clients equated it to the love she feels for her partner: "I love her unconditionally, no matter what she looks like," she told me. "Because I love her, I try to care for her and respect her. So loving myself therefore means that I can care for and respect myself."

Body love and body positivity don't necessarily mean that you love every single part of your body or that you feel positive about your body every day. Instead, it can mean that you love and respect yourself, no matter how you feel about your body.

The concept of "body love" can feel inaccessible to people who can't imagine feeling such a strong emotion or deep affection toward their bodies. The result is often some binary thinking, where people who feel like they can't love their bodies assume they have no other way to move forward. Not to mention the fact that, in recent years, body love and body positivity have been co-opted by corporations and thin, white, cisgender, heterosexual women. For something that was meant to be inclusive, the fat women who started the movement have been all but erased from it. For many women who are fat, Black, and/or queer, body positivity no longer represents them.

Body Neutrality

When the idea of body love or body positivity feels out of reach, perhaps a goal of feeling more neutral about your body can be a place to start. As opposed to the black-or-white trap of either loving or hating your body, body neutrality can be thought of as landing in the gray. With body neutrality, you don't necessarily love your body, but you also don't feel intense loathing either. You can think of it as the bad hair day example I shared earlier. You may have a bad body image day, but it doesn't cause you to spiral downward or affect how you move about the world. Body neutrality can be thought of as a place where you care for and respect your body without having a strong emotional reaction to how you look or passing judgment.

Some people find that "body neutrality" doesn't sit well for them. For people who live in marginalized bodies, the world is not "neutral" about how it judges them. This may mean that neutrality feels invalidating. In this case, body neutrality may be a step in the body image process but not the end goal.

Body Acceptance

Body acceptance involves acknowledging what your body is, regardless of your feelings about it. Acceptance means that you are allowing your body just to be rather than trying to change it. Instead of focusing on your perceived flaws, you can step back and realize that much of what your body looks like is out of your control. You accept that your body may change over time, but, no matter what it looks like, you can still take care of your body and live your life in accordance with your values.

Some people find the term "body acceptance" unhelpful because it can feel like they must be "okay" with everything. For transgender or nonbinary folks, accepting a body that does not match your gender identity may not be an option—and that is okay.

Body Appreciation

As I described in Chapter 12, body appreciation can be considered a component of body respect. Appreciating your body means that you pay attention to what your body can do for you rather than what it looks like or what you aren't able to do. Appreciation means that you notice and have gratitude for all of the ways your body shows up for you each day. Research has found that people with greater body appreciation feel more satisfied with their bodies and have better self-esteem (independent of their body image). Body appreciation can help you view your body in a different light. Rather than something that you love, you can instead appreciate it for the ways it allows you to live your life.

Body Peace

Making peace with your body can mean declaring a truce. Body peace happens when you stop fighting your body and allow it to just *be*. Body peace means letting your body communicate its wants and needs and that you listen to that communication without judgment. It means taking care of your body without trying to fix, change, optimize, or improve it. Body peace means getting back to the peaceful relationship with your body that you may have had as a child, free from outside expectations, beliefs, or judgments.

Body Liberation

Many people from the original body positive movement have moved toward using the term *body liberation*. To me, this term best expresses how to redefine your relationship with your body outside of social constructs and external approval. Like the fat acceptance movement, body liberation is rooted in social justice. As Jes Baker, from whom I first heard the term, explains, "Liberation is freedom from all outside expectations, even our own. Liberation is not having to love your body all the time. Liberation is not asking permission to be included in society's ideal of beauty. Liberation is bucking the concept of beauty as currency altogether. Liberation is recognizing the systemic issues that surround us and acknowledging that perhaps we're not able to fix them all on our own. Liberation is personally giving ourselves permission to live life."[18]

Body liberation represents more than just opting out of diet culture or loving how you look. It acknowledges the very real fact that society attempts to oppress marginalized bodies in a variety of ways every single day. Although the idea of loving your body or feeling positive about your body is great, it can be really difficult to do in our fatphobic, racist, sexist, ableist world. Liberation, on the other hand, lies in allowing yourself to be fully you—no matter how you feel about your body. Body liberation is rooted in social justice and is intersectional. It involves dismantling your internalized oppression and bias, including any anti-fat, anti-Black, ableist, sexist beliefs. As you liberate yourself from these internalized beliefs, you get to reclaim yourself and your body.

Body image is a systemic issue that goes far beyond an individual loving themselves. The goal of body liberation is not just liberation of the individual but of the collective. Liberating *all bodies* means that the systems of oppression would be destroyed, and everyone would be valued and treated equally. Shifting the culture and getting rid of the social constructs would naturally filter down into body peace for all people. Yes, we need individuals to liberate themselves, but we also need liberation at the collective level. The more people who reclaim their bodies and embody *liberation*, the more social and political effect we can have—both individually and collectively. Until all bodies are liberated and free from oppression, none of us will ever fully be.

Define Body Image Healing

I encourage you to define for yourself what body image healing and reclaiming your body means to you. Consider the following questions:

- How do you want to feel in your body?
- What does "body image healing" mean to you?
- What might "reclaiming your body" look like or mean to you?
- What words or descriptors feel inspiring or hopeful to you?

Practical Body Image Tools

At this point, you may be wondering how you actually start this process of body image healing. Here's the good news: If you've gotten this far in the book and worked through the reflection exercises I've suggested throughout the chapters, you've already started! A huge part of the process is unearthing and examining all of society's body constructs and the beliefs that you've internalized from years of swimming in this culture. As you continue to learn about the roots of body oppression and our culture's body ideals, you can then suss out for yourself what is a true belief (hint: very few of them probably are) and what is an arbitrary cultural expectation.

Use Mindfulness

Strengthening your mindfulness skills, which I discussed in Chapter 6, helps you to be more aware of the thoughts, feelings, beliefs, or situations that cause you to feel badly about your body. Once you are aware of which experiences cause you distress or pain, you can create some space to be able to observe what is happening. Aim to reduce the number of times that you try to act on or fix negative body image thoughts. Instead, allow yourself to feel, process, and work through the emotions that come up. The more and more you practice "sitting in the suck," the more you are able to come out on the other side and respond rather than react.

Practice Self-Compassion

Your response to a bad body image moment can include self-compassionate thoughts, statements, and/or actions. This is where you can pull out the self-compassion toolbox that you created in Chapter 11 and show yourself some kindness. It can also help to remind yourself that you are not alone in this experience. We must not turn body image difficulties into something that is "wrong" with you. It is normal to struggle with body image in a patriarchal, racist, ableist, capitalist society that profits off of body shame and oppression. This means that it is *not* your fault or your body's fault. The problem lies outside of your body: The blame rests squarely on the shoulders of society (and the socially constructed body ideals).

Deconstruct Bad Body Image Moments

Going along with what I mentioned earlier about mindfulness, notice when you are feeling bad about your body, and get curious. What was going on in that moment or on that day? What was happening to you or around you? What were you feeling? For example, my client Rochelle discovered that during the week of her period, she always felt awful about her body. For several days during that week, she'd pick her body apart and feel so much shame. Once she realized that it was linked to her menstrual cycle, and therefore was hormonal-related, she was able to ride the wave of those feelings without attaching to them as much.

Assess Body Image Cues _____

What cues (situations, people, experiences, thoughts, feelings) cause you to feel bad about your body? This may include looking at photos of yourself, comparing yourself to others, being in a bathing suit, weighing yourself, being around certain people, and more. Making a list will help you begin to anticipate these bad body image moments. Then, the next time you are in one of these situations, you can practice mindfulness and self-compassion.

Shift Your Language

Notice when you use the words "I am" or "My ____ is/are..." to describe your body. For example, you may find yourself saying things like, "I am so hideous," or, "My stomach is so huge and awful." Notice when this occurs and shift your language to terms of acknowledgment: "I am having a tough body image day," or, "I feel sad about my body today." Feelings are valid, but they are temporary. You can acknowledge them without letting them dictate how you treat yourself or care for yourself. Recognize your feeling, name it, and then reframe your initial unhelpful body image thought to something more helpful. What is something about your body that you do like, appreciate, or feel grateful for? For example, "I am grateful that my body allows me to play with my nephew," or, "I appreciate that my body gets me where I want to go." Professing appreciation or gratitude can help to take the focus off of how your body looks.

Find Community

When I first started doing anti-diet work, I noticed a recurring theme in my client sessions. Everyone would have huge breakthroughs in session and leave feeling hopeful and empowered. Then, without fail, they'd arrive back in my office a week or two later upset and spiraling downward. The culprit: A friend, family member, healthcare worker, or even a stranger who had commented about their weight or a social media influencer or coworker who was touting some new diet. "I'm literally the only one of my friends not dieting right now," they'd tell me. "All I hear about is dieting, weight loss, and how much people hate their bodies. It is so hard to be surrounded by people like this while I'm trying to stop dieting and accept myself."

Divesting from diet culture and redefining your relationship with your body outside of weight or body size can often feel like swimming upstream in a fast-moving river. Although intuitive eating and body positivity has made inroads in the past few years, the vast majority of people continue to diet and pursue weight loss. Even when you are the best boundary setter (which I'll touch more on in Chapter 16) or perfect the art of changing the topic of conversation, it's not easy.

An essential part of this process involves finding a community of people who are also on a body liberation journey. When diet culture comes roaring back to pull the rug out from under you (as it most likely will), having people to fall back on becomes invaluable. A community offers support and can help you to feel safe and secure enough to continue on your journey. Find people you can surround yourself with who can lift you and allow you to be your truest, most authentic self. As Audre Lorde writes in her book of essays, *Sister Outsider*, "Without community there is no liberation...Interdependency between women is the way to a freedom which allows the *I* to *be*, not in order to be used, but in order to be creative."[19]

Although it may be tough to find people in your day-to-day life who understand what you are going through, luckily dozens of incredible online communities exist—fat activist blogs, free Facebook groups, Instagram communities, and paid online support groups. In many of these spaces, you can find hundreds (if not thousands) of people on similar journeys who are being vulnerable and supportive and are working to lift each other up. For example, just this week in a free Facebook community that I run, members shared their fears of a changing body during pregnancy, opened up about the shame about the size of their newborn babies, and posted about body ideals they were terrified of parting with. Within no time, each post had dozens of comments providing support, advice, and encouragement. Those who join the group share that it helps them feel less alone and gives them a place to turn when they have no one else to talk to about their struggles. As one of the new members recently shared, "I am so happy I found this group, I could cry. I've felt so alone this past year, allowing food and working toward self-acceptance while everywhere I turn, diet culture is right there. I'm so tired of it. And I'm so grateful for this space."

As you continue forth in this process, surround yourself with people of all body sizes, shapes, colors, identities, and abilities who are on the same journey. Follow fat activists online. Seek role models in the size acceptance space. Consume podcasts, books, blogs, and articles written by people of all identities who have reclaimed their bodies (see the resource section at the end of this book for some recommendations). If you are in a fat body, a community run by a thin dietitian (like me) may not be the most helpful place for you. It is extremely valuable to be able to learn from and work with someone who can relate to your experience of living in a fat body. I encourage everyone—regardless of body size—to seek out the work and communities run by the fat activists who have been doing this work for decades. Often, I (and other thin providers) can only take people so far. It is really important to widen your circle outside of young, thin, white practitioners and work with people who hold similar identities to you. I've included a variety of online communities and other resources at in Appendix B.

Write a Letter to Your Body

This activity can help you gain insight on how you can move forward in redefining your relationship with your body. Write a letter to your body. In this letter, address your prior relationship with your body. You may apologize for how you may have treated it in the past and explain what societal beliefs or constructs affected your relationship with it. You may also include things about your body that you feel grateful for. At the end of your letter, tell your body how you hope to move forward in redefining your relationship with it. What will you spend less time *doing to* your body? What will you spend more time *doing for* your body?

Moving from Feeling to Growing

In the end, you have body autonomy. You get to decide how you want to define—and redefine—your life. This doesn't necessarily mean that you are happy all the time or that you always feel great about your body. It can be really hard to live in a body that society has told you is not worthy, should be different, or is just plain wrong. If you feel ambivalent, skeptical, or worried; this is okay. Rather than trying to change the way you feel, try to allow yourself to "sit in the suck" and show yourself compassion.

It takes time to unlearn the biases you've been indoctrinated into; it takes time to learn new truths. Bad body image days will come and go, so how can you deal with these so that you can pick yourself back up? Instead of fixating on your physical body, what does it mean to enjoy yourself, take care of yourself, and pursue a more meaningful, connected life? If you're not sure exactly what this means for you yet, that's okay, I'm going to guide you through some self exploration work in the next chapter.

PART 4

Growing

CHAPTER 14

Self-Exploration and Self-Discovery

When Tora was growing up, her parents and grandparents were always on her to be "better." Whether the subject was grades, sports, friends, or a job, "It was never good enough," she told me. By thirty-five, Tora was married and had two young children and a successful career. Yet every life or career goal she had hit, she'd never feel like what she had done was sufficient. "There is always a voice in the back of my head going, 'You can still do better,'" Tora said to me one day. For decades she had done the same with food and her body, aiming for "perfection" and improvement in every way possible. To Tora, that had meant maintaining a lower weight, having smaller thighs, only eating "clean" and "natural" food, and doing a specific amount of daily exercise. "I always feel like I need to be improving. Even when I meet my goal, it's still never good enough," Tora shared. "It's this constant striving for more and more, even though it makes me miserable in other ways." Tora realized that she had a fear of losing her family's love and respect if she didn't keep moving up in her career or if she "let herself go." Yet she also recognized that the persistent goal of "be better"— whether with her diet, her body, or her career—was getting in the way of other parts of her life. "I know that I don't want to always be searching for 'more,'" she said, "but I'm not sure what it is that I *actually* want or how to get there."

It is human nature to seek meaning in our lives. Many people feel incomplete, unsatisfied, or even worthless if they're not working toward something. Often we aim for external rewards that we are taught to seek by society: money, status, prestige, power. We are often afraid to rest or pause for even a minute because of fear of getting behind, being replaced, or becoming irrelevant. Is that really what gives our lives meaning, though? Is that really what we want out of life? To constantly be checking things off a list, never finished or never getting "there" (wherever "there" is)? Or, as Tora realized, is what we *actually* want the love, respect, and value we think we'll get when we get "there"?

For many years, I felt like something was missing in my life. I couldn't put my finger on what it was. I was living in a city I loved; I had many friends, a wonderful partner, and a good relationship with my family; and I had built my dream business. Most days, I felt happy, but, despite all of this, I couldn't shake the sense that there was something *more* that I was missing. Then, while on a trip to visit a close friend, I had an epiphany: I was missing *connection*. Deep, full connection with other people but also with myself. There was always a part of me that felt like I was on the outside looking in. Living part of my life outside of myself and second-guessing what I was say-ing or doing. I was never fully in the present moment because my brain was always pulling me out of my body with one thought: *What would other people think?* Even as I hugged my friend, I could feel that I was not fully present in the hug. I was instead thinking about what *she* was feeling. Thoughts ran through my head: *Is this too long to hug? Does she want to stop? How long should I hold on for?* I was all up in my head, which was not only keeping me disconnected from other people but disconnecting me from myself as well.

I had spent years self-silencing as I suppressed myself and my true thoughts and desires a thousand times a day. Whenever I thought about saying or doing something, I ran it through a filter in my brain: *Should I say this? Should I do this? What will other people think?* I second-guessed everything I wanted to say before it even came out of my mouth. And the thing was, *I never even realized I was doing this.* I had internalized all of the messages I received from society about what a woman should—and should not—be. The thoughts in my head did not stem from me; they stemmed from society's impossible standards. I was asking myself what others wanted from me instead of asking myself what it was that I wanted. In doing that repeatedly for years, I'd lost myself. I had become disconnected from my true self. This internal disconnection kept me always at arm's reach from others. In trying to control myself, I never let others fully see *me*. Heck, I wasn't even allowing myself to see me fully! I was subconsciously holding back, never letting go and just *being*. No wonder I was missing out on connection.

But how could I get to that place where I felt connected to myself and to others? Was I even capable of deep connection? It always felt just out of reach, and I had no idea how to get "all the way there." I wasn't even sure what "all the way there" meant or that I would recognize it when I arrived. Just like Tora, I had a tiny voice inside of me that kept saying *Not this*. Knowing what we don't want is a start—but how do we figure out what it is that we do want? How do we get back to our inner selves—the people we were before we internalized what society told us we should be? If *not this*, then what?

If *Not This*, Then What?

The messages we receive from society about how we are supposed to eat, look, dress, and act are not all-encompassing truths. As we bring to light and examine all of the beliefs we hold about how we "should" be, we can begin to realize that these messages were never reality. Instead, they're social constructs that have been created to keep us small and easier to control. If we want to figure out who we are, where we are going, and who we are truly meant to be, we need to release all of these beliefs and discover what is inside of us. When we strip away societal expectations, *who are we, really?*

The process of self-discovery starts when you turn inward and go deeper into yourself—away from the noise of the external world and beyond the chaos in your mind. You tap into your inner self so that you can figure out who you really are and who you want to be. My friend Hana Jung, the founder of Re:Boot Experiences, runs collaborative retreats for leaders, entrepreneurs, and creatives. To help break down barriers and encourage connection, she created a deck of 100 connection cards. Each card has a question on it that requires you to think hard about who you are and who you want to be. When I attended one of Hana's retreats, answering these questions helped me begin to connect more deeply to myself. I was able to challenge what I'd been taught and figure out who I was underneath who I thought I "should" be.

As I read each question, I was aware that my brain wanted to "filter" my response. I noticed this, thanked my brain for trying to protect me, but reminded it that I was safe. By doing this, I was able to tap into my inner self and express my true thoughts and feelings. For example, on the day I drew a card with the question, "What are you pretending not to know?" my immediate reaction was, "That I want children and a family." Then my analytic brain jumped in to say, "But you'd be fine without them. Think of all the travel you can do and the freedom you'd have." My brain immediately tried to talk me out of my true gut response and sway me in another direction. Because I was afraid that I might never have a family, I didn't want to admit that it was a desire of mine. Plus, I was among a group of mostly single people, and I was worried that they'd judge me for that response. I shook off both fears, pushed the filter away, and said what my immediate gut response had been. "I want children and a family," I said. As soon as I said it aloud, I felt my entire body relax: a sign that I was connecting to the truth in that deeper part of me.

Another friend of mine had a similar experience to answering the question, "What are you pretending not to know?" except her gut instinct was that she actually did not want kids. "My whole life, I've been told, directly and indirectly, that the 'correct' path a woman should take is marriage and then children. So I've always just assumed that will be what I do. But the more I reflect and question, the more I realize that—deep down—I've known for a while that I do not want to have kids."

Asking yourself deep questions can be a way to get to know yourself better. In the following self-connection activity, I've included a selection of questions from Hana's connection deck. You can reflect on these questions on your own or with other people. If you are discussing your responses with others, I encourage you to make sure they are people you can trust to create a safe, nonjudgmental space for you to open up in.

Self-Connection Questions _____

The following questions are used with permission from Hana Jung's connection card deck. Before you begin, I recommend spending a few minutes using one of the meditation techniques on page 157 to help draw you deeper inward. Then pull out a piece of paper, ask yourself the following questions and write down whatever comes to mind. You can answer them all at once or create a daily ritual for journaling your response to one question per day.

- When was the last time you laughed really hard?
- How would your best friend describe you?
- What is something you are passionate about?
- What memory would you want to relive again?
- What can't you live without?
- How would you spend the last month of your life?
- How do you want others to feel when they meet you?
- What would your ten-year-old self say to you now?
- What do you wish people knew about you?
- If you were stranded on an island with a group of people, what would be your role?
- What do you appreciate most in others?
- Are you an introvert, extrovert, or ambivert?
- When do you feel the most at peace?
- What are you most proud of?
- When do you feel most inspired?
- What advice would you give your younger self?
- When are you "in your element"?
- What are three words to describe you?
- What are you most afraid to share with people?

Uncovering Your Core Values

A person's core values are their fundamental beliefs that guide the choices they make. As you reconnect to yourself, identifying and getting clarification about your values is an important part of the process. Values are personal. They are not society's beliefs, your culture's beliefs, or your family's beliefs; they're *your* beliefs.

Values are the things that are important to you in life. Often values describe the person you want to be and how you want to live your life. Values can be used as a gauge to tell if your life is turning out the way you want it to or not. If you feel satisfied and content most of the time, you're probably living life according to your values. But if there is any part of you that feels discontent, or if there is a little voice piping up to say, *Not this,* then the way you are living may not be aligned with your values. Often, personal values may be blocked by negative or unhelpful thoughts, feelings, or experiences about eating behaviors or body size. Living in misalignment with your values can create internal stress, conflict, and overall dissatisfaction and often creates a situation when things can feel "wrong" or—as I experienced—like something is missing.

Figuring out your core values will help give you direction and keep you moving toward what is important to you. It can help to answer the question, "If *not this,* then what?" Where is it you want to go in life? Perhaps you value relationships, connection (like me!), adventure, playfulness, or trust. When you know your core values, you can be fully present in your life. Working on identifying your values reduces feelings of being "stuck" and allows you to live a richer, more meaningful life. Uncovering your values will help you to get a better idea of who you are and how you'd like to be living, and they provide a framework for how you're going to get there. When you get clarity about what is truly important to you, you can take steps toward spending more time living according to your values.

Before you work on identifying your values, it's important to understand what values are *not:*

- Values are *not* feelings or emotions, such as happy or calm.
- Values are *not* about how others treat you or feel about you, like whether you are loved or appreciated.
- Values are *not* things that you have.
- Values are *not* goals with a specific end point.

Values are how you see *yourself* and who *you* want to be. They are *not* how other people see you or treat you, or who others want you to be. The point is not to make other people happy or to get external validation. You cannot control how others behave; you can control only how you choose to behave. Another way to think about this is that if nobody were watching or paying attention, would this value still be important to you? Would you still be doing what you're doing now? Take, for example, food and dieting. If you didn't live in a society that had certain beauty and body ideals, would you still try to control what you ate?

There is no end point or finish line with values. As much as the organized part of my brain dislikes this, values are not something that can be checked off of a list. We have to be always striving to live in a way that aligns with our values. For example, honoring your body cues and eating whenever you feel hungry is a goal, whereas respect (in this case, for your body) is the value. Honoring your hunger one day doesn't mean that you've achieved the value of respecting your body. You will need to find ways to respect your body consistently every day.

Step 1: Identifying Your Values

Begin by figuring out what your top values are. When confronted with a list of dozens of values, it can be hard to narrow your list down to just a couple, and many people struggle with this task because many values sound appealing. The goal is to home in on just the top few values to have more focus. It doesn't mean that all the other values are off-limits or that you can't live your life in alignment with them, but picking just two or three gives you an initial direction to take.

There are many different activities designed to help you identify your values. Here I describe four different exercises, which I adapted from *The Big Book of ACT Metaphors* by Jill Stoddard and Niloofar Afari.[1] The exercises each approach the identification of values in a slightly different way, so you may find it helpful to complete all four activities.

- **Values List:** Review the list of values in the appendix. Circle all of the values that you feel strongly about. Then go back through the ones you circled and put an X through those that you feel like you could let go of. Go back to the remaining circled values and put a star next to the top three or four values that really matter to you.
- **The Sweet Spot:** Think about a moment in your life where you felt fully present, engaged, or alive. It doesn't have to be a big experience; it could be something small and seemingly mundane. If you get stuck trying to choose the "right" moment, notice this. Can you let your mind settle on whatever experience shows up? Once you have this moment, spend some time recalling all of the details of that time. What

were you doing? What did you see? Was anyone with you? How did you feel at that moment? What else do you remember about the sights, sounds, smells, or tastes related to that moment? Write down all of the things that you remember. Don't get too caught up in explaining what was going on at that moment; instead, try to connect to that moment and express how you *felt*. Here's an example of my "sweet spot" moment: *I'm lying in the grass in a friend's backyard. I'm by myself, but I can hear my friends chatting while they make lunch. My eyes are closed. I feel the soft grass under my arms and legs. The sun is shining, heating up my skin. My friend's dog runs over and curls up next to me. I can feel his chest rising and falling underneath my hand. I am fully present in the moment, in my body. I'm not worrying about what just happened or what is coming next. I feel warm, relaxed, and safe.*

- **Autobiography Exercise:** Imagine yourself years from now after you've lived a long, fulfilling, meaningful life. You've been the person you wanted to be and stood for what was important to you. Focus on that image of how you lived and who you became. Now imagine you are writing your life story as an autobiography. What would you want to share about yourself? What would you want readers to learn about you? What would you write about how you spent your time and who you were? As you reflect on your story of your imagined life, write down the values that the story expresses.

- **Tombstone Exercise:** What do you want written on your tombstone? Another way to imagine this is by asking yourself how you want people to remember you. What would people say at your funeral? Do you hope that people remember your ability to skip dessert? Or how good you looked in your jeans? "She did a damn good job of counting her macros and fitting into her skinny jeans." My guess is no; these are probably not the things you want to be remembered for. How sad would a life be if that were all it amounted to? When I do this exercise, I hope that people will talk about my strong relationships, my ability to put people at ease, my inclusiveness, and how playful and silly I was.

After working through the activities, you will end up with three or four top values. Make sure you've come up with values and not qualities that have to do with how other people respond to you. Review the list to verify that all of these values come from your authentic self. Is there potential that one or more of them are actually societal values coming from what you were taught in our appearance-focused, sexist, racist, fatphobic world? Could some of these values be coming from diet culture or healthism? Or perhaps some of these values came from your family experiences growing up? Try to figure out if there is a discrepancy between what diet culture values, what your family values, or what your culture values versus what feels authentically true to you. For example, when Tora was going through this activity, the values of *appearance* and *beauty* stood out to her. When she dug a bit deeper, she realized that her mother placed a huge emphasis on good looks and attractiveness. All of her life, she remembered her mother commenting on other women's appearances, including hers and her sisters'. To this day, Tora's mother still highly values beauty—so it's no wonder it was also on Tora's list. But was "beauty" a value that actually would lead her in the direction of becoming the person she wanted to be? (Her answer: nope!)

If you're struggling to choose your values, that's okay. Later in Step 4, when I explain how to act on your values, you can experiment with the ones you *think* are your authentic values. When you start to practice behaviors and actions that align with these values, you will learn over time which values feel important to you and which don't.

Step 2: Assessing Where You Are Versus Where You Want to Go

Take a look at the three or four core values you selected. For each of the values, answer the following questions:

- Are you living in alignment with this value?
- Are your behaviors today moving you in the direction you want to go?
- Where are your behaviors consistent with this value?
- Where are your behaviors out of alignment with this value?

Consider life in general, as well as how you are taking care of yourself and your body using food, movement, and other coping tools. Often there is a big gap between our life values and our relationship to food and our bodies. For example, Tora ended up listing her values as courage, compassion, creativity, and equality. She realized that her attempts to restrict her food, exercise excessively, and pursue weight loss were not in alignment with any of her values:

- *Courage*: "It doesn't take courage to make my body smaller; it is actually the opposite. Being willing to go against the tide, against society's standards, is what really takes courage. Playing into them doesn't feel courageous to me," Tora reflected.
- *Compassion*: "All my thoughts are judgmental. I speak really harshly to myself, which is not at all compassionate."
- *Creativity*: "Dieting and pursing a certain body stifles my creativity. I'm so focused on what others are thinking of me that I'm not doing the creative things that I want."
- *Equality*: "I really do believe in and value equity, justice, and equality," Tora said. "That means all bodies are worthy and valuable, and all bodies have access to what they need. Dieting and pursing weight loss is not in alignment with this, as diet culture is not equality."

If you notice any discrepancies between your values and how you've been behaving, don't beat yourself up. Shaming yourself for living in a way that doesn't uphold your values is not helpful. Instead, show yourself some compassion and begin to get curious about why there may be a discrepancy (see Step 3).

You also may find that your values are shifting. This is completely normal. Our values change over time, and this change is often a necessary part of learning and growing. In my mid-twenties, I would have listed "organization" as a top value. I was moving up the ladder in my corporate hospital job, and it was something I put a lot of effort into achieving. Now, a decade later, I realize that organization is not what I want out of life. I still value it, but it's not where I'm trying to steer my life. You may also notice a shift in your values once you begin to unpack what you were doing for external reasons—based on the social messages you've absorbed—and what you are doing for internal reasons. When we stop thinking about what the world wants from us and instead focus on what *we* want from *ourselves,* our values will shift.

As Glennon Doyle asks in her book *Untamed,* "What is the truest, most beautiful story about your life you can imagine?"[2] Set aside what society insists is "the only way." Step back from what you've been taught to conform to or what you've been told is "good." What is it that *you* want from your life? Your relationships? Your world? And what about your current life, or current relationships, are *not* "true and beautiful" enough for you? How can you begin to let go of what is not serving you so that you can take steps toward the life, the relationships, and the world that *you* want?

Valued Living Reflection ⎯⎯⎯⎯⎯⎯

Reflect upon your values. How might living in alignment with these values support healing your relationship to food, with your body, and with yourself?

Step 3: Identifying Barriers to Valued Living

If there is a discrepancy between your values and the way you are living, begin to explore what barriers are getting in your way. Consider the following questions:

- Why may you not be living in alignment with all of your values?
- Where are you getting stuck?
- Are you clear on your "why"? (If not, go back and review Chapter 7.)
- Are you getting attached to your thoughts or feelings about your body?
- Are diet culture and society's messages dictating or influencing your behaviors?
- What thoughts, emotions, physical sensations, or experiences might you be trying to avoid?
- Are you at a point in your life where your values are shifting? (This is normal; values can change as we age.)

Barriers to living out your values can take many forms. Your thoughts, feelings, memories, urges, and fears can keep you stuck and out of alignment. For example, when I was examining what was keeping me from feeling connected to others, I realized it went back to childhood experiences of wanting to fit in, be liked, and be accepted, and having a period of time in elementary school when I felt abandoned by my friends. There was still a part of me that worried that others wouldn't accept the full me, so I wasn't letting all of myself be seen. These fears were also rooted in my socialization as a white, middle-class woman, which taught me the message that women shouldn't be "too much." I had a fear of being labeled bossy, bitchy, angry, etc. These thoughts and feelings were keeping me stuck, unable to connect to my true self or other people. In other words, the thoughts, feelings, and fears were keeping me out of alignment with my values.

In my work with clients, an internal barrier I often see is a fear of their bodies changing. They want to live out their values, yet there is also a part of them that is afraid of letting go of control and the potential weight changes that may occur. Some people have memories of being treated better when they were in smaller bodies. A desire to lose weight can stem from very real difficulties like trauma and oppression, which means wanting to lose weight may mean wanting to feel safe in your body. These fears can be very real and difficult to face. Our patriarchal, racist, queerphobic society has programmed all sorts of messages and beliefs into our minds. It's common to feel caught up in society's expectations, our experiences in our bodies, and our personal shame.

There may also be external barriers to living out your values, such as in the form of an unsupportive partner or family, going through a traumatic event, or not having the resources to pursue your values. For example, one of my clients was working on eating more consistent meals throughout the day but sometimes didn't have enough money to eat whatever or whenever she wanted. You may also find that some of your values are seemingly in conflict. A value of self-care, for example, may seem hard to take action to-ward if you also value spending time with your loved ones and have only so many hours in the day. In this case, know that your values are not mutually exclusive. Although you may not be able to do goal-related actions for every value every day, you can still live out your values over time.

As you analyze for any real or potential barriers, think about how you might be able to encounter those experiences and take action toward your values despite the obstacles. Very real systemic oppression exists for people who live in marginalized bodies, yet you can still challenge these thoughts, and your reaction to them, without invalidating them. These be-liefs, thoughts, and feelings may never totally go away, but in doing the work to unpack and examine them, you can begin to refuse to use them to guide your life choices. Remember, just because a thought occurs to you doesn't mean that you have to do what it says. Your skills of mindfulness and self-compassion will come in handy as you work through these barriers and con-tinue to practice taking small, supportive steps toward valued living.

What Are Your Barriers to Valued Living? _____

Make a list of all of the barriers—both internal and external—that are getting in the way of your living out your values. These could be real barriers or potential barriers that you foresee popping up.

Step 4: Acting on Your Values

It is one thing to get clarity around your core values; it's another thing to change your behaviors and take action to align with those values. Identifying your values is the fun part. It's a pretty simple exercise, and completing it can feel good because you're "doing something." That's true—in a way, you are. Values identify which direction you want to go. But the real growth comes from following through and taking action to *move* in that direction. Although many of us would love for personal growth to be quick and painless, it never is. Taking steps to act on your values is much more difficult and often much less fun. It takes a lot of bravery and inner strength. It is *hard*. But this is where the real, painful, magical, joyful expansion happens. This is where you start to unlock your true self. This is where you start to live more authentically.

Once you've assessed where you want to go (your values) and where you are right now, you can establish goals to help you move toward your values. If values are the direction you are going, goals are stops along the road, and actions are behavior steps that you take to get to those goals. For example, for Tora's value of *compassion,* she set the following goals and action steps:

- Goal: Do at least one self-compassionate action every day.
  Action step: Come up with a list of at least five self-compassionate actions.
- Goal: Record five to ten affirmations and listen to it at least once a week.
  Action step: Brainstorm a list of affirmations that feel authentic.
- Goal: Buy two new pairs of pants that fit comfortably.
  Action step: Research online clothing stores that carry my size.

When setting goals, it helps to have concrete objectives to work toward in the hopes of more valued living. Goals might aim either to increase or decrease a behavior. For example, decreasing the use of compensatory exercise or increasing the amount of "off-limits" food that you keep in the house. Goals are ideally SMART: specific, measurable, achievable, realistic, and time-bound. They should also be small. Many people overestimate what they can successfully do and then feel disappointed or upset when they don't achieve the goal. Start with the actions or behavior changes that feel the easiest and most attainable. Then gradually move toward the more difficult behavior changes.

While specific goals increase the chance that you make changes, it's also important to be flexible. The point is not to check the box and be done with it. It is the experience that is important. As you identify your values and practice making changes to align with that value, some of them may not go well. This is okay! Rather than looking at it as pass/fail, try to view your action steps as experiences that will teach you something.

If the thought of making changes brings up any feelings of resistance, this is understandable. It's common to want to feel "ready" to make changes before taking action. The reality is that if you try to wait until you are fully "ready," the changes may never happen. Changing actions and behaviors precede shifting feelings. You need to act first by changing your behavior, and then over time your feelings will catch up. Once you start changing your behaviors and seeing the improvement, it can feel more doable. My client Carolyn was really resistant to allowing herself unconditional permission to eat sweets. She was afraid of feeling out of control and wanted to wait until she felt more "ready." When I asked her what she might be *willing* to do instead, she agreed to keep a certain type of candy in her house. It felt scary, but after a little while of allowing herself to eat it—and using mindfulness to explore her experience—Carolyn noticed a change. She didn't feel as out of control around the candy and didn't feel the same amount of urgency to eat it. This experience gave her the confidence to know that she could handle these changes. Generally behavior change comes first; then your thoughts change; then your feelings catch up and begin to shift.

As you continue to take action, revisit your "why" and your core values. Remind yourself that every action is a choice that either leads you *toward* or *away* from where you want to be. Which direction do you want to go?

Instead of pouring time and energy into changing your body, can you put energy toward the things that you value most?

Commit to Action

For each of your core values, write down at least two specific goals and associated actions you can take to help you live out those values. These goals and actions should be specific, realistic behaviors that you can commit to in the short term. Make them workable, actionable, manageable, and something that you know you can do. Don't worry if these actions don't seem like "enough." You will revisit your actionable goals periodically and gradually build in more and more actions that bring you closer to valued living.

Use your values to remember what you are fighting for, whether that be connection, growth, relationships, adventure, justice, or compassion. Your values are your North Star, guiding you on your path. You may not be able to see what is right in front of you. You're taking a new direction, so there may not even be a path, hence your greater life vision becomes your inner compass. Distractions may come up, your mind might be pulled outside of your body, and you may be tempted to step back onto the well-worn path of your past. Continue to come back to your purpose and your vision of what you want your life to be like.

Coming Back to Your Intuition

We weren't born distrusting ourselves—we were taught. Many of us have been trained to believe that who we are in our natural state is wrong. We are often taught to fear our intuition in every aspect of our lives, which means we may not trust our bodies. Instead, we doubt. We doubt our hunger, our curiosity, our personalities, our judgment, our experiences, our ambition. We ignore our gut instinct. We make decisions based upon our external training rather than our internal knowing. We chase success and happiness by following other people's directions rather than our own. We spend our lives contorting ourselves to be what we think others want us to be. The more energy we spend focusing on how we are perceived, the more we lose who we really are.

But your intuition, your deep inner knowing, is still there. Intuition exists in all of us, regardless of whether we hear it, acknowledge it, or listen to it. Intuition is our quick, instinctual response that occurs in a matter of seconds. This differs from our analytical, conscious brain—the one that has been trained to ignore intuition. Yet the intuitive part of our bodies often knows what is best for us long before our analytical brain jumps in. Underneath all the thoughts and beliefs and feelings that the world has taught you, your core essence exists. Some people think of this as their soul, their spirit, their inner self. No matter what you call it, you can rebuild your connection, your trust, your relationship with yourself. The more you can get back to that inner knowing, the more you can use it to lead your truest, most beautiful, unapologetic life.

How do you figure out what your intuition, or your gut, is telling you? It starts with listening. Turning inward, ask *yourself* the question. It can start small: What do *I* feel like eating? What do *I* want to wear today? Then it gets bigger: What do *I* want out of life? Ask yourself the question, be still, and listen. What does your body tell you? Not your rational brain, or your intellect, or the messages the world has taught you. Not what you think you "should" or "shouldn't" do or what you think is "right" or "wrong" or "good" or "bad." But what does your soul, your inner self want? This requires some silence and stillness. If you are always going-going-going, you are probably not going to be able to tune in to what your intuition is telling you.

Try to find some silence and stillness and feel into your body. What sensations do you notice? I'll share more about how to feel into your body in Chapter 15, but for now, see what you can feel. Signs that your intuition is saying *yes* can include feelings of openness, expansiveness, lightness, powerfulness, and/or excitement. On the other hand, feeling tight and stuck with a sense of dread may mean your intuition is telling you *no*. For example, a company recently reached out to me with a business opportunity that—on paper—sounded great. Although my mind was saying, "You *should* go for this," when I tapped into my body, I noticed that my shoulders had tightened, my neck was tense. I now know that my body's signals are often a sign that something is not in line with my gut instinct. When I pressed send on the email saying "no," I immediately felt a sense of relief, and my body relaxed. This response confirmed for me that I had listened to my intuition.

Now, you may notice that feelings of openness and excitement are also accompanied by fear or anxiety. This doesn't necessarily mean your intuition is saying *no*; it may just mean that you have internalized beliefs that are getting in the way of your intuition or you may have some nervous anticipation. Try to tap into the fear and anxiety and figure out whether it stems from a gut reaction or a brain reaction. A gut reaction may mean the answer is *no*, whereas a brain reaction may mean that you go ahead and say *yes* despite the fear.

It's okay if you're not exactly sure what your body is feeling or what your gut instinct is. Feel around, and then do what you think your intuition is telling you. No apologies, no explanation, no justification. Just act based on what you're feeling and see what happens. Then check in with yourself. Over time, you'll know if you decided based on your intuition. "Deep down, I'll know" can be a helpful phrase to repeat over and over and over. The more you check in with yourself, the easier it becomes to know *your* answer. As you get more comfortable with your inner knowing and allow yourself to dream up the best, most authentic, unapologetic life you can imagine, you can then begin to feel more free. You may not know exactly where life will take you, but you are learning, you are growing, and you are becoming.

Rebuilding your relationship to food is the first step toward throwing out all the rules that you've been taught and starting to write your own, not just about food or your body, but about who you are and who you get to be. What you wear. Who you love. The work that you do (or don't do). The life you live. It can start with turning inside and figuring out what it is you really want to eat. In the end, though, it's so much more. By finding freedom with food, you can find freedom in life. When you don't have to be in control, when you don't have to follow the rules, when you don't have to rebel, you can be free to be yourself. No explanations, no justifications, no apologies. In the next chapter, we'll take a look at how the process of embodiment can help you to do this.

CHAPTER 15

Becoming Embodied

Reconnecting to your authentic, unapologetic self involves getting out of your head and into your body. The first time someone told me I needed to "get into my body," my immediate reaction was, "WTF does that even mean? Aren't I *in* my body already?" Technically, yes, but in many ways, no. I was living in my body, but I wasn't connected to it. I was letting my head make all the decisions without any consultation with my body. I was *thinking* things through rather than *feeling* things through. What I didn't realize at the time is that this is very common.

Our bodies communicate so much wisdom and information to us all day long. Taking in that information and listening to that wisdom is essential for our personal growth, learning, and connection. However, the vast majority of us spend most of our time in our heads, listening to our thoughts. When our attention becomes focused mainly on external tasks or problems or getting things done, it can make it easy to ignore—or even silence—any cues that the body is sending. Many of us tend to pay way more attention to the information in our heads than to the information in our bodies.

It can be a challenge to stay present in the body. Every day you may encounter thousands of thoughts, feelings, and experiences that encourage you to tune out, numb, and disconnect. Many people disassociate from their bodies because, at some point in their lives, they had to. This disassociation or disconnection can help to lessen feelings of pain (at least in the short term), but it also can shut you off from feeling joy and connection. Over time, this numbing out can become a type of "functional freeze" response.

You may disconnect from your internal sensations and emotions while you stay outwardly functional—working, eating, parenting, etc. It's become so normalized in our culture that it's hard to notice when it is happening. Here are some signs that you may be disconnected from your body:

- You often feel numb, flat, or lethargic.
- You are constantly trying to keep yourself busy to avoid feeling.
- You feel like something is missing and there should be something more.
- You often put others' thoughts and opinions before your own.
- You fear the judgment of others.
- You worry about not being "enough" or being "too much."
- You aren't sure how to feel your full range and depth of emotions.
- You often feel like you're on the outside, looking in.
- You have no idea what it is that you are feeling.

Some of the issues from the list could be signs of a more serious mental health concern. Consider reaching out to a therapist or counselor.

One of my clients, Vanessa, explained the sensation of disconnection this way: "From the neck down, I feel totally disconnected from my body. It's like my brain and my body are two different entities. And 99 percent of the time, I disconnect from my body, existing only in my head. I consider my body an entirely separate entity from 'me.'"

If you experience disconnection with your body, it doesn't make you wrong or broken or less than. Most of us are not taught how to connect to our bodies; in fact, we often learn the exact opposite. Noticing these signs of disconnection is an invitation to begin to explore, learn, and grow. When did this disconnection from your body begin? What experiences or feelings have caused you to disconnect? How may have this disconnection protected you over the years? As you begin to understand your history with your body, you can then work toward becoming more present in your body.

How Disconnection Occurs

People disconnect from their bodies for all sorts of reasons, often out of necessity. Those who experience trauma often note that disconnecting from their bodies is a matter of survival. "I was in my head trying to survive and had to disconnect from my body in order to do so," Vanessa told me. "I couldn't pay attention to my body because I was so busy trying to just make it through the day."

Very often, internal emotions can feel like they're too much or too painful, so disconnecting from the body functions as a means of protection. This response may be due to trauma, chronic stress, and more. Here's a (very) simple example from one of my clients: "I hate my stomach, so I disconnect from it." This disconnection is often not a conscious decision but rather an instinctive reaction. It can be really hard to feel discomfort, no matter whether it comes from an external source or one's internal feelings. To avoid the discomfort, many people direct all the attention into their heads. Some experiences that can lead to body disconnection include

- Going through puberty
- Dealing with a developing or changing body that betrays who you feel like inside
- Experiencing chronic pain
- Constantly being told that you are "too fat" and should lose weight
- Intergenerational trauma
- Facing daily micro- and/or macroaggressions
- Experiencing racism, ableism, sexism, transphobia, or homophobia
- Getting severely injured in an accident and spending months in a hospital
- Being diagnosed with cancer and undergoing multiple invasive medical procedures
- Encountering toxic shame, like being told you're not good enough or that you need to "toughen up"
- Having difficulty moving about in a world that wasn't built for your body
- Chronic dieting, restricting food intake, and ignoring body hunger cues
- Experiencing emotional, physical, or sexual abuse

Many of my clients tell me that they feel like their body has betrayed them. As a thin, white, able-bodied, cisgender woman, I have little personal experience with this, but I've learned so much from my clients about the deep sense of shame and disconnection that comes from living in a body that has betrayed their trust in some way. As one of my clients, a cancer survivor in her mid-thirties, said to me, "It's hard to connect to a body that recently tried to kill me. My illness made me have to separate myself from my body in order to get through treatment. Because why would I want to be in my body when terrible things were happening to my body?"

Navigating this sense of betrayal, shame, and disconnection is difficult. The culture we live in doesn't make it any easier on us. As Virgie Tovar writes, "Our culture is set up to make us not feel things, because injustice is an unbearable state for an embodied person. There is no conceivable way for people to be in their bodies in a culture that is so committed to violence against its most vulnerable."[1] It is one thing to know injustice from an intellectual standpoint, but it is another thing to feel it in your body. As Virgie says, feeling it can be unbearable. So we instead may push it away and take cover in our minds.

Even people who have never experienced significant trauma can find themselves disconnected from their bodies. Recall that even dieting is a form of trauma. Consider how your time dieting and ignoring your body cues may have caused body disconnection. Or perhaps your disconnection occurred through your socialization, as much of mine did. I was so concerned with what others thought of me that I spent the vast majority of my time living in my head, not my body. The trip to visit my friend was when I first realized that every thought or action that I wanted to take first had to go through a filter. *Is this okay to say? What will other people think? Are they going to think I'm weird/too much/not ____ enough?* I was so trained to seek external validation and approval that I was never fully connecting to my body.

Our culture's obsession with "busyness" often adds to our disconnection. In our capitalistic, profit-driven world, the bottom line is what's most important. This means that our society measures success upon how hard a person works and how much they produce. Busyness is often seen as a status symbol. In my twenties, the running joke was that friends—and potential dates—had to book me at least three weeks in advance to get any time on my calendar (and this was something I was proud of). Even outside of work, many of us are constantly plugged in. The average adult in the United States consumes more than twelve hours of media *per day*. We are often plugged into our phones at all hours of the day (and night). Social media has turned many of us into a generation of performers. The focus can become what we look like to others (or what will be "Instagram-worthy") rather than being fully present and experiencing the moment. No wonder so many of us are always in our heads!

Although disconnection may have once been a tool for survival, at some point, it can do more harm than good. The body carries much knowledge and wisdom. When we ignore, dismiss, or try to silence that wisdom, we can lose out on opportunities for learning and growth. As I shared in Chapter 12, not listening to your body can be a sign of disrespect, which only makes the chasm between your body and mind grow wider.

Disconnecting from your body inevitably means disconnecting from yourself. Where has that led you? For me, it meant that I was caught up in a comparison game. I never fully trusted myself or felt like I could be my true self. Instead, I looked to external sources to get feedback about what I should or shouldn't do, say, wear, be. The result is that I often felt like I was outside of myself, looking in. I didn't feel connected to my body; thus, I wasn't able to fully connect with others.

For Vanessa, who had spent years trying to diet and couldn't figure out why she kept "failing," disconnecting from her body made her feel like it was a separate entity. Part of her blamed her body for changing, for gaining weight, for being fat. "I'm so sick of it," she told me, speaking about her body. "I feel like my body has done me wrong." In that moment, Vanessa realized that the feelings of disconnection and betrayal caused her to use food subconsciously as a way to punish her body. It's not that she was "failing" at the diet by bingeing or eating foods that she knew would make her feel awful. It was happening because, subconsciously, part of her wanted to retaliate against her body. "I know what I eat will cause me pain, but I still do it. For so long, I believed this was because of my lack of willpower, as I just couldn't stick to a diet. Now I realize that I'm eating this way to punish my body for betraying me."

Physical and emotional disconnection from our bodies can lead us to treat ourselves and our bodies in a multitude of harmful ways. Body disconnection, or *disembodiment*, makes it next to impossible to experience life fully. When we are present in our bodies, we can get more clarity around what matters to us and how we can create a deep, meaningful life. To be our full, unapologetic selves, we must become *embodied*.

What Does It Mean to Be *Embodied*?

As you are sitting here reading this book, how present do you feel in your body? Can you feel your feet on the floor (or—as mine are currently—on the couch)? Do you notice the sensation of your butt making contact with whatever surface you are sitting on? Are you able to feel your chest rise and fall as you breathe?

Being embodied means being present in your body and feeling all your body sensations, even when—or especially when—you are engaged with the world in some way. As you are walking, can you notice the sensation of your feet on the ground? Are you aware of where your body is in space? How does your body feel? Embodiment is a feeling of connectedness to your body. When you are embodied, you can notice, sense, and listen to what your body has to say rather than going through the day without having any idea of what your body is communicating. It is not about thinking; it is about your body becoming more aware of itself. Embodiment is often described as the sense of *being at home* in your body, which is the direct opposite of what Vanessa described about her body being a separate entity from herself.

Most people exist solely in their heads, spending very little, if any, time feeling into their bodies. Those who do practice being present tend to reserve their embodiment practices for specific chunks of time, such as during yoga class as they're cued to listen to their breathing or during a guided meditation that includes prompts to draw attention to various parts of the body. However, true embodiment means integrating both body *and* mind so that you may feel each experience fully. It isn't either/or—your head *or* your body—rather, it is both/and. Connection to both your head knowing *and* your body knowing. Becoming embodied means opening yourself—both body and mind—to the entirety of what you are experiencing. Fully inhabiting your sense of *knowing* as bodymind (or mindbody) together as one.

The idea of being present in the body might sound a little woo-woo to you. I say this because I once thought the same thing. I would internally roll my eyes whenever I heard someone mention the idea of "being grounded" or "noticing your feet." So if you had the same response a few paragraphs back, I feel you. But try to stick with me here for a minute. To better illustrate "embodiment," let me share a story about the first time I really felt this sensation. I had to set aside my instinctual eye roll as I realized, "Ohhh, this is what they meant."

It happened just a few years ago on the visit to my friend Hana, whom I mentioned in Chapter 14. As a reminder, this was the same trip where I first put two and two together and realized that what I was missing was connection, and the reason I had been missing it was because I was always filtering everything I said or did through my brain. I had had glimpses of what it was like to feel into my body, but I still was all up in my head the vast majority of the time.

On the last day of my trip, we went to the beach with a few other friends. After playing in the water for a bit, everyone got out to eat lunch, yet I had the strongest urge to stay and sit on the sand. Part of me felt like I "should" go with the group, but I leaned into what my body was feeling and sat down. I sat there for who knows how long, the gentle waves crashing over me and then retreating. I noticed the other people around me but, for the first time in as long as I could remember, I didn't hear that voice in my head, worrying about what they were thinking about me. I surrendered to the moment and the feeling. The water rushing over me and pulling at my limbs as it receded. The feeling of the retreating sand swirling against my skin. My whole body felt loose and open; my breath slowed. Although I was still aware of the presence of other beach goers, the tape in my head was (mostly) still and silent. It felt so nice to just sit and feel rather than think. This experience was the first time I felt fully in my body, fully present, fully me. I finally understood getting "out of your head and into your body."

Later that day, Hana said to me, "You came into this week looking worn down, under pressure, and overworked. But now I can see a light in your eyes—a spark that wasn't there before." She was right; I did feel different. But why? What about this experience had allowed me to open up and finally feel what it was like to be embodied?

Strengthening Your *Felt Sense*

Philosopher Eugene Gendlin coined the term *felt sense*.[2] He described it as a person's ability to experience the physical sensations of their body in a noncognitive way. To notice the sensations and feelings coming from the body rather than analyzing them via the brain. You may *feel* sad, anxious, or happy, but how do those feelings reveal themselves in your body? Turning inward and listening with your felt sense allows your body to guide you toward deeper self-knowledge. This is similar to the concept of interoceptive awareness that I spoke about in Chapter 8, or the ability to be aware of the sensations arising within the body. The awareness of what is being felt in the body can ground you in the present moment.

Your felt sense lies beyond your thoughts and feelings. For example, you may express the thought of "I feel stressed," which is your brain talking. What does "stressed" feel like in your body? What sensations are present in your body that let you know that you are stressed? Perhaps your jaw is clenched, your tongue glued to the top of your mouth, or your shoulders feel tight and hunched. Once you have that felt sense in focus, and it is clear what you are feeling, try not to react to it. Your inclination might be to push the feeling away, judge the sensations, or resist the sensations. Instead, try to use your mindfulness skills to create that "pause" between the noticing and reacting. You can then *respond* (rather than react) with what Gendlin calls *asking*.

Asking is bringing your attention to the physical sensations you are experiencing (i.e., your *felt sense*) and checking in with them. What are you stressed about? Is it what you are working on or doing in that moment, or is there something deeper going on? If this sensation feels uncomfortable, why is that? Ask yourself—including your body—"What do you need right now?" Then sit and wait. What comes up? What answer or insight do you perceive in your bodymind?

You can work on strengthening your felt sense at any time of day. Practice pausing, dropping into your body, and noticing what sensations arise. Then begin to ask questions to get clearer about what is going on and what your body is trying to tell you. It's okay if you're unsure what your body is feeling. (In fact, you may not know what your body is feeling the first several times you try this—this is okay!) The act of *responding* and *questioning* takes practice, but it will help you begin to connect more with your felt sense and learn what it is communicating to you.

Becoming Embodied

Learning how to inhabit all of your bodily experiences fully is not easy, especially for folks who have disconnected from their bodies or their feelings as a matter of survival. Before we can be *in* our bodies, we need to feel safe. That safety is essential (and yet another reason why liberation for *all bodies* is so important). Unresolved traumas—of any magnitude—remain in the body. That means that for some people, the practice of feeling into the body can be activating or upsetting.

If you do not feel safe in your body, or safe feeling certain body sensations, then I highly recommend working with a therapist who is trained in trauma-specific modalities. *Psychology Today* offers a list of therapists who specialize in this area: https://www.psychologytoday.com/us/therapists/ trauma-focused/.

Becoming more embodied is not something that happens overnight. After my experience on the beach, I did not immediately go from being in my head to always being present in my body. In fact, one week after that experience, I was dancing at an event and was acutely aware of how in my head I was. But that was the key: I was now aware of it. I had an experience to connect to that I could remind myself of. And using that awareness, I could continue to practice working toward being in my body more consistently.

Embodiment Practices

There are a number of things you can try to do to bring yourself back to your body and into the present moment. None of these practices are "one and done." Embodiment ebbs and flows. All of us will become momentarily disconnected from our bodies from time to time, whether out of necessity or just because life gets busy or chaotic. This is part of being human. The important thing is that you can start to recognize that the disconnection is occurring and take steps to bring your body back online. This could be through regular therapy (being all up in my head is often a sign for me that it's been too long since my last therapy appointment) or through consistent practice of some of the following activities.

Practice Body Respect

When you respect your body—by listening, serving, being kind, and appreciating—you show care, love, and acceptance. This can increase feelings of safety and trust in your body, which may make it easier to connect to body sensations. For many of the people I work with, embodiment starts when they strengthen their interoception skills or their ability to answer the question, "How do I feel?" Interoception can apply to feelings of hunger and fullness but also occurs when you notice the sensation of having to go to the bathroom, changes in body temperature, or any feelings such as stress, anxiety, excitement, or sadness. As you strengthen those skills and take action based on what you're feeling, you can begin to practice body respect consistently. Body respect builds body trust and safety, which then can allow you to feel more ready and willing to connect to other sensations in your body.

Check In with Your Body

Try to take a minute to pause each day (or several times throughout the day) to check in with your body. Ask yourself questions like:

- How is my body doing today?
- How is my body feeling today?
- What sensations am I feeling in my body right now?

These check-ins allow you to practice feeling your body's response to both your internal and your external environments. For example, I have learned that when I work, my shoulders automatically tighten and move toward my ears. When I'm in the depths of a busy workday, I often don't notice this, which usually means that by the end of the day, my neck, shoulders, and sometimes my head are throbbing in pain. When I make time for a quick body check-in during the day, I can bring my attention to my shoulder tightness and remind myself to unclench and relax (or, as my partner says, "wiggle").

The body scan meditation described on page 157 is another way that you can connect to your body during the day. You don't need to practice it as a "formal" meditation; you can simply take a few minutes and scan your body from head to toe to notice how each body part feels. The goal here is not to judge or react but to be present and notice: What is your body communicating to you? The more consistently you practice this, the easier it will become to feel connected to your body throughout the day, even when you are engaged in another task.

Build Body Curiosity

If you struggle to check-in somewhat "blindly" throughout the day, try instead to notice how your body feels during certain daily activities. You might be vacuuming, gardening, or washing dishes. While you do the activity, get curious: How does it make your hands feel? How does it make your legs feel? How does it make your shoulders feel? How intense are the feelings on a scale of 1 to 10? If this type of assessment feels too abstract, you may try offering yourself choices instead: Do your legs feel heavy or light? Does your brain feel focused or distracted? Do your shoulders feel tight or loose?[3] Practice staying present with yourself and your body as you notice different sensations. As you work on this, try to go deeper. What type of emotions might your body sensations be conveying? For example, if you are washing dishes and your legs feel heavy, what emotion could that be expressing? It's okay if you don't have an "exact" answer (watch for that perfectionism!). Just the practice of noticing, observing, and getting curious can help you start to become more aware of your body in different ways throughout the day.

Explore Your Body

Avoiding mirrors and halting body-checking can be helpful early in this process to calm your nervous system and prevent disordered eating or exercise behaviors. When you've gotten to a point where you are more relaxed and feel ready to explore your body, looking at and touching your body is a helpful part of the embodiment process. You are the expert of your body, and embodiment means allowing yourself to explore and know every part of it. Building a loving, trusting relationship means getting to know your body, just as you might with a partner, which may happen through both observation and touch.

Observe

One observation exercise that can be helpful is something called *mirror exposure*. Stand in front of a full-length mirror while wearing minimal or fitted clothing so that you can see your body. Start at the top of your head and observe. What do you see? Use neutral, objective descriptors to identify what you notice. For example, "My hair is brown and curly. My eyes are blue. Bangs cover part of my forehead." When a criticism or analysis pops up, you have reached the end of the exercise.

At first, you may be able to get only to your eyebrows before a critical thought invades; this is okay (and totally normal). The benefits of the mirror exercise can come when you repeat it regularly (at least two or three times per week). As you get used to objectively observing your body, you may find it easier to get through the exercise without as many negative thoughts bubbling up. Here is how one of my clients described the process of doing the mirror exercise: "The more I did it, the longer I could go before an uncomfortable emotion or thought arose. It felt almost like a meditation, where I was neutrally observing without judgment. I didn't love what I saw, and at certain points a little disappointment would come through, like 'Oh, that is what I look like.' But there was no longer that intense self-hatred or negativity."

You can also explore your body through observation without using a mirror. Spend some time examining your skin, noticing the different textures, colors, moles, lumps, or bumps. Again, practice doing this examination objectively and neutrally. Use your mindfulness skills to notice when a negative or uncomfortable thought comes up and try to create a "pause" to observe and respond rather than react.

Touch

Embodiment can include feeling a sense of intimacy with your body. This familiarity may come from looking at, feeling, and understanding it. Touching your body—both in sexual and nonsexual ways—can be an important part of getting to know your body and improving your body image. Nonsexual touch can include some of the self-compassionate actions that you brain-stormed in Chapter 11: gently rubbing your arms, massaging your shoulders, holding your belly, or hugging yourself. As you touch your body, try to stay in the moment and focus on how it feels. Again, use mindfulness to notice when a negative thought, judgment, or analysis arises. Bring your focus back to the sensations that you feel under your hands and on your skin. How would you describe those sensations in a nonjudgmental way?

When you practice exploring your body in a nonjudgmental way, it may help to think about how toddlers and young children interact with the world. Before kids are indoctrinated with society's negative body messages, they love exploring the textures and sensations of bodies—both their own and their parents'. One of my clients hated her belly and couldn't stand to look at it or feel it; she was so uncomfortable with it that she often wouldn't let her husband touch it either. One day, the woman's two-year-old daughter put her head in her mother's lap and said, "Mommy, your stomach is like a fluffy cloud. I love how soft and squishy it feels." Hearing her child use these descriptors and profess her love for it allowed something to shift. Things that are soft and squishy *do* feel good to many people. Think about how much people love pillows, stuffed animals, Play-doh, memory foam mattresses, and gel shoe inserts. Yet many people feel such intense, nega-tive thoughts about their soft, squishy bellies. Although these thoughts or feelings won't disappear overnight, beginning to touch these parts of your body can help to foster intimacy, relationship, and embodiment.

Exploring your body through sensual self-touch may also be helpful. Mas-turbation—especially when it comes to a woman's pleasure—is such a taboo topic in our society. If even reading that word made you feel somewhat un-comfortable, know that you are not alone. You may even be wondering what a book about food and body image is doing talking about *sensual self-touch*. But here's the thing: As I dove more into body image work, it became abun-dantly clear to me how important our sexuality is when it comes to our re-lationships to food, with our bodies, and ultimately with ourselves. Women who are more self-conscious of their bodies have fewer orgasms than women who report better body image (now, if that's not a reason to work on your body image...). On average, women who are more body-conscious orgasm only 42 percent of the time compared to women who are less self-conscious, who orgasm 73 percent of the time. Overall research shows that at least one-third of all women struggle to reach orgasm because they're worried about how they look.[4] The ability to be *in* your body, including during sex, can be improved. Sensual self-touch can help to increase your awareness of and connection to your body. Our bodies are designed for pleasure, yet many of us don't often permit ourselves to feel it. We are often taught by society that pleasure is shameful, whether pleasure through food, self-touch, or someone or something else. Really, though, pleasure is awareness, connection, and—ultimately—a form of self-care. If it feels right for you, go ahead and set aside some time to practice body self-exploration and sensual self-touch. (That's right; I encourage you to masturbate.)

Belly Breathe

When people are busy, stressed, or in their heads, their breathing can become shallow and short. Belly breathing, on the other hand, can help you get deeper into your body. This involves taking longer, deeper breaths to breathe into your stomach and fill yourself fully with air. Here's how you can practice this: Breathe in through your nose to a count of four, imagining a balloon in your stomach filling with air. Then hold your breath for a second at the top. Exhale out of your mouth as if you're breathing through a straw as you count to four; then hold for a second at the end. Continue taking these deep, slow, even belly breaths five to ten times. If it feels comfortable, you can close your eyes and place your hands gently on your belly so that you can feel it expanding and filling with air. If you are new to belly breathing, you may want to try to do it while lying flat on your back, which may make it easier for your diaphragm to expand.

The beauty of belly breathing is that it is available and accessible to you at any time throughout the day. You can even do it while sitting at your desk because it takes less than a minute. Bonus: Deep belly breathing also helps to lower stress. Just the simple act of taking slow, deep breaths signals to your body to lower your stress hormones, which can make you feel more calm, relaxed, and connected to your body.

352

Meditate

Whereas informal body check-ins are available to you at any point in the day, as described earlier, developing a more formal meditation practice can also help increase feelings of embodiment. Mindfulness and other forms of meditation have been shown to help improve interoceptive awareness (presumably as a result of neuroplasticity changes[5]). Meditation, especially mindfulness meditation, teaches you how to focus intentionally on body sensations. It also can help you learn how to redirect your focus to your body whenever your mind wanders. This continued noticing and redirecting can, over time, increase your ability to be aware of any physical or emotional sensations that arise within your body. Increased body awareness then can persist not only while you meditate but throughout the rest of the day even as your mind becomes busy with other things. Refer to Chapter 6 for more resources on starting a meditation practice.

Ground Yourself

Anyone who's taken a yoga class has probably been invited to "ground down" through the soles of the feet or via their "sit bones." *Grounding* is one of those esoteric terms that many people (like me) hear and sort of understand, but they aren't exactly sure what they are supposed to be feeling (or doing). It didn't click for me until I experienced that "out of my head/into my body" moment on the beach because feeling "grounded" involves letting go of what is in your head and coming back to the physical feelings in the body. The practice of grounding down can help connect you to the present moment. As you connect to the feeling of being in touch with the ground beneath you, you can come back to yourself and your body. Feeling your feet on the floor, or your back on the ground, reminds you that you are still *here*. Grounding may also enable you to feel how your body is physically supporting you, which can cultivate a sense of self-trust and stability.

You don't have to take a yoga class to feel more grounded (though you certainly can). There are many ways to "ground down" and this practice can be accessible to you all day long. The key is to find what way(s) works best for you so that you can return to it whenever you notice that your attention is focused up in your head. The more you direct your focus from your mind to your body, the more you can remain embodied and in the present moment. Here are a few grounding techniques to try:

- **Lie down:** (Note: You also can do this seated in a chair if that feels better or is more accessible to you.) Begin by lying down somewhere that feels comfortable—a couch, the bed, or (my personal favorite) on a patch of grass. Spread your arms and legs so that as much of your body is touching the ground as possible. If it feels comfortable, close your eyes. Take a few deep breaths and notice how your belly rises and falls. Bring your attention to your body. Notice the contact between your body and the ground. You may press your arms and legs into the ground for a few seconds and notice how that feels. Imagine your energy going from your body into the ground, and vice versa. Try to let your body feel heavy and relax into the ground. Notice any body sensations that arise.

- **Do a yoga pose:** You don't need to complete an entire yoga class to get the benefits of grounding. One of my favorite grounding techniques involves doing a few sets of cat/cow pose. I love that I can do this anytime throughout the day, and it takes just a few minutes to bring myself back into my body. Some other poses that can feel especially grounding include mountain pose, chair pose, child's pose (my second favorite), and savasana (which is basically lying on the ground as I described in the first bullet). If you're doing a standing pose, bring your awareness to the entire surface of the bottoms of your feet. Put more pressure down through the ball of your foot and notice how that feels. You can also make a slight bend in your knees, which may allow you to feel your body holding you up. When you're in a pose like cat/cow, spread your fingers wide on the ground. When you press into your hands, notice the pressure of the ground beneath you and how your limbs support your body. Remember to breathe into your belly as you do the pose.

- **Stand or walk barefoot (ideally outdoors):** Take off your shoes and socks and go outside. You can stand in one place or walk around. The key is to make contact with the ground, whether that is grass, sand, dirt, or stone. If you don't have easy access to a safe outdoor spot (hello, to all my fellow Manhattanites!), you can go barefoot indoors instead. Either way, stand or walk mindfully for a few minutes. Bring awareness to your feet making contact with the ground. How does that feel? As you stand or walk, what do you notice in your feet, in your legs, and further up your body? Can you feel any energy moving in your body? If you can't, that is okay. If I'd tried this five or ten years ago, I know I wouldn't have either. But as you build greater body awareness, you may find that you can notice and observe more subtle sensations in your body.

- ◆ **Spend time in nature:** I grew up in the woods, but after moving to New York City more than a decade ago, my time in nature became limited. For the first half dozen years, I was so caught up in experiencing all the things the city offered that I didn't even notice. Then a few years ago, I started experiencing this "pull" to be in nature. I resisted it for almost a year. "I'm a New Yorker; I love the city!" I thought (in my head, naturally). But my body felt differently. I finally planned a trip that would have me experiencing nature daily. For a week, I walked barefoot, hiked through the woods, swam in lakes and streams, lay in the grass, and sat outside watching the clouds. I couldn't believe how different I felt. A friend pointed out to me that being in nature is *grounding*. You don't need a vacation to experience this grounding. The next time you're outdoors, bring your attention to all of your senses. Look around you, what do you see? What do you feel? Notice the sun on your skin, the breeze through your hair, the ground beneath you. What do you smell? If you can't go outside, open a window. Look at the clouds, let in the breeze. Connecting to nature can help you reconnect to your body.

Move

Any form of movement can allow you to feel embodied, but more so if you are allowing yourself to be present and feel. So many people distract themselves during movement—exercising with headphones on, biking while talking to a friend, or running while watching TV or listening to a podcast. Although these things can be enjoyable to do, it often doesn't allow you to be fully in the moment when you are moving. Also, so many exercise classes or fitness studios focus on teaching you to master your body rather than inhabit it. Common phrases like "no pain, no gain" or "push through this, keep going!" effectively teach you the opposite of embodiment. Your mind then wills your body to perform and potentially go against any signals it may be sending.

Now, I'm not saying you have to stop going to fitness classes or that you always have to unplug while running. Instead, try to build some form of movement into your week that allows you to be present and connect with your body. Moving your body can help you explore what it means to be embodied and inhabit your body. Certain yoga classes can be a great way to start because they often include both meditation and focused breathing.

Unfortunately, some yoga classes or teachers put the focus on "performing" each pose perfectly. If you don't feel like you can do that, you may feel like giving up. Instead, look for a yoga practice that allows you to be in *your* body and notice how *you* are feeling. You can actually do this in any yoga or fitness class, even if the instructor is focused on teaching certain moves. Listen to your body and notice when a certain position doesn't feel right to you. Then do what feels better. Depending on how my body feels, I might spend a large chunk of a yoga class in child's pose. I felt embarrassed at first; then I realized that the embarrassment was just me comparing myself to others when my body clearly wanted to do something different. Keep practicing putting the focus back into your body, listening and honoring what it is telling you.

You can work on building body awareness during any type of movement. As you are moving—whether that's walking, running, biking, swimming, etc.—bring your awareness to your body. You can even do a body scan to check on how each part of your body feels. Notice all the sensations. At first, you may notice certain body parts, like the backs of your legs or the weight in your feet. As you notice these sensations, try to go deeper. If there are parts of you that you feel "nothing," what does "nothing" feel like? Explore both the sensations and the lack of sensation. In this way, you can use movement not as a means to burn calories or increase stamina and strength but as a way to experience your body.

Play

Many children fully inhabit their bodies. They run and jump and play, completely present in the moment. As adults, so often we stop playing, and I tend to think one result is that we get caught up in our heads. *Playing* is all about finding ways to enjoy being in your body. You're not thinking about what you're doing; instead, you're experiencing it fully through your body. Play is naturally more about feeling than thinking, which is why it can be such a powerful part of embodiment work. As my friend Hana—who I give credit to for bringing out my inner playfulness—says, "Sometimes our 'inner work' looks more like play."

What does this "play" thing look like for adults? (If you're like me, you want concrete examples. If so, I've got you.) Here are a few ideas of how to incorporate more play.

- **Dance:** Put on your favorite music and dance. No excuses or apologies about not being a "good dancer." You don't have to be "good" at something to enjoy it or get the benefits from it. Dancing is a fantastic way to practice getting out of your head and into your body. If you struggle with worrying about what others are thinking of you (like I sometimes do), find a place where you can be alone. It helps me to close my eyes, so I can stop focusing on what is around me and instead turn inside. While it may feel awkward at first, try to push through that initial feeling. Keep moving—jump, twirl, swing your arms around. Try not to worry about what you look like; instead try to do whatever your body wants to do. You also can search for an in-person ecstatic dance event or try an online "class" from 5rhythms.com.

- **Sing:** Once again, it doesn't matter what your voice sounds like. Even if you're like me and you believe that you can't sing, do it anyway. (My partner would like me to note here that while I "stubbornly refuse to admit" that I am a singer, I sing all the time.) Singing not only gets you out of your head but it can also help lower stress and anxiety. Studies have found that singing releases endorphins, the brain's "feel good" chemicals.[6] People who sing regularly—whether on their own, as part of a group, or even in the shower—tend to be happier. Singing, as well as dancing, can allow you to use your body as a conduit for self-expression, creativity, and playfulness. Again, if it is easier, start by singing along to your favorite songs while you are alone. If a judgment arises, try to bring your attention back to your body and notice what you feel in your body as you do so.

- **Create:** For most of my adult life, one of the stories I told myself was that I was "not creative." I spent so much time tapping into my scientific brain that I assumed I was "bad" at art and creativity. My perfectionism was creeping in: I felt that I had to be good at something to do it, and now I know that this is total BS. As with the two other suggestions I've given, you don't have to be "good at art" to create. Creativity is not about the output; it's about the process. When you create with no end goal in mind (and no intention of being "perfect"), you can get out of your head and let whatever is within you come out.

Creating doesn't have to take the form of a huge art project—it can be small things. Try doodling on a piece of paper, take fifteen minutes to color (there are some great "adult" coloring books out there—and no, I'm not talking about dirty coloring books, though I'm sure there are some of those, too), try a new recipe, write a short poem, or take some photos. The key is to just start making something. Whenever you notice a judgment pop into your mind, try to shut it down and remind yourself why you are doing this. I tell myself, "You are not doing this to make something beautiful. You're doing it to enjoy the process and allow your body to be in the moment."

- **Roll down a hill:** Or do whatever else your heart is calling out to you. The last time I rolled down a hill, I was probably about nine years old. But recently, I was driving through a beautiful part of Vermont, and I said to my partner, "That looks like a really great hill to roll down." Part of me felt embarrassed to say it aloud, but once I did, I realized that, yup, I really wanted to roll down that hill. So we stopped, and I did! I know it may sound ridiculous, but I've never felt as in my body as I did while I was rolling through the grass. (I've also never laughed harder.) Maybe rolling down a hill isn't for you, but there's probably something your body and your heart are prompting you to do. Listen, and then go do it.

The options for play are endless. When you think of play as "enjoying being in your body," what does that mean for you? Playing—or doing something you enjoy without becoming attached to the outcome—can help undo a perfectionistic mindset. It also can enable you to sink into the "doing" rather than focus on the "done."

It takes consistent, intentional practice to become embodied. While embodiment is both body and mind, for those of us who tend to let our heads be in control, embodiment starts when we get back into our bodies. Start by choosing one or two of the practices I've described and try to integrate them into your weekly routine. Experiment to find which ones you most enjoy. Over time, you can build more connection to—and with—your body.

Dealing with Discomfort

Although embodiment can feel incredible, it's not all hearts and rainbows. I once heard someone joke that as we start to become aware of body sensations, we quickly realize why we have been disconnected from them. Feeling all of the emotions in our bodies can be an uncomfortable sensation, especially when it comes to difficult emotions. It's one thing to feel happiness, acceptance, or comfort; it's another thing to allow yourself to feel anger, sadness, or heartbreak. Those emotions are often *not* fun to face. But being human doesn't mean feeling good or happy all of the time. We have to face our difficult emotions to get to the other side. Yes, being embodied means you may feel the difficult emotions more, but you may also feel the pleasurable emotions and sensations more, too.

Give yourself grace as you move through this process. Remember that even when things are difficult, you can still show up for yourself kindly, gently, and patiently. No matter what, you can take steps to care for your body. Prioritize self-care and coping tools to help regulate your nervous system. If you are really struggling, consider seeking more support from a therapist. As you practice connecting more with your body, and bring awareness to all of its sensations, you can learn to trust your body's ability to feel and ride it out. When you lean in and feel the full range of your body's experiences, you can become more embodied, more connected, more alive, and more empowered.

CHAPTER 16

Embracing Your Power

In Western cultures, power is often conflated with individual success, private wealth, and getting closer to those with privilege. This type of power is rooted in the patriarchy and white supremacy. In our current system, power requires you to dominate another person in some way. If we try to strive for power in this environment without questioning the people and the systems that benefit from this type of power (or those who are oppressed by it), then our empowerment ends up oppressing others. In *Sister Outsider*, Audre Lorde writes, "The master's tools will never dismantle the master's house. They may allow us to temporarily beat him at his own game, but they will never enable us to bring about genuine change."[1]

When we view empowerment through a patriarchal, racist lens, our version of empowerment upholds the same systems of oppression. What we need instead is more women and folks with marginalized identities *empowered* to challenge the status quo and dismantle the current systems of power. *Empowered* to take up space and openly share their feelings, ideas, hopes, dreams, and desires. *Empowered* to let go of society's expectations and instead look inward for guidance and validation. *Empowered* to sit with uncertainty and discomfort while letting go of perfectionism and shame. *Empowered* to know and trust themselves. *Empowered* to say and do whatever it takes to live out their vision of their most authentic, beautiful life. *Empowered* to celebrate and embrace diversity and use their differences as a source of power. *Empowered* to live without apologizing, asking for permission, or offering explanations. Imagine what our world would look like if more of us felt *empowered* to take up space and use our power in this way to change societal systems, and ultimately, the world.

Empowerment must be defined through an intersectional feminist lens. Feminism is about working toward ending discrimination against and the oppression of women. It does *not* mean hating men or trying to make women be the gender in power. Rather, it's about guaranteeing equality for *all* genders. Intersectionality is important when we talk about feminism because if we aren't taking into consideration the ways different identities affect oppression, then feminism just becomes equality for white, thin, cisgender, heterosexual, able-bodied women. Intersectional feminism is *inclusive* feminism. It argues for the rights and equality of *all* people and considers issues of race, ethnicity, class, religion, nationality, ability, and—yes—gender.

As you've read throughout this book, diet culture is an offshoot of both the patriarchy and white supremacy. Men (specifically white men) benefit from women and other marginalized folks being preoccupied with dieting and conforming to body and beauty ideals. We cannot do the work of resisting (and dismantling) diet culture and liberating all bodies if we aren't talking about intersectional feminism. As one of my clients says, "Respecting and embracing my body, promoting the acceptance of diverse bodies, and rejecting diet culture are all ways of smashing the patriarchy and raising up women and under-represented people in our society." Using an intersectional feminist lens, *empowerment* looks like people of all identities working to abolish the systems of oppression that affect them and other human beings. Empowerment must be about bringing change and collective liberation *outside* of the current patriarchal, white supremacist framework; otherwise, it will end up leaving others behind.

Empowerment: Taking Up Space

Those in power stay in power when others stay quiet and small. The system has been set up to make you feel "less than" so that people in power benefit from your lack of confidence and low self-worth. When you stay small—physically, emotionally, intellectually—you are less likely to challenge their power, which is what they want. But when you take up space and express your emotions, you demand to be seen; you demand equality and justice.

Taking up space means being the best, fullest version of yourself—physically, emotionally, and intellectually. It means making your presence known and taking up *physical space* by not trying to shrink your body. Ever notice how men often sit with their knees wide and legs splayed? When a man sits with his legs so wide that they encroach on the seat next to him, we often apply the term *manspreading*. A New York City subway campaign even targeted this penchant for sprawling. (The ads implored: "Dude, stop the spread, please." I love my city.) Meanwhile, I watch women on the subway curl into themselves as they try to make their bodies as small as possible. And it's not simply an issue of anatomy. In general, men feel entitled to take up space and are unapologetic about doing so. Whenever I've asked a man to please move his legs so I can sit down, they typically glare at me, grumble, or outright refuse. While I'm not advocating that women start encroaching into others' space (because this would mean exerting power in the way of our patriarchal society), I am encouraging you to practice spreading out when possible. How can you unapologetically start to make your existence known?

Taking up space also means fully occupying *emotional space* and *intellectual space*. Emotional space may involve expressing your feelings (yes, even the big ones) rather than keeping them inside. It also can involve protecting and holding space for the emotions of others, especially the most vulnerable among us. Taking up intellectual space can mean sharing your opinions, thoughts, and ideas and not filtering yourself because you worry about how others may react (more on this shortly). It is your inherent right as a human to take up space and be your most authentic self (so long as it is not oppressing others or infringing on their right to be themselves). You get to be everything and anything that you want to be. You don't need to be small, shrink yourself, or stay silent to keep others comfortable. You don't owe anyone smallness—in body, mind, or soul.

Empowerment: Living in Alignment with Your Knowing

Dieting and staying caught up in how our bodies look pull us outside of who we really are. Struggling with your relationship to food and your body may have caused you to partake in things that are not in alignment with your values. Stepping into your power means that you stop doing anything that takes you away from yourself. Consider this: If no one else was around, would you still be doing what you are doing right now? You can contemplate this both from the perspective of your food and exercise behaviors (in other words, if the size of your body had no effect on what people thought of you, would you still eat and move this way?), as well as all the other ways in which you interact with the world.

For Nadia, one of my former clients, living in alignment with her values meant going out more, meeting new people, making more friends, and taking the initiative to ask people to hang out. "I used to put a veil over myself when I met people, never letting them see my full self. Now I'm approaching people fully, standing in my power and my knowing," she said. When you stop doing the activities or behaviors that don't align with your values, you free up time and energy for the things that matter most. Empowerment can mean showing up, even when you're afraid or insecure, and going after your desires. When you refuse to contort yourself to live by someone else's rules, you get to prioritize yourself.

Empowerment: Letting Go of People-Pleasing

Girls and women are often socialized to please others. Perhaps you were taught from a young age that you were expected to make others happy. Or maybe you were raised with an emphasis on the importance of being liked. Most often, people-pleasing behavior comes at the sacrifice of a person's own wants, needs, and desires. When you put everyone else first, you are less likely to have your needs met. You may think you're being agreeable, nice, or low-drama, but really you're just keeping your true self hidden below the surface. This doesn't do anyone any favors, least of all yourself.

While the need for external validation isn't all bad, there is a difference between enjoying validation for things like doing a good job at work or being a compassionate partner or a good friend, and your entire idea of self and self-worth being dependent on the opinions of others. (Shout out to James Rose, who regularly does validations on Instagram (@jamesissmiling) and has an entire highlight dedicated to normalizing the idea of wanting validation. They speak so well to the difference between, as they say, "Your entire self worth being dependent on the affirmation of others and the little stuff.") If your life revolves around external validation, you will never feel "good enough" or never feel as though you are enough. Seeking validation from others is a short-term fix that feels good for only so long before you need a hit of validation again. If and when you don't get the response that you were hoping for, you can end up feeling not good enough. When you free yourself from the need for external approval, you get to live your life by your internal beliefs and values. Realizing that it is not your job to make others happy can be liberating. When you let go of the need to manage other people's expectations or perceptions of you, you can honor yourself and your needs.

Empowerment can also come from not reacting to or internalizing everything that is said about you and instead sitting back, observing, and critically considering whether something is worth listening to. Other people's opinions have little, if anything, to do with you. Their opinions are not based on your beliefs but on theirs. If they make a negative or hurtful comment to you, it tells you something about their values—not yours. Most of us will have just a small circle of people whom we trust and who know our values. In terms of everyone else, it's usually not worth the time to listen to—or try to change—their opinions of you.

Part of stepping into your power is learning to be okay with other people misunderstanding you or having strong opinions about how you live your life. This is especially true for all of us who are out there questioning the status quo and going against the mainstream tide. Some people are threatened by those who are unapologetically themselves and see a person with a marginalized identity showing up in their power as a personal affront. It won't always be comfortable to be fully yourself, and you may risk a negative response from certain people. For some folks, the fear of judgment from others is a very real concern, and you may have some trauma around past experiences with the judgment or opinions from other people. These fears may be very valid, but at the end of the day, it can be helpful to remind yourself that the only person you need to answer to is you. Try to do things because you want to do them, not because you are trying to please others. Instead of looking externally for guidance or approval, turn inward. Eat what you want, wear what you want, speak your truth, and live your best life. The way others respond is not your business; your business is to stay loyal to you.

Empowerment: Setting Boundaries

The first time my therapist asked me about my boundaries, I stared at her with a blank face. "What boundaries have you set with your partner?" she asked me. I literally had no idea what she was talking about. (No wonder I wasn't getting what I wanted out of that relationship.)

Boundaries are essential for navigating both personal and professional relationships. Setting boundaries involves telling others how you want to be and expect to be treated. When you don't set boundaries, or don't hold those boundaries, burnout, anger, or resentment can occur. Knowing your boundaries means that you're aware of what you need to thrive mentally, emotionally, and physically. You then can set guidelines or limits about the ways in which people can behave around you. You can set boundaries for your time, energy, emotions, personal space, sexuality, and more. Personal boundaries help to protect you and are a form of self-care. When you put yourself first, you can maintain your time, energy, and well-being for the things (and the people) that really matter to you. For example, in my last month of writing this book, I put up an email auto-responder that clearly spelled out that I would not be checking email more than once a week. I needed to set that boundary to finish my manuscript on time.

Boundaries are personal and can vary from person to person. They are not rigid or permanent rules; they're flexible guidelines that may change over time. Note that *flexible* doesn't mean that you compromise your boundaries but that you may reassess them as needed. Boundaries are shaped by your life experiences, your values, and your intuition or gut instincts. Start by defining the types of boundaries you want to set both personally (with friends, family members, and partners) and professionally (with clients, coworkers, and your boss). Then communicate those boundaries, explaining clearly why this is important to you. "I" or "I feel" statements work best for keeping the focus on you rather than blaming someone ("You make me...") for something they did. For example, you might say to your coworker, "I need a few minutes to myself at lunch today, so please don't interrupt me."

Setting boundaries often involves learning how—and when—to say no. If you're someone who struggles with this, it may be easier to start with small things like declining dessert at a restaurant or letting your partner know when you'd rather read a book than watch a movie (did this one myself yesterday!). When you say "no," you do not need to apologize or explain yourself. A simple "no" or "no, thank you" suffices. This was difficult for me at first. I would end up giving some long-winded explanation because I felt so guilty for saying no. It took self-awareness and practice to get to the point where I'm now able to reply with a direct "no." Because I am clear on my values, my worth, and what is important to me, I find it easier to say no to things that don't serve me. I have grown to trust my gut instinct, which also helps me do what feels best. The more you practice setting boundaries—of any kind—the easier it becomes.

If you struggle with saying "no," here are a few situations and people to consider starting with:

- Something that doesn't align with your values
- Something you don't want to do
- Something (or someone) that will harm your mental health
- Something (or someone) that takes up a lot of negative energy
- Something that is inconvenient or will require you to go out of your way
- People who continue to let you down
- When your gut instinct is "no"

Chapter 16: Embracing Your Power

Setting Boundaries with Food and Body Comments

Most people in our society are so used to measuring health and success by dieting and weight that you may get pushback or confusion at best and defensiveness or anger at worst when you opt out of dieting. In our diet-obsessed culture, intuitive eating and body liberation can be a completely foreign concept to many people. When you've made so much progress, a well-meaning (or not so well-meaning) person making a comment can be really difficult to handle. Statements like, "Oh, wow. You're really going to eat all that food?" or, "You look bigger than the last time I saw you," may send you spiraling back into negative food or body image thoughts.

Setting boundaries with friends and family related to food, diet, and weight or body talk is an act of self-care and self-respect. You have the right to ask people not to talk about dieting or weight loss around you. This is especially important to do with the people in your life with whom you used to discuss these things because they may still expect you to want to talk about those topics. Start by explaining to your friend or family member why comments about food or weight are harmful to you. They may not be aware of the effect of their words until you bring it up. It can also be helpful to let those close to you know about the journey you're on. This can be an isolating process, and it's important to share it with the people you trust. You may explain that you are no longer dieting and are focusing on your health instead of your weight.

If a person seems open to learning more, you may direct them to this book or another anti-diet resource. If they are not open, that's okay, too. They may not entirely understand, but it is not on you to "fix" them (as much as you may want to). Don't try to force them to give up dieting; if they're not ready for this type of change, they're not ready. Instead, communicate how you feel. Set a boundary by asking them not to talk about their diets or weight when they are around you. If they continue to bring it up, remind them of your position by saying something like

- I'm asking you not to make comments about what I'm eating or my appearance.
- My body and food choices are not up for discussion.
- This isn't something I want to talk about.

Stand in your power and communicate clearly. You do not need to apologize or offer explanations. If they continue to make diet-y comments, show them some compassion. Diet culture and fatphobia is ingrained in everybody, and you've been there before, too. You still can continue to remind them of your boundary.

What should you do when diet talk comes up in casual settings? In this instance, you have a few choices:

- If you don't feel like explaining yourself or sharing what you're doing (or rather, not doing), you can shut down the conversation by saying something like, "It sounds like you found something that works for you," and then change the topic.
- If the conversation is really triggering and bothering you, you don't have to stay there. Go to the bathroom or step into another room to give yourself a break from the diet talk.
- If you feel comfortable and ready to talk about what you're doing, you can share more about why you're no longer dieting, what you're doing instead, and how you have been feeling so far.

You may find it helpful to have some go-to phrases ready when someone starts talking about their diet or comments on your food or weight. Here are some suggestions:

- I'd rather talk about something other than diets. How was your trip to see your family?
- I work out because of how it makes me feel; I don't pay attention to the number on the scale.
- I'm still hungry, so I'm going to have some more.
- That was delicious, but I'm satisfied—how about we take it to go?
- I'm glad you've found something that works for you, but I'm focusing on listening to my body.

No matter what, remember that you are under no obligation to share more than you feel comfortable with. You don't always have to have your anti-diet culture advocacy hat on, though some people find it helpful to advocate and speak to this journey once they are further along in the process. You're not always going to have the perfect thing to say, and it's okay if you say the "wrong" thing. When in doubt, change the subject! Then go to your anti-diet community for support and reassurance.

Dealing with the Doctor's Office

The doctor's office can be a traumatic experience for many people, especially those in fat bodies. While there are more and more physicians who have taken the Health at Every Size Pledge (you can find a list of those doctors at www.haescommunity.org), the vast majority resort to prescribing weight loss no matter what you went into their office for. If there is not a HAES® physician in your area, you can advocate for yourself with your doctor. I know that this is not easy, especially for people in fat bodies. Our society tends to think of doctors as the be-all and end-all when it comes to health, but they are humans who were raised—and educated—in diet culture. While it should not come down to you having to advocate for compassionate, ethical, evidence-based care, unfortunately, it often does. Ragen Chastain, a speaker, writer, and activist who blogs at danceswithfat.org, developed a set of cards that people can take with them to their appointments to read or give to the doctor. The cards include statements and requests such as

- Do thin people get this health problem? What do you recommend for them?
- The research I've seen shows that the vast majority of people who attempt weight loss fail.
- Please don't prescribe weight loss as a health intervention.
- Don't weigh me unless medically necessary.[2]

As Ragen states, you have the right to refuse to be weighed at the doctor's office. There are very few reasons why a doctor would have to know your weight; most record it as a matter of routine. For the majority of medications, doctors don't need your weight to determine the proper dosage. Insurance companies don't require a weight either; most just ask for two measurements at any given visit, which could be your temperature, blood pressure, heart rate, or height. Start by asking the doctor (or nurse because that's often the person who ends up weighing people) if it's okay not to be weighed. You may also ask if you can self-report your weight or if they can just use the same weight as your last visit. You do not need to offer any explanation or apologize for your refusal to be weighed. If they ask, you can say something like, "I am working to heal my disordered eating behaviors, and seeing my weight is very triggering." If they do require you to get on the scale, ask them to take a blind weight, which means you turn around so you can't see the number. Having this conversation can feel awkward or uncomfortable, so it can help to practice with a friend or family member or in front of the mirror before trying with the doctor. If you are working with an anti-diet dietitian or therapist, you may also consider asking that person if they'd be willing to advocate for you by calling and speaking to your doctor. Most of us are happy to do so.

Maintaining Your Boundaries

The last thing to remember with boundaries is that you are in charge of holding people to them. If someone crosses your boundary, ask yourself if you had clearly communicated your boundary. Or did you just assume they knew? I used to get so frustrated with one of my exes for always interrupting me when I was working. Then my therapist asked me the boundary question, and I realized that I had never communicated to my partner that I needed quiet during certain times of the workday. Boundary conversations can be uncomfortable at first, but the long-term gains are indisputable. One client really struggled with people-pleasing, especially with her mom. However, she also struggled mentally and emotionally as her mom continued to make comments about her body size and weight gain. When she finally set a boundary with her mom and asked that she not comment on her body, she felt so much better. "Not only did I feel like I was standing up for myself, but it opened up a great conversation between my mom and me."

If someone repeatedly crosses your boundaries, and you've clearly communicated your boundaries, then perhaps consider whether this person is someone who you want or need in your life. Do they add value to your life? If no (or even if yes), are you okay tolerating continued boundary-crossing and disrespect? You may take this chance to rebuild trust with this person, or you may decide that you need to end your relationship. The people who matter most are those who are willing and able to respect your boundaries and—therefore—respect you.

Empowerment: Resting, Being Quiet, and Reflecting

Stepping into your power requires that you take time to rest and replenish. If you are exhausted, drained, burnt out, or miserable, it can become hard to stand in your power. Society trains us to be go-go-go. There is pressure to be productive all the time, meet goals, to accomplish something. When any downtime does arise, we are often quick to fill it up with external noise. Sometimes this "noise" includes consuming helpful, educational, and powerful content, but we reach a point when perpetual consumption—without rest, quiet, and reflection—becomes useless. When we fill up all of our days and hours with consumption, there is no space for us to find and hear the inner wisdom.

Empowerment involves protecting your time and energy. It means making time to rest, rejuvenate, and recharge. It also means allowing yourself time and space to reflect and explore. The ability to sit with your thoughts in the quiet is powerful. Although not always easy or comfortable, stillness and reflection are where the real growth occurs. Slow down. Rest. Be bored. Do nothing. Sit with the silence of your mind. Journal. Process the thoughts and feelings that come up. Allow your intuition—your inner voice—space to speak and guide you. Rest, reflect, replenish, recharge, and embrace your power.

Empowerment: Letting Go of What Doesn't Serve You

To fully step into your power, try to start letting go of the things—and the people (refer to the earlier section about setting boundaries)—that don't serve you. Where in your life do you feel stress? Where do you feel discontent? Where do you feel a sense of overwhelm? What aspect(s) of your life are not serving you right now?

Throughout this book, you've had a chance to reflect on your thoughts, feelings, beliefs, and behaviors. Which of these do not serve you? Which are not helping you live your most authentic, empowered life? Examine your beliefs about food, body size, beauty ideals, and exercise. Which beliefs come from your cultural conditioning, and which are your true inner knowing? Think about your behaviors; how may these not be serving you? Consider eating behaviors like dieting, food restriction, or rigid food rules as well as movement behaviors like grueling workouts or attempts to exercise your body into submission. Reflect upon other actions or behaviors that you do throughout your day, such as body-checking, only wearing certain clothes (or avoiding certain clothes), or following social media accounts that cause you to feel bad about yourself.

One of my former clients, Nyah, was a dedicated runner; it was her main form of exercise. She had been running several days per week for years. During our work together, Nyah realized that she didn't enjoy her runs. She often would dread them, and she felt super unmotivated, but a part of her was resistant to letting that activity go. She still attached running to making her body look a certain way. So we started with an intermediate step: letting go of running for one month. During that month, Nyah discovered several new types of activities that she really loved. "A cloud lifted once I didn't have my daily run looming over my head," she told me. "It was so much more clear that running, at least on a regular basis, is not what I need right now."

If you identify as a perfectionist, now is the time to let that shit go. Embracing your power involves feeling and accepting all the discomfort, missteps, and uncomfortable learnings that come out of this process. Perfectionism, which puts the focus on the individual *being* a mistake rather than *making* a mistake, gets in the way of true growth. This leaves little room for reflection or self-improvement. Let go of the desire for perfectionism and learn to be comfortable with "good enough." When you let go of things that do not serve you, you have more space to attract and go after the things that bring you happiness and joy, and you can step into your power and take action to live in alignment with your core values. What can you begin to let go of today?

Empowerment: Understanding, Uplifting, and Advocating for Others

Power in our society often involves tearing others down or stepping over others to get to the top. We are taught that resources are scarce and that there is not enough space, time, money, or love for all of us. This idea couldn't be further from the truth. True empowerment means standing in your power while embracing, uplifting, and advocating for others. You don't need to shrink yourself or your power to support someone else. It is not either/or—*either* you have power *or* someone else does—it can be both/and.

The world needs more folks with varying identities who unapologetically own themselves and embrace their power. The more you do that, the more you can inspire and advocate for others to do the same. Those of us who hold various privileged identities—be that thin, white, able-bodied, cisgender, etc.—must deprogram ourselves from the biases we hold against bodies and identities not like our own. We must acknowledge the unearned privileges or advantages that we get in society because of our bodies. We don't have this privilege because we asked for it or because it's fair but because this is how our society is currently set up. Having privilege doesn't mean that you haven't struggled; it just means that certain aspects of your identity are not the cause of your struggle. Recognizing this privilege means acknowledging the very real imbalance of power between groups of people.

Empowerment means educating yourself on the various forms of oppression, unlearning your indoctrinated beliefs, and using your privilege to advocate for all bodies. We must all stop commenting not just on our own bodies but upon others' bodies as well. We must consider the effect of our words and actions and communicate in ways that convey understanding. We can have the best of intentions, but that doesn't mean we aren't negatively affecting someone else (always consider *impact* over *intention*). Those of us in thin bodies must learn to reject fatphobia and stop judging others based on their size. Those of us who are white must learn to recognize our implicit bias and speak out against racism. Those of us who are able-bodied must learn how ableism makes life challenging for those with disabilities and seek ways to help provide support. Those of us who are cisgender must learn the difference between sex and gender, use people's pronouns correctly, and correct others when they misgender someone.

Empowerment is taking up space so that we can then share that space with others. We must not focus on just the individual experience; we must focus on the collective. We cannot turn away from these injustices, even if they are something that does not directly affect us. Because none of our bodies are free until all bodies are free.

Empowerment: Being Unapologetic

So many of us have been taught to be apologetic for what we eat, how our bodies look, the space we take up, the ideas that we have, the decisions that we make. Empowerment is being bold and unapologetic, no matter how society (mis)labels you. Empowerment is refusing to apologize for being *yourself*.

I hope that this book enables you to get one step closer to figuring out who you are and what is important to you. One step closer to caring less about what other people think of you and more about what you think of yourself. One step closer to being unapologetic about how you show up and take up space in the world. One step closer to living a life where you feel so unwavering in your power that you can eat, move, speak, and act without apology. One step closer to being unapologetically *you*.

Acknowledgments

This book rests upon the decades of work by all of the fat activists who have been in the trenches fighting for the rights and liberation of all people, all while dealing with abuse and vitriol. Without your work, this book, and so many others, would not exist. I am so grateful for the work of Ragen Chastain, Your Fat Friend, Lisa DuBreuil, and Virgie Tovar, who were my first introductions into fat-positivity and fat activism. You have all taught—and continue to teach—me so much.

To the entire team at Victory Belt Publishing, thank you for believing in my (very vague) initial book pitch, letting me run with it, and helping me bring this book to life in a way that stayed true to my values and intention. A huge thanks to my editor Charlotte for being just as detail-oriented as I am (if not more), really "getting" the concept of this book, and making sure my voice and message shone through.

Thank you to Lindley Ashline and McKensie Mack and the Radical Copy team for your thoughtful input and suggestions while helping me root out my bias to make this book as inclusive and anti-oppressive as possible.

Thank you to Ashley Rust for sharing all of your book publishing and marketing expertise with me. "Assuming the book is a bestseller" (or even if not), I'll have all my ducks in a row because of you.

Thank you to all of my colleagues, mentors, and supervisors who continue to inspire me and help me learn and grow into a better practitioner (and person). I am so grateful for this community; you all have made such a difference in my life and the lives of so many others.

A special thank you to Fiona Sutherland for all of your wise words (many of which appear in this book!) that I will forever use and practice daily; Marci Evans for your kindness and compassion and for being the kind of practitioner that I aspire to be; Kelly Diels for helping me overcome my impostor syndrome throughout the writing process, proposing the concept of equity readers, and inspiring me to be a culture maker and keep showing up to my spot on the wall; Lindsay Stenovec, who years ago provided me with the framework for this work that allowed me to lean into the unknown and not run back to diet culture; Evelyn Tribole, without whom I would have never started on this journey; Christy Harrison for introducing me to so many of the different facets of this work and being a constant inspiration; and Brianna Campos for teaching me about body grief (and so much more) and being one of my favorite "Instagram friends." I appreciate you all so much!

Thank you to Carol Guizar for being my unofficial "work wife" and always being just a text or video call away whenever I needed to talk through anything book-related (or otherwise). You were the first person I trusted to read the early versions of my book chapters, and I'll always appreciate your input, support, and friendship.

Thank you to Hana for helping me embrace uncertainty and rediscover play and for always "seeing" me—all of me. There's no way I'd be where I am, or who I am, today without you and your friendship (and that Re:Boot beach trip). I'm so grateful for you (and to Craigslist for bringing us together!) and can't wait for our next adventure.

To my family, thank you for all of your unconditional love and support, always. Thank you for always trusting me and allowing me to be who I am and who I am becoming, even when you don't completely understand. Dad, your inquisitive mind, enthusiasm for learning (who else starts teaching online courses in their eighties?), and willingness to sit and ponder anything—even things you don't agree with—will forever be inspiring to me. Mom, thank you for being my biggest cheerleader and support system, whether that involved proofreading all of my written work, being my unofficial "virtual assistant," or answering my (often panicked) phone calls at all hours of the night: I don't know what I'd do without you.

To Pete, thank you for being a constant source of support, compassion, and love. From doing all the grocery shopping and errands, to cooking me three meals per day for months (and, let's be real, probably forever), to reminding me to "wiggle" and move after hours of writing, to always providing a judgment-free sounding board, this process would have been so much harder (and hangrier) without you. I could never have imagined finding a partner whose response to me freaking out about a dream where I shave my head says, "That actually sounds like it would be really liberating." Thank you for giving me the space to experiment, play, learn, and grow. I love doing life with you.

And last but not least, to all of my clients, thank you for trusting me with your stories and sharing your lived experiences so openly and vulnerably. Your bravery and willingness to challenge the status quo in your search for *something more* is truly inspiring. Thank you for allowing me to share your stories within these pages; you have helped everyone who reads this book. You've been my greatest teachers and have changed my life in so many ways, both personally and professionally. You are the reason this book exists, and for that I am eternally grateful.

Examples of Personal Values

Acceptance	Devotion	Innovation	Risk
Achievement	Discovery	Integrity	Satisfaction
Adventure	Empathy	Intelligence	Security
Amusement	Empowerment	Intuition	Self-care
Authenticity	Energy	Joy	Self-respect
Authority	Enjoyment	Justice	Sensitivity
Autonomy	Enthusiasm	Kindness	Service
Awareness	Equality	Knowledge	Simplicity
Balance	Ethics	Leadership	Solitude
Beauty	Exploration	Learning	Spirituality
Boldness	Fairness	Logic	Spontaneity
Bravery	Faith	Love	Stability
Candor	Family	Loyalty	Success
Challenge	Freedom	Meaning	Support
Comfort	Friendship	Openness	Surprise
Commitment	Fun	Optimism	Sustainability
Communication	Generosity	Order	Teamwork
Community	Grace	Organization	Tolerance
Compassion	Gratitude	Originality	Toughness
Confidence	Growth	Passion	Tranquility
Connection	Happiness	Patience	Truth
Consistency	Harmony	Peace	Understanding
Contentment	Health	Playfulness	Uniqueness
Courage	Honesty	Pleasure	Wealth
Creativity	Hope	Purpose	Wisdom
Curiosity	Imagination	Reason	Wonder
Dedication	Improvement	Recognition	
Dependability	Influence	Respect	

Resources

The books, podcasts, social media accounts, online communities, and websites I share here are some of my favorite resources for furthering knowledge and supporting a journey of unapologetic eating and living. To the best of my knowledge, I have included only resources that are weight-inclusive. However, I am not responsible for the content on these sites, so if you come across something that feels "off" or unhelpful, feel free to skip it. An essential part of this process involves finding a community of people who are also on a body liberation and body peace journey, and I hope that these resources will help you begin to build this community for yourself.

Books

- *Anti-Diet: Reclaim Your Time, Money, Well-Being and Happiness Through Intuitive Eating* by Christy Harrison
- *The Beauty Myth: How Images of Beauty Are Used Against Women* by Naomi Wolf
- *Beyond Beautiful: A Practical Guide to Being Happy, Confident, and You in a Looks-Obsessed World* by Anuschka Rees
- *Big Girl: How I Gave Up Dieting and Got a Life* by Kelsey Miller
- *The Body Is Not an Apology: The Power of Radical Self-Love* by Sonya Renee Taylor
- *Body Kindness: Transform Your Health from the Inside Out—And Never Say Diet Again* by Rebecca Scritchfield
- *Body Respect: What Conventional Health Books Get Wrong, Leave Out, and Just Plain Fail to Understand About Weight* by Linda Bacon and Lucy Aphramor
- *A Burst of Light and Other Essays* by Audre Lorde
- *Eat to Love: A Mindful Guide to Transforming Your Relationship with Food, Body, and Life* by Jenna Hollenstein
- *The Eating Instinct: Food Culture, Body Image, and Guilt in America* by Virginia Sole-Smith
- *Fat Activism: A Radical Social Movement* by Charlotte Cooper

- *Fat Politics: The Real Story Behind America's Obesity Epidemic* by J. Eric Oliver
- *The Fat Studies Reader* by Esther Rothblum and Sandra Solovay
- *FAT!SO?: Because You Don't Have to Apologize for Your Size* by Marilyn Wann
- *Fattily Ever After: A Black Fat Girl's Guide to Living Life Unapologetically* by Stephanie Yeboah
- *Fearing the Black Body: The Racial Origins of Fat Phobia* by Sabrina Strings
- *The F*ck It Diet: Eating Should Be Easy* by Caroline Dooner
- *Hunger: A Memoir of (My) Body* by Roxane Gay
- *I Thought It Was Just Me (But It Isn't): Making the Journey from "What Will People Think?" to "I Am Enough"* by Brené Brown
- *Intuitive Eating: A Revolutionary Program That Works*, 4th Ed. by Evelyn Tribole and Elyse Resch
- *The Intuitive Eating Workbook: Ten Principles for Nourishing a Healthy Relationship with Food* by Evelyn Tribole and Elyse Resch
- *Landwhale: On Turning Insults into Nicknames, Why Body Image Is Hard, and How Diets Can Kiss My Ass* by Jes Baker
- *Lessons from the Fat-o-sphere: Quit Dieting and Declare a Truce with Your Body* by Kate Harding and Marianne Kirby
- *Self-Compassion: The Proven Power of Being Kind to Yourself* by Kristin Neff
- *Sister Outsider: Essays and Speeches* by Audre Lorde
- *Thick and Other Essays* by Tressie McMillan Cottom
- *Things No One Will Tell Fat Girls: A Handbook for Unapologetic Living* by Jes Baker
- *Unashamed: Musings of a Fat, Black Muslim* by Leah Vernon
- *You Have the Right to Remain Fat* by Virgie Tovar

Podcasts

- The Body Image Podcast: corinnedobbas.com/podcast/
- Body Kindness: bodykindnessbook.com/podcast
- The BodyLove Project: jessihaggerty.com/blppodcast
- The Chenese Lewis Show: cheneselewisshow.com/
- The Embodied & Well Mom Show: intuitiveeatingmoms.com/podcast
- Every Body Podcast: everybodypodcast.org
- Fat Girls Club: buzzsprout.com/187520
- Fierce Fatty: fiercefatty.com/podcast
- Food Confidence: andreapaulrd.com/podcast
- Food Heaven: foodheavenmadeeasy.com/podcast
- Food Psych: christyharrison.com/foodpsych
- The F*ck It Diet: thefuckitdiet.com/category/podcast/
- Going Beyond the Food: stephaniedodier.com/podcast-episodes/
- Intuitive Bites: theintuitiverd.com/podcast
- Intuitive Eating for the Culture: encouragingdietitian.com/category/podcast/
- Love, Food: juliedillonrd.com/lovefoodpodcast/
- The Mindful Dietitian: themindfuldietitian.com.au/podcast

- My Black Body Podcast: myblackbody.org/
- Nourishing Women: nourishingwomenpodcast.libsyn.com/
- RD Real Talk: heathercaplan.com/rd-real-talk-podcast/
- Rebel Eaters Club: rebeleatersclub.com/
- She's All Fat: shesallfatpod.com/podcast
- Unpacking Weight Science: unpackingweightscience.com/shop
- Woman of Size: womanofsize.com/

Social Media

- Alissa Rumsey: @alissarumseyrd
- Anna Sweeney: @dietitiananna
- Ashlee Bennett: @bodyimage_therapist
- Ayana Habtemariam: @thetrillrd
- Beauty Redefined: @beauty_redefined
- Brianna M. Campos: @bodyimagewithbri
- Cara Harbstreet: @streetsmartrd
- Carolina Guizar: @eathority
- Christyna Johnson: @encouragingdietitian
- Dalina Soto: @your.latina.nutritionist
- Dani Adriana: @iamdaniadriana
- The Fatphobia Slayer: @thefatphobiaslayer
- Gabi Gregg: @gabifresh
- Haley Goodrich: @hgoodrichrd
- Ivy Felicia: @iamivyfelicia
- James Rose: @jamesissmiling
- Jessamyn Stanley: @mynameisjessamyn
- Julie Duffy Dillon: @foodpeacedietitian
- Kimmie Singh: @bodypositive_dietitian
- Lauren Leavell: @laurenleavellfitness
- Lindley Ashline: @bodyliberationwithlindley
- Maria Paredes: @with_this_body
- Meg Boggs: @meg.boggs
- Monique Melton: @moemotivate
- The Nap Ministry: @thenapministry
- Nicola Salmon: @fatpositivefertility
- Patrilie H.: @the_bodylib_advocate
- Rachael Hartley: @rachaelhartleyrd
- Sam Dylan Finch: @samdylanfinch
- Sassy Latte: @sassylatte
- Shira Rose: @theshirarose
- Sonya Renee Taylor: @sonyareneetaylor
- Stephanie Yeboah: @stephanieyeboah
- Tiffany Ima: @tiffanyima
- The Unplug Collective: @theunplugcollective
- Virgie Tovar: @virgietovar
- Your Fat Friend: @yrfatfriend

For more social media recommendations, visit alissarumsey.com/socialmedia.

Online Resources and Websites

- My website: alissarumsey.com
- All Bodies Are Good Bodies Facebook Group: facebook.com/groups/allbodiesaregoodbodies
- Association for Size Diversity and Health: sizediversityandhealth.org
- The Body Is Not An Apology: thebodyisnotanapology.com
- Certified Intuitive Eating Counselor Directory: intuitiveeating.org/certified-counselors
- Dances with Fat: danceswithfat.org
- Ditch the Diet Support Facebook Group: facebook.com/groups/DitchTheDietSupport
- Eating Disorder Help and Support: nationaleatingdisorders.org/help-support
- Everyday Feminism: everydayfeminism.com
- Fat Acceptance Cloud Facebook Group: facebook.com/groups/FAcloud
- Fat Women of Color Collective: collective.fatwomenofcolor.com
- Find a Therapist: psychologytoday.com/us/therapists
- Health at Every Size Provider Registry: haescommunity.com/search
- Intuitive Eating Crash Course: alissarumsey.com/shop
- Latinx Health Collective: latinxhealthcollective.com
- Made on a Generous Plan: generousplan.com
- The Militant Baker: themilitantbaker.com
- Nalgona Positivity Pride: nalgonapositivitypride.com
- PCOS Body Liberation: pcosbodyliberation.com

Cooking and Recipe Resources

- *Gentle Nutrition: A Non-Diet Approach to Healthy Eating* by Rachael Hartley
- *How to Cook Vegetables: Essential Skills and 90 Foolproof Recipes* by Kim Hoban
- Kara Lydon Blog: karalydon.com/recipes
- Rachael Hartley Nutrition Blog: rachaelhartleynutrition.com/recipe-index
- *Salt, Fat, Acid, Heat: Mastering the Elements of Good Cooking* by Samin Nosrat
- Smitten Kitchen Blog: smittenkitchen.com/
- Streetsmart Nutrition Blog: streetsmartnutrition.com/recipes/

Endnotes

Introduction

1. B. Campos, Instagram direct messages to the author, September 10 and 25, 2020.

2. S. Latte, "Black lives over wh-te comfort." Instagram photo, September 28, 2020. https://www.instagram.com/p/CFsPTOZlk8g/.

3. C. A. Carruthers, *Unapologetic: A Black, Queer, and Feminist Mandate for Radical Movements* (Boston, MA: Beacon Press Books, 2018), x.

4. C. Frisby in "Where Did BIPOC Come From?" by S. E. Garcia, *New York Times*, June 17, 2020, https://www.nytimes.com/article/what-is-bipoc.html.

5. M. Laws, "Why We Capitalize 'Black' (and not 'white')." *Columbia Journalism Review Online*, June 16, 2020, https://www.cjr.org/analysis/capital-b-black-styleguide.php.

6. Associated Press, "AP Changes Writing Style to Capitalize 'b' in Black," AP News, June 19, 2020.

7. S. Yeboah, *Fattily Ever After: A Black Fat Girl's Guide to Living Life Unapologetically* (London: Hardie Grant, 2020), 231.

8. K. Crenshaw, "Demarginalizing the Intersection of Race and Sex: A Black Feminist Critique of Antidiscrimination Doctrine, Feminist Theory and Antiracist Politics," *University of Chicago Legal Forum* 1989, no. 1 (1989): http://chicago-unbound.uchicago.edu/uclf/vol1989/iss1/8.

9. G. L. Palmer, J. S. Fernández, G. Lee, H. Masud, S. Hilson, C. Tang, D. Thomas, L. Clark, B. Guzman, and I. Bernai, "Oppression and Power" in *Introduction to Community Psychology*, eds. L. A. Jason, O. Glantsman, J. F. O'Brien, and K. N. Ramian, Rebus Community, https://press.rebus.community/introductiontocommunitypsychology/chapter/oppression-and-power/.

Chapter 1

1. "Fast Facts: Media's Effect on Body Image," Teen Health and the Media, accessed August 21, 2020, https://depts.washington.edu/thmedia/view.cgi?section=bodyimage&page=fastfacts.

2. "Children, Teens, Media, and Body Image: A Common Sense Research Brief," Common Sense Media website, accessed August 21, 2020, https://www.commonsensemedia.org/research/children-teens-media-and-body-image#.

3. C. Harrison, *Anti-Diet* (New York: Little, Brown Spark, 2019), chap. 1.

4. S. Strings, *Fearing the Black Body: The Racial Origins of Fat Phobia* (New York: New York University Press, 2019), Kindle edition, Introduction.

5. N. Wolf, *The Beauty Myth* (New York: Harper Collins ebooks, 2010), ePub edition, chap. 6.

6. S. R. Taylor, *The Body Is Not An Apology* (Oakland, CA: Berrett-Koehler Publishers, 2018), 25.

7. Kelly Diels to Sunday Love Letter mailing list, April 12, 2020.

8. I. Coelho, Twitter post, December 29, 2015, 1:36 a.m., https://twitter.com/ines_opcoelho/status/681725407591284736.

9. J. Baker, *Things No One Will Tell Fat Girls* (Berkeley, CA: Seal Press, 2015), 28.

10. American Society of Plastic Surgeons, "New Statistics Reveal the Shape of Plastic Surgery," March 1, 2018, https://www.plasticsurgery.org/news/press-releases/new-statistics-reveal-the-shape-of-plastic-surgery.

11. American Society of Plastic Surgeons, "2018 Plastic Surgery Statistics Report," accessed August 21, 2020, https://www.plasticsurgery.org/documents/News/Statistics/2018/plastic-surgery-statistics-full-report-2018.pdf.

12. J. S. Wong and A. M. Penner, "Gender and the Returns to Attractiveness," *Research in Social Stratification and Mobility* 44 (2016): 113–23.

13. R. F. Baumeister and M. R. Leary, "The Need to Belong: Desire for Interpersonal Attachments as a Fundamental Human Motivation," *Psychological Bulletin* 117, no. 3 (1995): 497–529.

14. *Sex and the City*, "Models and Mortals." Directed by Alison Maclean. Written by Darren Star. HBO, June 6, 1998.

15. Carolina Guízar, email message to author, May 13, 2020.

Chapter 2

1. "Methods for Voluntary Weight Loss and Control. NIH Technology Assessment Conference Panel. Consensus Development Conference, 30 March to 1 April 1992," *Annals of Internal Medicine* 119, no. 7 pt. 2 (1993): 764–70.

2. *Merriam-Webster Dictionary Online*, s.v. "diet," accessed October 1, 2020, https://www.merriam-webster.com/dictionary/diet.

3. Marketdata LLC, "The U.S. Weight Loss & Diet Control Market," February 2019, https://www.researchandmarkets.com/research/6sb283/united_states?w=5.

4. C. B. Martin, K. A. Herrick, N. Sarafrazi, and C. L. Ogden, "Attempts to Lose Weight Among Adults in the United States, 2013–2016," *NCHS Data Brief* 313 (2018), https://www.cdc.gov/nchs/products/databriefs/db313.htm.

5. T. Harris, "Disordered Eating: The Disorder Next Door," *Self Online*, April 21, 2008, https://www.self.com/story/eating-disorder-risk.

6. Statista Research Department, "U.S. High School Students Trying to Lose Weight in 2017, by Gender and Ethnicity," Statista, September 16, 2020, https://www.statista.com/statistics/871927/us-students-who-are-trying-to-lose-weight/; A. M. Gustafson-Larson and R. D. Terry, "Weight-Related Behaviors and Concerns of Fourth-Grade Children," *Journal of the American Dietetic Association* 92, no. 7 (1992): 818–22.

7. C. L. Kurth, D. D. Krahn, K. Nairn, and A. Drewnowski, "The Severity of Dieting and Bingeing Behaviors in College Women: Interview Validation of Survey Data," *Journal of Psychiatric Research* 29, no. 3 (1995): 211–25.

8. C. Harrison, "How to Avoid Falling for the Wellness Diet," Christy Harrison (blog), April 9, 2018, https://christyharrison.com/blog/the-wellness-diet.

9. "What Is Whole30," Whole30, accessed October 1, 2020, https://whole30.com/.

10. "Methods for Voluntary Weight Loss and Control. NIH Technology Assessment Conference Panel. Consensus Development Conference, 30 March to 1 April 1992," *Annals of Internal Medicine* 119, no. 7 pt. 2 (1993): 764–70.

11. T. Mann, A. J. Tomiyama, E. Westling, A. Lew, B. Samuels, and J. Chatman, "Medicare's Search for Effective Obesity Treatments: Diets Are Not the Answer," *The American Psychologist* 62, no. 3 (2007): 220–33.

12. M. L. Dansinger, A. Tatsioni, J. B. Wong, M. Chung, and E. M. Balk, "Meta-Analysis: The Effect of Dietary Counseling for Weight Loss," *Annals of Internal Medicine* 147, no. 1 (2007): 41–50; A. E. Field, J. E. Manson, C. B. Taylor, W. C. Willett, and G. A. Colditz, "Association of Weight Change, Weight Control Practices, and Weight Cycling Among Women in the Nurses' Health Study II," *International Journal of Obesity and Related Metabolic Disorders* 28, no. 9 (2004): 1134–42.

13. T. Mann et al., "Medicare's Search for Effective Obesity Treatments"; J. W. Anderson, E. C. Konz, R. C. Frederich, and C. L. Wood, "Long-Term Weight-Loss Maintenance: A Meta-Analysis of US Studies," *American Journal of Clinical Nutrition* 74, no. 5 (2001): 579–84.

14. L. M. Gianini, B. T. Walsh, J. Steinglass, and L. Mayer, "Long-Term Weight Loss Maintenance in Obesity: Possible Insights from Anorexia Nervosa?" *International Journal of Eating Disorders* 50, no. 4 (2017): 341–2.

15. T. Mann et al., "Medicare's Search for Effective Obesity Treatments."

16. T. Harris, "Disordered Eating: The Disorder Next Door."

17. J. Robison, C. Cool, E. Jackson, and E. Satter, "Helping Without Harming—Kids, Eating, Weight, and Health," *Absolute Advantage: The Workplace Wellness Magazine* 7, no. 1 (2007): 2–15.

18. K. M. Culbert, S. E. Racine, and K. L. Klump, "Research Review: What We Have Learned About the Causes of Eating Disorders—A Synthesis of Sociocultural, Psychological, and Biological Research," *Journal of Child Psychology and Psychiatry, and Allied Disciplines* 56, no. 11 (2015): 1141–64.

19. E. W. Diemer, J. M. W. Hughto, A. R. Gordon, C. Guss, S. B. Austin, and S. L. Reisner, "Beyond the Binary: Differences in Eating Disorder Prevalence by Gender Identity in a Transgender Sample," *Transgender Health* 3, no. 1 (2018): 17–23.

20. The Trevor Project, "Eating Disorders Among LGBTQ Youth: A 2018 National Assessment," accessed October 1, 2020, https://www.nationaleatingdisorders.org/sites/default/files/nedawi8/NEDA%20-Trevor%20Project%20 2018%20Survey%20-%20Full%20Results.pdf.

21. K. H. Gordon, M. M. Brattole, L. R. Wingate, and T. E. Joiner, Jr., "The Impact of Client Race on Clinician Detection of Eating Disorders," *Behavior Therapy* 37, no. 4 (2006): 319–25.

22. G. Lucas in "Centering the Voices of People of Color in the Fight Against Eating Disorders," National Eating Disorders Association (blog), accessed October 1, 2020, https://www.nationaleatingdisorders.org/blog/centering-voices-people-color-fight-against-eating-disorders.

23. D. Burgard in "Recognizing and Resisting Diet Culture," R. Chastain, National Eating Disorders Association (blog), accessed October 1, 2020, https://www.nationaleatingdisorders.org/blog/recognizing-and-resisting-diet-culture.

24. J-P. Montani, Y. Schultz, and A. G. Dulloo, "Dieting and Weight Cycling as Risk Factors for Cardiometabolic Diseases: Who Is Really at Risk?" *Obesity Reviews* 16, no. Suppl 1 (2015): 7–18; T. L. Tylka, R. A. Annunziato, D. Burgard, S. Daníelsdóttir, E. Shuman, C. Davis, and R. M.

Calogero, "The Weigh-Inclusive Versus Weight-Normative Approach to Health: Evaluating the Evidence for Prioritizing Well-Being over Weight Loss," *Journal of Obesity* 2014 (2014).

25. L. Bacon and L. Aphramor, "Weight Science: Evaluating the Evidence for a Paradigm Shift," *Nutrition Journal* 10, no. 9 (2011).

26. *Merriam-Webster Dictionary Online*, s.v. "willpower," accessed October 1, 2020, https://www.merriam-webster.com/dictionary/willpower.

27. R. E. Keesey and T. L. Powley, "Body Energy Homeostatis," *Appetite* 51, no. 3 (2008): 442–5; C. Logel, D. A. Stinson, and P. M. Brochu, "Weight Loss Is Not the Answer: A Well-Being Solution to the 'Obesity Problem,'" *Social and Personality Psychology Compass* 9, (2015): 678–95.

28. J. M. Friedman, "Modern Science Versus the Stigma of Obesity," *Nature Medicine* 10 (2004): 563–569.

29. A. Fildes, J. Charlton, C. Rudisill, P. Littlejohns, A. T. Prevost, and M. C. Guiliford, "Probability of an Obese Person Attaining Normal Body Weight: Cohort Study Using Electronic Health Records," *American Journal of Public Health* 105, no. 9 (2015): e54–9.

30. L. Bacon and L. Aphramor, *Body Respect: What Conventional Health Books Get Wrong, Leave Out, and Just Plain Fail to Understand About Weight* (Dallas, TX: BenBella Books, 2014), 60.

31. D. L. Johannsen, N. D. Knuth, R. Huizenga, J. C. Rood, E. Ravussin, and K. D. Hall, "Metabolic Slowing with Massive Weight Loss Despite Preservation of Fat-Free Mass," *Journal of Endocrinology and Metabolism* 97, no. 7 (2012): 2489–96; M. Rosenbaum and R. L. Leibel, "Adaptive Thermogenesis in Humans," *International Journal of Obesity* 34 (2010): S47–55.

32. L. H. Epstein, K. A. Carr, M. D. Cavanaugh, R. A. Paluch, and M. E. Bouton. "Long-Term Habituation to Food in Obese and Nonobese Women," *American Journal of Clinical Nutrition* 94, no. 2 (2011): 371–6; L. H. Epstein, J. L. Temple, J. N. Roemmich, and M. E. Bouton, "Habituation as a Determinant of Human Food Intake," *Psychological Review* 116, no. 2 (2009): 384–407.

33. G. Rasmusson, J. A. Lydecker, J. A. Coffino, M. A. White, and C. M. Grilo, "Household Food Insecurity Is Associated with Binge-Eating Disorder and Obesity," *International Journal of Eating Disorders* 52, no. 1 (2019): 28–35.

34. "About Us," Overeaters Anonymous, accessed October 1, 2020, https://oa.org/about-us/.

35. H. Ziauddeen and P. C. Fletcher. "Is Food Addiction a Valid and Useful Concept?" *Obesity Reviews* 14, no. 1 (2013): 19–28.

36. M. L. Westwater, P. C. Fletcher, and H. Ziauddeen. "Sugar Addiction: The State of the Science," *European Journal of Nutrition* 55, Suppl 2 (2016): 55–69.

37. T. M. Furlong, H. K. Hayaweera, B. W. Balleine, and L. H. Corbit, "Binge-Like Consumption of a Palatable Food Accelerates Habitual Control of Behavior and Is Dependent on Activation of the Dorsolateral Striatum," *Journal of Neuroscience* 34, no. 14 (2014): 5012–22.

38. R. L. W. Corwin, "The Face of Uncertainty Eats," *Current Drug Abuse Reviews* 4, no. 3 (2011): 174–81.

Chapter 3

1. J. M. Hunger, J. P. Smith, and A. J. Tomiyama, "An Evidence-Based Rationale for Adopting Weight-Inclusive Health Policy," *Social Issues and Policy Review* 14, no. 1 (2020): 73–107.

2. A. J. Tomiyama, D. Carr, E. M. Granberg, B. Major, E. Robinson, A. R. Sutin, and A. Brewis, "How and Why Weight Stigma Drives the Obesity 'Epidemic' and Harms Health," *BMC Medicine* 16 (2018): 123.

3. R. M. Puhl and C. A. Heuer, "The Stigma of Obesity: A Review and Update," *Obesity* 17, no. 5 (2009): 941–64; M. Roehling, "Weight-Based Discrimination in Employment: Psychological and Legal Aspects," *Personnel Psychology* 52, no. 4 (1999): 969–1016.

4. A. R. Sutin, Y. Stephan, H. Carretta, and A. Terracciano, "Perceived Discrimination and Physical, Cognitive, and Emotional Health in Older Adulthood," *American Journal of Geriatric Psychiatry* 23, no. 2 (2015): 171–9; Hunger, Smith, and Tomiyama, "An Evidence-Based Rationale for Adopting Weight-Inclusive Health Policy"; K. S. O'Brien, J. D. Latner, R. M. Puhl, L. R. Vartanian, C. Giles, K. Griva, and A. Carter, "The Relationship Between Weight Stigma and Eating Behavior Is Explained by Weight Bias Internalization and Psychological Distress," *Appetite* 102 (2016): 70–6.

5. M. R. Hebl and J. Xu, "Weighing the Care: Physicians' Reactions to the Size of a Patient," *International Journal of Obesity and Related Metabolic Disorders* 25, no. 8 (2001): 1246–52; K. D. Bertakis and R. Azari, "The Impact of Obesity on Primary Care Visits," *Obesity Research* 13, no. 9 (2005); 1615–23.

6. Tomiyama et al., "How and Why Weight Stigma Drives the Obesity 'Epidemic' and Harms Health."

7. Tomiyama et al., "How and Why Weight Stigma Drives the Obesity 'Epidemic' and Harms Health."

8. A. R. Sutin, Y. Stephan, M. Luchetti, and A. Terracciano, "Perceived Weight Discrimination and C-Reactive Protein," *Obesity* (Silver Spring) 22, no. 9 (2014): 1959–61; B. Major, D. Eliezer, and H. Rieck, "The Psychological Weight of Weight Stigma," *Social Psychological and Personality Science* 3, no. 6 (2012): 651–8; B. Major, J. M. Hunger, D. P. Bunyan, and C. T. Miller, "The Ironic Effects of Weight Stigma," *Journal of Experimental Social Psychology* 51 (2014): 74–80.

9. A. R. Sutin, Y. Stephan, and A. Terracciano, "Weight Discrimination and Risk of Mortality," *Psychological Science* 26, no. 11 (2015): 1803–11.

10. P. Muennig, "The Body Politic: The Relationship Between Stigma and Obesity-Associated Disease," *BMC Public Health*, 8 (2008): 128; J. Tomiyama, "Weight Stigma Is Stressful. A Review of Evidence for the Cyclic Obesity/Weight-Based Stigma Model," *Appetite* 82 (2014): 8–15.

11. M. Daly, E. Robinson, and A. R. Sutin, "Does Knowing Hurt? Perceiving Oneself as Overweight Predicts Future Physical Health and Well-Being," *Psychological Science* 28, no. 7 (2017): 872–81.

12. R. M. Puhl and C. A. Heuer, "Obesity Stigma: Important Considerations for Public Health," *American Journal of Public Health* 100, no. 6 (2010): 1019–28.

13. R. M. Puhl and K. D. Brownell, "Confronting and Coping with Weight Stigma: An Investigation of Overweight and Obese Adults," *Obesity* (Silver Spring) 14, no. 10 (2006): 1802–15.

14. R. M. Puhl, C. A. Moss-Racusin, and M. B. Schwartz, "Internalization of Weight Bias: Implications for Binge Eating and Emotional Well-Being, *Obesity* (Silver Spring) 15, no. 1 (2007): 19–23.

15. G. Eknoyan, "Adolphe Quetelet (1796–1874)— The Average Man and Indices of Obesity," *Nephrology, Dialysis, Transplantation* 23, no. 1 (2008): 47–51.

16. H. Blackburn and D. Jacobs, Jr., "Commentary: Origins and Evolution of Body Mass Index (BMI): Continuing Saga," *International Journal of Epidemiology*, 43, no. 3 (2014): 665–9.

17. J. E. Oliver, *Fat Politics: The Real Story Behind America's Obesity Epidemic* (Oxford, United Kingdom: Oxford University Press, 2005).

18. Blackburn and Jacobs, Jr., "Commentary: Origins and Evolution of Body Mass Index (BMI): Continuing Saga."

19. The Endocrine Society, "Widely Used Body Fat Measurements Overestimate Fatness in African-Americans, Study Finds," ScienceDaily, June 22, 2009, https://www.sciencedaily.com/releases/2009/06/090611142407.htm; R. V. Burkhauser and J. Cawley, "Beyond BMI: The Value of More Accurate Measures of Fatness and Obesity in Social Science Research," *Journal of Health Economics* 27, no. 2 (2008): 519–29.

20. N. R. Shah and E. R. Braverman, "Measuring Adiposity in Patients: The Utility of Body Mass Index (BMI), Percent Body Fat, and Leptin," *PLoS ONE* 7, no. 4 (2012): e33308.

21. Oliver, *Fat Politics*.

22. A. J. Tomiyama, J. M. Hunger, J. Nguyen-Cuu, and C. Wells, "Misclassification of Cardiometabolic Health When Using Body Mass Index Categories in NHANES 2005–2012," *International Journal of Obesity* 40 (2016): 883–6; R. P. Wildman, P. Muntner, K. Reynolds, A. P. McGinn, S. Rajpathak, J. Wylie-Rosett, and M. R. Sowers, "The Obese Without Cardiometabolic Risk Factor Clustering and the Normal Weight with Cardiometabolic Risk Factor Clustering: Prevalence and Correlates of 2 Phenotypes Among the US Population (NHANES 1999–2004)," *Archives of Internal Medicine* 168, no. 15 (2008): 1617–24.

23. Oliver, *Fat Politics*.

24. K. M. Flegel, B. K. Kit, H. Orpana, and B. I. Graubard, "Association of All-Cause Mortality with Overweight and Obesity Using Standard Body Mass Index Categories," *JAMA* 309, no. 1 (2013): 71–82; D. K. Childers and D. B. Allison, "The 'Obesity Paradox': A Parsimonious Explanation for Relations Among Obesity, Mortality Rate and Aging?" *International Journal of Obesity* 34 (2010): 1231–8.

25. L. Bacon and L. Aphramor, "Weight Science: Evaluating the Evidence for a Paradigm Shift," *Nutrition Journal* 10 (2011): 9.

26. Tomiyama, Hunger, Nguyen-Cuu, and Wells, "Misclassification of Cardiometabolic Health When Using Body Mass Index Categories in NHANES 2005–2012."

27. Tomiyama, Hunger, Nguyen-Cuu, and Wells, "Misclassification of Cardiometabolic Health When Using Body Mass Index Categories in NHANES 2005–2012."

28. Oliver, *Fat Politics*.

29. A. M. Wolf and G. A. Colditz, "Current Estimates of the Economic Cost of Obesity in the United States," *Obesity Research* 6, no. 2 (1998): 97–106.

30. Oliver, *Fat Politics*, x.

31. T. K. Kyle, E. J. Dhurandhar, and D. B. Allison, "Regarding Obesity as a Disease: Evolving Policies and Their Implications," *Endocrinology & Metabolism Clinics of North America* 45, no. 3 (2016): 511–20.

32. Hunger, Smith, and Tomiyama, "An Evidence-Based Rationale for Adopting Weight-Inclusive Health Policy."

33. L. Bacon and L. Aphramor, *Body Respect: What Conventional Health Books Get Wrong, Leave Out, and Just Plain Fail to Understand About Weight* (Dallas, TX: BenBella Books, 2014).

34. E. M. Matheson, D. E. King, and C. J. Everett, "Healthy Lifestyle Habits and Mortality in Overweight and Obese Individuals," *Journal of the American Board of Family Medicine* 25, no. 1 (2012): 9–15; P. McAuley, X. Sui, T. Church, J. Hardin, and S. Blair, "The Joint Effects of Cardiorespiratory Fitness and Adiposity on Mortality Risk in Men with Hypertension," *American Journal of Hypertension* 22, no. 10 (2009): 1062–9.

35. P. Caudwell, M. Hopkins, N. A. King, R. J. Stubbs, and J. E. Blundell, "Exercise Alone Is

Not Enough: Weight Loss Also Needs a Healthy (Mediterranean) Diet?" *Public Health Nutrition* 12, no. 9A (2009): 1663–6.

36. S. Klein, L. Fontana, V. L. Young, A. R. Coggan, C. Kilo, B. W. Patterson, and B. S. Mohammed, "Absence of an Effect of Liposuction on Insulin Action and Risk Factors for Coronary Heart Disease," *New England Journal of Medicine* 350, no. 25 (2004): 2549–57; B. S. Mohammed, S. Cohen, D. Reeds, V. L. Young, and S. Klein, "Long-Term Effects of Large-Volume Liposuction on Metabolic Risk Factors for Coronary Heart Disease," *Obesity* 16, no. 12 (2008): 2648–51.

37. D. Ciliska, C. Kelly, N. Petrov, and J. Chalmers, "A Review of the Weight Loss Interventions for Obese People with Non-Insulin-Dependent Diabetes Mellitus," *Canadian Journal of Diabetes Care* 19 (1995): 10–15.

38. R. Hartley, *Gentle Nutrition* (Las Vegas, NV: Victory Belt Publishing, 2021).

39. "HAES® Principles," Association for Size Diversity and Health, accessed October 2, 2020, https://www.sizediversityandhealth.org/content.asp?id=152.

40. E. Choi, J. Sonin, D. Reeves, B. Wong, Hrothgar, and K. Kittelson, "Determinants of Health," GoInvo, last updated April 14, 2020, https://www.goinvo.com/vision/determinants-of-health/.

41. World Health Organization, "Social Determinants of Health," World Health Organization, accessed October 2, 2020, https://www.who.int/social_determinants/sdh_definition/en/.

42. E. S. Spatz and J. Herrin, "Cardiovascular Outcomes in the Wake of Financial Uncertainty," *Circulation* 139, no. 7 (2019): 860–862.

43. C. Blackstock, "The Emergence of the Breath of Life Theory," *Journal of Social Work Values and Ethics* 8, no. 1 (2011).

44. R. Crawford, "Healthism and the Medicalization of Everyday Life," *International Journal of Health Services* 10, no. 3 (1980): 365–88.

Chapter 4

1. E. Tribole and E. Resch, *Intuitive Eating*, 4th ed. (New York: St. Martin's Press, 2020).

Chapter 5

1. D. Neumark-Sztainer, K. W. Bauer, S. Friend, P. J. Hannan, M. Story, and J. M. Berge, "Family Weight Talk and Dieting: How Much Do They Matter for Body Dissatisfaction and Disordered Eating Behaviors in Adolescent Girls?" *Journal of Adolescent Health* 47, no. 3 (2010): 270–6.

2. R. Poínhos, D. Alves, E. Vieira, S. Pinhão, B. M. P. M. Oliveira, and F. Correia, "Eating Behaviour Among Undergraduate Students. Comparing Nutrition Students with Other Courses," *Appetite* 84 (2015): 28–33.

3. D. Drummond and M. S. Hare, "Dietitians and Eating Disorders: An International Issue," *Canadian Journal of Dietetic Practice and Research* 73, no. 2 (2012): 86–90.

4. C. M. Handford, R. M. Rapee, and J. Fardouly, "The Influence of Maternal Modeling on Body Image Concerns and Eating Disturbances in Preadolescent Girls," *Behaviour Research and Therapy* 100 (2018): 17–23.

5. J. M. Berge, R. MacLehose, K. A. Loth, M. Eisenberg, M. M. Bucchianeri, and D. Neumark-Sztainer, "Parent Conversations About Healthful Eating and Weight: Associations with Adolescent Disordered Eating Behaviors," *JAMA Pediatrics* 167, no. 8 (2013): 746–53; J. M. Berge, A. Trofholz, S. Fong, L. Blue, and Dianne Neumark-Sztainer, "A Qualitative Analysis of Parents' Perceptions of Weight Talk and Weight Teasing in the Home Environments of Diverse Low-Income Children," *Body Image* 15 (2015): 8–15.

6. Berge et al., "Parent Conversations About Healthful Eating and Weight."

7. J. M. Berge, M. R. Winkler, N. Larson, J. Miller, A. F. Haynos, and D. Neumark-Sztainer, "Intergenerational Transmission of Parent Encouragement to Diet from Adolescence into Adulthood," *Pediatrics* 141, no. 4 (2018): e20172955.

8. Berge et al., "Parent Conversations About Healthful Eating and Weight"; Handford et al., "The Influence of Maternal Modeling on Body Image Concerns and Eating Disturbances in Preadolescent Girls."

9. Statista Research Department, "U.S. High School Students Trying to Lose Weight in 2017, by Gender and Ethnicity," Statista, September 16, 2020, https://www.statista.com/statistics/871927/us-students-who-are-trying-to-lose-weight/.

10. M. O'Connor, D. Warren, G. Daraganova, "Eating Problems in Mid-Adolescence," *LSAC Annual Statistical Report 2017* (2018), accessed May 21, 2020, https://growingupinaustralia.gov.au/research-findings/annual-statistical-report-2017/eating-problems-mid-adolescence.

11. Centers for Disease Control, "2 to 20 Years: Girls: Stature-for-Age and Weight-for-Age Percentiles," last updated November 21, 2000, https://www.cdc.gov/growthcharts/data/set2clinical/cj41c072.pdf.

12. M. Ehman in "Disney Told 'We Need a Fat Princess' by Body Positive Bloggers" by O. Petter, *Independent*, December 16, 2017, https://www.independent.co.uk/life-style/body-positivity-disney-fat-princess-shaming-diversity-scarred-not-scared-a8114066.html.

13. "The See Jane Top 50: Gender Bias in Family Films of 2016," Geena Davis Institute on Gender in Media, accessed October 7, 2020, https://seejane.org/the-see-jane-top-50-gender-bias-in-family-films-of-2016/.

14. C. Heldman et al., "See Jane 2020 Report," Geena Davis Institute on Gender in Media at Mt.

St. Mary's (2020), https://seejane.org/research-informs-empowers/2020-film-historic-gender-parity-in-family-films/.

15. J. J. Brumberg, *The Body Project: An Intimate History of American Girls* (New York: Vintage, 2010), Kindle edition.

16. Dictionary.com, s.v. "socialization," accessed May 23, 2020, https://www.dictionary.com/browse/socialization.

17. K. H. Karraker, D. A. Vogel, and M. A. Lake, "Parents' Gender-Stereotyped Perception of Newborns: The Eye of the Beholder Revisited," *Sex Roles* 33 (1995): 687–701.

18. C. N. Adichie, "We Should All Be Feminists." Filmed December 2012. TED video. Posted April 14, 2017, https://www.ted.com/talks/chimamanda_ngozi_adichie_we_should_all_be_feminists?language=en.

19. "Ban Bossy: What's Gender Got to Do with It?" Center for Creative Leadership, accessed October 7, 2020, https://www.ccl.org/articles/white-papers/bossy-whats-gender-got-to-do-with-it/.

20. B. Brown, *I Thought It Was Just Me (But It Isn't): Making the Journey from "What Will People Think?" to "I Am Enough"* (New York: Avery Publishing, 2007), 17.

21. G. Kaufman, *Shame: The Power of Caring* (Rochester, VT: Schenkman Books, 1992), viii.

22. Brown, *I Thought It Was Just Me*.

Chapter 6

1. J. Kabat-Zinn, "Some Reflections on the Origins of MBSR, Skillful Means, and Trouble with Maps," *Contemporary Buddhism* 12, no. 1 (2011): 281–306.

2. R. Harris, *The Single Most Powerful Technique for Extreme Fusion* (self-pub., 2016), PDF.

3. "Getting Started with Mindfulness," Mindful, accessed October 8, 2020, https://www.mindful.org/meditation/mindfulness-getting-started/.

Chapter 7

1. L. L. Birch, S. L. Johnson, G. Andresen, J. C. Peters, and M. C. Schulte, "The Variability of Young Children's Energy Intake," *New England Journal of Medicine* 324 (1991): 232–5.

2. "Intuitive Eating Studies," The Original Intuitive Eating Pros, accessed October 8, 2020, https://www.intuitiveeating.org/resources/studies/.

3. T. L. Tylka and A. M. K. Van Diest, "The Intuitive Eating Scale-2: Item Refinement and Psychometric Evaluation with College Women and Men," *Journal of Counseling Psychology* 60, no. 1 (2013): 137–53.

4. H. Caplan, "Changes to RD Real Talk!" podcast audio, August 27, 2020, https://rdrealtalk.libsyn.com/158-changes-to-rd-real-talk.

5. "The Principles of Mindful Eating," The Center for Mindful Eating, accessed October 8, 2020, https://www.thecenterformindfuleating.org/Principles.

6. "Appendix 2: Estimated Calorie Needs Per Day, by Age, Sex, and Physical Activity Level," Dietary Guidelines 2015–2020, Health.gov, accessed October 8, 2020, https://health.gov/our-work/food-nutrition/2015-2020-dietary-guidelines/guidelines/appendix-2/.

7. Institute of Medicine, *Dietary Reference Intakes for Energy, Carbohydrate, Fiber, Fat, Fatty Acids, Cholesterol, Protein, and Amino Acids* (Washington, DC: The National Academies Press, 2005).

8. J. A. Lydecker and C. M. Grilo, "Food Insecurity and Bulimia Nervosa in the United States," *International Journal of Eating Disorders* 52, no. 6 (2019): 735–9; C. B. Becker, K. Middlemass, B. Taylor, C. Johnson, and F. Gomez, "Food Insecurity and Eating Disorder Pathology," *International Journal of Eating Disorders* 50, no. 9 (2017): 1031–40.

9. E. Satter, "Hierarchy of Food Need," *Family Meals Focus Newsletter*, no. 56, accessed October 8, 2020, https://canberra.libguides.com/c.php?g=599301&p=4149450.

Chapter 8

1. "What Is Body Trust?" Be Nourished, accessed September 26, 2020, https://benourished.org/about-body-trust/.

2. B. M. Herbert, J. Blechert, M. Hutzinger, E. Matthias, and C. Herbert, "Intuitive Eating Is Associated with Interoceptive Sensitivity. Effects on Body Mass Index," *Appetite* 70 (2013): 22–30.

3. Hunger-Fullness scale adapted from E. Tribole and E. Resch, *Intuitive Eating*, 4th ed. (New York: St. Martin's Press, 2020).

4. E. Tribole. 2020. "If you hold your breath for a long time and finally take your first panicked inhale, no one calls it 'loss of control breathing' or 'binge breathing'! We need that perspective for eating." Instagram photo, January 24, 2020. https://www.instagram.com/p/B7tDlHDlFlS/.

5. *Merriam-Webster Dictionary Online*, s.v. "satisfaction," accessed June 26, 2020, https://www.merriam-webster.com/dictionary/satisfaction.

6. R. Hartley, "Why Am I Feeling Hungry After Eating? Satisfaction vs. Fullness in Intuitive Eating," Rachael Hartley Nutrition (blog), October 21, 2019, https://www.rachaelhartleynutrition.com/blog/2017/6/11/satisfaction-vs-fullness.

7. "Dietary Guidelines," The Japan Dietetic Association, accessed October 9, 2020, https://www.dietitian.or.jp/english/health/.

8. C. Boyd, S. Abraham, and J. Kellow, "Psychological Features Are Important Predictors of Functional Gastrointestinal Disorders in Patients with Eating Disorders," *Scandinavian Journal of Gastroenterology* 40, no. 8 (2005):

929–35; R. Satherley, R. Howard, and S. Higgs, "Disordered Eating Practices in Gastrointestinal Disorders," *Appetite* 84 (2015): 240–50.

9. J. R. Biesiekierski, S. L. Peters, E. D. Newnham, O. Rosella, J. G. Muir, and P. R. Gibson, "No Effects of Gluten in Patients with Self-Reported Non-Celiac Gluten Sensitivity After Dietary Reduction of Fermentable, Poorly Absorbed, Short-Chain Carbohydrates," *Gastroenterology* 145 (2013): 320–8.

Chapter 10

1. B. Campos. 2020. "You can't bypass body grief and go straight to body acceptance." Instagram photo, January 30, 2020. https://www.instagram.com/p/B78uYg_limp/?igshid=b1e50ebvn88y.

2. A. Lorde, *A Burst of Light and Other Essays* (Mineola, NY: Ixia Press, 2017), 130.

3. R. Helfferich, Instagram message to author, July 2020.

4. R. Scritchfield, Body Kindness website, accessed November 11, 2020, https://www.bodykindnessbook.com/the-philosophy.

5. R. Scritchfield, *Body Kindness* (New York: Workman Publishing, 2016), 5.

6. R. Scritchfield, Body Kindness website, accessed November 11, 2020, https://www.bodykindnessbook.com/get-started/.

7. R. Hartley, "Emotional Eating in Intuitive Eating: How to Build a Self Care Toolbox," Rachael Hartley Nutrition (blog), July 22, 2020, https://www.rachaelhartleynutrition.com/blog/2017/03/self-care-toolbox-for-emotional-eating.

8. "Body Image Online Training for Clinicians,"Marci RD Nutrition website, accessed November 11, 2020, https://marcird.teachable.com/p/body-image.

9. Dictionary.com, s.v. "grief," accessed October 9, 2020, https://www.dictionary.com/browse/grief.

10. J. Courtney, "Size Acceptance as a Grief Process: Observations from Psychotherapy with Lesbian Feminists," *Journal of Lesbian Studies* 12, no. 4 (2008): 347–63.

11. M. Noble, "Body Acceptance Begins with Grieving the Thin Ideal," Made on a Generous Plan, accessed October 9, 2020, https://www.generous-plan.com/body-acceptance-grieving-thin-ideal/.

Chapter 11

1. K. Jones and T. Okun, "The Characteristics of White Supremacy Culture," in *Dismantling Racism: A Workbook for Social Change Groups* (ChangeWork, 2001), https://www.showingupforracialjustice.org/white-supremacy-culture-characteristics.html.

2. E. Tribole and E. Resch, *Intuitive Eating*, 4th ed. (New York: St. Martin's Press, 2020).

3. T. Hersey, "Observations from My Month-Long Sabbath," The Nap Ministry, December 1, 2019, https://thenapministry.wordpress.com/2019/12/01/observations-from-my-month-long-sabbath/.

4. T. Hersey, "What We Believe," The Nap Ministry, August 21, 2018, https://thenapministry.wordpress.com/2018/08/21/what-we-believe/.

5. T. Hersey in "It's a Right, Not a Privilege: The Napping Resistance Movement," by M. Kroth, Elemental, August 19, 2019, https://elemental.medium.com/its-a-right-not-a-privilege-the-napping-resistance-movement-54fc147ba32b.

6. T. D. Braun, D. L. Park, and A. Gorin, "Self-Compassion, Body Image, and Disordered Eating: A Review of the Literature," *Body Image* 17 (2016): 117–31.

7. K. Neff, *Self-Compassion: The Proven Power of Being Kind to Yourself* (New York: William Morrow and Company, 2011).

8. K. Neff, "The Space Between Self Esteem and Self Compassion." TEDx Talks video. Posted February 6, 2013, https://www.youtube.com/watch?v=IvtZBUSplr4.

9. K. Neff, "Exercise 4: Supportive Touch," Self-Compassion.org, accessed October 9, 2020, https://self-compassion.org/exercise-4-supportive-touch/.

Chapter 12

1. Lexico, s.v. "respect," accessed October 8, 2020, https://www.lexico.com/en/definition/respect.

2. J. Baker, *Landwhale: On Turning Insults into Nicknames, Why Body Image Is Hard, and How Diets Can Kiss My Ass* (New York: Seal Press, 2018), 84.

3. Baker, *Landwhale*, 86.

4. E. Tribole and E. Resch, *Intuitive Eating*, 4th ed. (New York: St. Martin's Press, 2020), 229.

5. Measuremake, "Why Clothing Sizes Aren't Standard," ExtraNewsfeed, March 5, 2016, https://extranewsfeed.com/why-clothing-sizes-aren-t-standard-8134acdd6e9c.

Chapter 13

1. Dictionary.com, s.v. "perception," accessed September 30, 2020, https://www.dictionary.com/browse/perception.

2. J. Mond, D. Mitchison, J. Latner, P. Hay, C. Owen, and B. Rodgers, "Quality of Life Impairment Associated with Body Dissatisfaction in a General Population Sample of Women," *BMC Public Health* 13, no. 920 (2013); D. Garner, "Body Image in America: Survey Results," *Psychology Today Online*, last reviewed September 14, 2017, https://www.psychologytoday.com/us/

articles/199702/body-image-in-america-survey-results#:~:text=Fifty%2Dsix%20percent%20of%20women,muscle%20tone%20(58%20percent).

3. S. R. Taylor, *The Body Is Not an Apology* (Oakland, CA: Barrett-Koehler Publishers, 2018), Kindle edition, Introduction.

4. C. A. Brownell, S. Zerwas, and G. B Ramani, "'So Big: The Development of Body Self-Awareness in Toddlers,'" *Child Development* 78, no. 5 (2007): 1426–40.

5. S. R. Damiano, S. J. Paxton, E. H. Wertheim, S. A. McLean, and K. J. Gregg, "Dietary Restraint of 5-Year-Old Girls: Associations with Internalization of the Thin Ideal and Maternal, Media, and Peer Influences," *International Journal of Eating Disorders* 48, no. 8 (2015): 1166–9; S. A. McLean, E. H. Wertheim, and S. J. Paxton, "Preferences for Being Muscular and Thin in 6-year-old Boys," *Body Image* 26 (2018): 98–102.

6. National Eating Disorders Association, "What Are Eating Disorders," accessed September 30, 2020, https://www.nationaleatingdisorders.org/sites/default/files/ResourceHandouts/GeneralStatistics.pdf.

7. K. Crenshaw, "Demarginalizing the Intersection of Race and Sex: A Black Feminist Critique of Antidiscrimination Doctrine, Feminist Theory and Antiracist Politics," *University of Chicago Legal Forum* 1989, no. 1 (1989): http://chicagounbound.uchicago.edu/uclf/vol1989/iss1/8.

8. V. Tovar. *You Have the Right to Remain Fat* (New York: The Feminist Press at CUNY, 2018); V. Tovar, "Take the Cake: The 3 Levels of Fatphobia," Ravishly, October 19, 2017, https://ravishly.com/3-levels-of-fatphobia.

9. V. Tovar in "Body Positivity Has Lost All Meaning in 2020," by M. S. Ospina, Vice, July 27, 2020, https://www.vice.com/en_uk/article/ep45qa/what-does-body-positivity-mean-in-2020.

10. S. Rosenbluth, "Can we stop making body image about personal choice?" Instagram photo, July 15, 2020, https://www.instagram.com/p/CCrchnxphpR/.

11. Anonymous, "In Defense of Fat Sadness," Your Fat Friend (blog), August 15, 2018, https://www.yourfatfriend.com/home/2018/5/10/in-defense-of-fat-sadness.

12. C. Johnson, "Ways that racial trauma affect body image and experience." Instagram photo, June 15, 2020. https://www.instagram.com/p/CBdNM9ep_6D/.

13. C. Johnson, email message to the author, July 27, 2020.

14. C. Cooper, *Fat Activism* (Bristol, England: HammerOn Press, 2016), e-book edition, location 3479.

15. L. Louderback, "More People Should Be FAT," *The Saturday Evening Post* (November 4, 1967).

16. C. Cooper, *Fat Activism*, location 2393.

17. V. Tovar in "Body Positivity Has Lost All Meaning in 2020."

18. J. Baker, "Why I've Chosen Body Liberation over Body Love," The Militant Baker (blog), June 25, 2018, http://www.themilitantbaker.com/2018/06/why-ive-chosen-body-liberation-over.html.

19. A. Lorde, *Sister Outsider* (New York: Crossing Press, 2007), 111–2.

Chapter 14

1. J. A. Stoddard and N. Afari, *The Big Book of ACT Metaphors: A Practitioner's Guide to Experiential Exercises and Metaphors in Acceptance and Commitment Therapy* (Oakland, CA: New Harbinger Publications, 2014).

2. G. Doyle, *Untamed* (New York: The Dial Press, 2020), 68.

Chapter 15

1. V. Tovar. 2020. "Our Bodies Crave and Desire Justice." Instagram photo, June 9, 2020. https://www.instagram.com/p/CBORtzIsBjh/.

2. E. T. Gendlin, "Quotations from the Book *Focusing* (1978)," Eugene T. Gendlin, accessed October 5, 2020, https://www.eugenegendlin.com/quotation.

3. K. Mahler, *The Interoception Curriculum: A Step-by-Step Framework for Developing Mindful Self-Regulation* (self-pub., 2019), PDF.

4. T. Cash, *The Body Image Workbook: An Eight-Step Program for Learning to Like Your Looks*, 2nd ed. (Oakland, CA: New Harbinger Publications, 2008).

5. J. Gibson, "Mindfulness, Interoception, and the Body: A Contemporary Perspective," *Frontiers in Psychology* 10 (2019): 2012.

6. J. R. Keeler, E. A. Roth, B. L. Neuser, J. M. Spitsbergen, D. J. M. Waters, and J-M. Vianney, "The Neurochemistry and Social Flow of Singing: Bonding and Oxytocin," *Frontiers in Human Neuroscience* 9 (2015): 518; R. I. M. Dunbar, K. Kaskatis, I. MacDonald, and V. Barra, "Performance of Music Elevates Pain Threshold and Positive Affect: Implications for the Evolutionary Function of Music," *Evolutionary Psychology* 10, no. 4 (2012): 688–702.

Chapter 16

1. A. Lorde, *Sister Outsider* (New York: Crossing Press, 2007), 112.

2. R. Chastain, "What to Say at the Doctor's Office," Dances with Fat (blog), April 1, 2013, https://danceswithfat.org/2013/04/01/what-to-say-at-the-doctors-office/.

Index

Index